Artificial Intelligence/Machine Learning in Nuclear Medicine and Hybrid Imaging

Patrick Veit-Haibach · Ken Herrmann
Editors

Artificial Intelligence/ Machine Learning in Nuclear Medicine and Hybrid Imaging

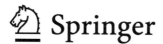

Editors
Patrick Veit-Haibach
Joint Department of Medical Imaging
University Health Network
Toronto, ON, Canada

Ken Herrmann
Deptartment of Nuclear Medicine
Universitätsmedizin Essen
Essen, Nordrhein-Westfalen, Germany

ISBN 978-3-031-00121-5   ISBN 978-3-031-00119-2   (eBook)
https://doi.org/10.1007/978-3-031-00119-2

This Springer imprint is published by the registered company Springer Nature Switzerland AG
The registered company address is: Gewerbestrasse 11, 6330 Cham, Switzerland

Foreword

It is such a pleasure to write the foreword for this visionary and timely book on the role of artificial intelligence (AI)/machine learning (ML) in nuclear medicine and hybrid imaging—including molecular imaging and theranostics. Discussions of the role of AI/ML are increasingly *en vogue* in all areas of medicine, from pathology and laboratory medicine to imaging, surgery, neurology, and cardiology, to name a few [1, 2]. In the world of medical imaging, examples of meaningful applications of AI/ML include distinguishing normal from abnormal findings (without necessarily providing a diagnosis or a list of differentials); computer-assisted disease detection and scoring to inform patient management (e.g., in the assessment of coronary calcium [3], detection and management of thyroid nodules [4], evaluation of the prostate by MRI [5], or staging of lung cancer or lymphoma with ^{18}F-FDG PET [6]); computer-enhanced image reconstruction [7]; and lesion tracking, quantification, and categorization for the assessment of treatment response (e.g., with RECIST or PERCIST).

Enthusiasm about the many potential applications of AI/ML is not unmitigated. Concerns have been raised about the lack of explainability [8] and reproducibility [9] of ML-generated data, as well as the lack of validation and proof of applicability in real-life scenarios and under varying conditions (e.g., across age groups and ethnicities). Importantly, to be clinically meaningful, AI/ML models should obviate the need to perform a currently routine task or provide some other advantage, such as an improvement in diagnostic performance or prediction of risk and patient outcome; a reduction in errors (e.g., in exam selection or interpretation); or increased throughput in the clinic. To their credit, Drs. Veit-Haibach and Herrmann have assembled an outstanding international group of authors, who address these issues head-on. The text examines both the challenges of applying AI/ML and the wide range of benefits AI/ML will likely provide for workflow and clinical care. While the potential of AI/ML for advancing healthcare has been touted for quite a while, advances in technology are now bringing this potential closer to realization. AI and ML will have a tremendous impact on nuclear medicine and hybrid imaging on both the front and the back end. Many functions will be automated, improving efficiency while ensuring much better quality control.

The book is divided into several main parts. Part I focuses on the technical aspects of AI and ML and includes a much-needed chapter on repeatability, reproducibility, and standardization of techniques. Lack of reproducibility and an unwillingness to share codes or other programmatic details have been pervasive in the field of AI and ML [9], and a lack of standardization has also stymied the field for many years. It is now time for investigators and vendors to address these issues. Part II lays out current and potential clinical applications. While modern computational techniques are essential to contemporary applications of AI/ML, the groundwork for some of the projects described in this section started decades ago, without using the terms AI and ML; for example, early attempts at computer-assisted recognition, characterization, and description of imaging patterns led to the generation of standardized reports in nuclear cardiology. In this book, Slomka et al. discuss some of the more recent work in this area, all ultimately aimed at the generation of images of better diagnostic quality, with shorter acquisition times or lower injected activities, as well as the prediction of cardiovascular risk. In oncology, different ML methodologies, and the use of radiomics and radiogenomics, can be expected to enhance lesion characterization tremendously, allowing the assessment of much more than the standardized uptake value. In addition, the ability to automatically extract total tumor volume quickly and with high reproducibility will be extremely helpful. The clinical application of AI/ML should also lead to the development of novel imaging biomarkers with predictive and prognostic value far exceeding that of currently available imaging biomarkers. Of note, the value of these markers will be maximized when they are *integrated* with each other and with other forms of data (clinical, laboratory, etc.) with the help of AI and ML. Beyond diagnostics, AI and ML are expected to play growing roles in theranostics, aiding in appropriate patient selection, dosimetry, and response assessment. Finally, as enormous amounts of data are being gathered in medical imaging, as in all areas of modern life, ethical and legal questions have been raised regarding the ownership of these data and their appropriate use. It is therefore very timely that the editors invited Prof. Prainsack, a political scientist, and coauthors to contribute a chapter that helps put these pertinent issues into perspective and offers potential solutions.

We remain optimistic about applications of AI/ML in nuclear medicine and hybrid imaging. While the future is unpredictable, we do not expect these techniques to replace physicians; rather, we expect changes in the nature of our work, reducing or eliminating some time-consuming tasks, while adding or enhancing others. In closing, we congratulate the editors on contributing this valuable treatise on AI/ML to the literature and hope it reaches the ample audience it deserves.

References

1. Rajpurkar P, Chen E, Banerjee O, et al. AI in health and medicine. Nat Med. 2022;28:31–8.
2. Topol EJ. High-performance medicine: the convergence of human and artificial intelligence. Nat Med. 2019;25:44–56.
3. Atkins KM, Weiss J, Zeleznik R, et al. Elevated coronary artery calcium quantified by a validated deep learning model from lung cancer radiotherapy planning scans predicts mortality. JCO Clin Cancer Inform. 2022;6:e2100095.

4. Peng S, Liu Y, Lv W, et al. Deep learning-based artificial intelligence model to assist thyroid nodule diagnosis and management: a multicentre diagnostic study. Lancet Digit Health. 2021;3:e250–9.

5. Hosseinzadeh M, Saha A, Brand P, Slootweg I, de Rooij M, Huisman H. Deep learning-assisted prostate cancer detection on bi-parametric MRI: minimum training data size requirements and effect of prior knowledge. Eur Radiol. 2021;32(4):2224–34. https://doi.org/10.1007/s00330-021-08320-y.

6. Sibille L, Seifert R, Avramovic N, Vehren T, Spottiswoode B, Zuehlsdorff S, Schäfers. 18 F-FDG PET/CT uptake classification in lymphoma and lung cancer by using deep convolutional neural networks. Radiology. 2020;294(2):445–52. https://doi.org/10.1148/radiol.2019191114.

7. McMillan AB, Bradshaw TJ. Artificial intelligence-based data corrections for attenuation and scatter in position emission tomography and single-photon emission computed tomography. PET Clinic. 2021;16(4):543–52. https://doi.org/10.1016/j.cpet.2021.06.010.

8. Holzinger A, Langs G, Denk H, et al. Causability and explainability of artificial intelligence in medicine. Wiley Interdiscip Rev. Data Min Knowl Discov. 2019;9:e1312.

9. Haibe-Kains B, Adam GA, Hosny A, et al. Transparency and reproducibility in artificial intelligence. Nature. 2020;586:E14–6.

Department of Radiology
Memorial Sloan Kettering Cancer Center,
New York, NY, USA
hricakh@mskcc.org

Hedvig Hricak

Molecular Imaging and Therapy Service,
Department of Radiology
Memorial Sloan Kettering Cancer Center,
New York, NY, USA
schoderh@mskcc.org

Heiko Schöder

Preface: Benefits and Challenges of AI/ML in Hybrid Imaging and Molecular Imaging

Artificial intelligence (AI) and machine learning (ML) are two buzz words which are currently electrifying multiple areas in medicine and beyond. As every new technology AI/ML can induce a complex mix of emotions and reactions in the medical community as well as in patients, ranging from euphoria and optimism to fear and rejection. In several medical disciplines, including but also certainly not limited to imaging specialties, the growing role of AI/ML brings more implicit and sooner implications than in other and maybe more "manual" medicine applications. Even well recognized magazines as *The Economist* recently titled "Why scan-reading artificial intelligence is bad news for radiologists" whereas other journals state "Doomsday predictions about AI replacing radiologists are unrealistic, dangerous."

There are many opinions when it comes to the use and integration of AI/ML and they range from just being considered toys for gadget heads all the way to being considered to provide true value for patients and physicians. This very heterogenous mix of views and perception as well as the lack of a dedicated view especially on how AI/ML potentially impacts Nuclear Medicine and Hybrid Imaging motivated us to initiate this book. Nuclear Medicine and Hybrid Imaging may not seem the first choice for artificial intelligence and machine learning applications since the main advantage of these techniques is prediction of specific patterns and not contextual diagnosis but there are actually a multitude of specific areas where those techniques can be used to our advantage.

Moreover, as many new technologies are prone to undergo the "Gartner hype cycle" with a steep increase of interest and expectations following a technical trigger and a deep decrease of interest due to disillusionment prior to a final slope of enlightenment and consecutive plateau of productivity, this book intends to provide information hopefully accelerating the arrival in the enlightenment and productivity phases.

Following this introduction a total of five chapters are dedicated to existing technologies setting the stage for a better understanding of clinical applications and its potential impact on molecular imaging and theranostics. Franc et al. highlight the role and influence of AI/ML in healthcare with a special focus on hybrid imaging and molecular imaging (Chap. 1). There give real-world examples where such technologies could have values in clinical practice. The Kleesiek group reviews and establishes definitions and applications for radiomics, radiogenomics, artificial intelligence, deep learning, and machine learning (Chap. 2). Rezai et al. provide a short overview of the current knowledge of robustness, reproducibility, and standardization of radiomics (Chap. 3). This is an especially important aspect to understand when evaluating current radiomics results being published. The following chapter by Schaeffertkoetter include the views of imaging device manufacturers highlighting steps of device evolution (Chap. 4). Afterwards, basic principles of neural networks are explained in (Chap. 5). The latter provides a broad overview on how networks are built, why they are built this way, and also explains their basic function.

The clinical applications part kicks off with a review of Bayarri et al. about imaging biomarkers and their meaning for molecular imaging (Chap. 6). By understanding the meaning of such biomarkers, readers, molecular imaging specialists, and referring physicians are able to connect the rather abstract imaging features with the underlying pathophysiology. Currie and coworkers tackle the question on how to integrate AI/ML into clinical routine of molecular imaging (Chap. 7) whereas the Bayarri group again discusses possibilities to integrate AI/ML into our databases (Chap. 8). The next three chapters discuss how AI/ML applications can be clinically implemented into neurodegenerative (Chap. 9), oncological (Chap. 10), and cardiac (Chap. 11) imaging applications.

The review of the potential impact of AI/ML on molecular imaging and theranostics clinically as well as technologically has high relevance. A total of four chapters are dedicated to reviewing the potential benefits and challenges of this new technology. Braren and coworkers discuss the potential impact of AI/ML from the perspective of how it influences therapeutic decisions and potential patient outcome (Chap. 12). Jurisica et al. elaborate why imaging data alone is not enough and what additional data is needed to make the most out of it (Chap. 13). This chapter points out the important aspect that imaging data should not be considered without clinical context and not without other available data (in vivo as well as in vitro) to get the most comprehensive overview of the patients' state of disease. Prainsack and collaborators discuss the legal and ethical issues involved with AI/ML and focus on the aspect whether (or not) the patient does now own his/her data (Chap. 14). This is internationally an increasingly debated topic since on one side there is the need for international collaboration to provide high-volume and high-quality data for studies, but on the other side there are different jurisdictions involved with different legal and ethical requirements. The remaining chapter by Hustinx et al. addresses two very timely and important questions not about the technology itself but about the human side of our profession: (1) how is AI/ML impacting the role of imaging specialists and what can we do to still attract the smartest people to our field, and (2) how are we best prepared to successfully handle the challenges of AI/ML (Chap. 15).

This compilation of chapters reviews the challenges and benefits of AI/ML in special regard to nuclear medicine and hybrid imaging. Despite the overall favorable mindset of the authors and editors towards AI/ML, this book also considers ethical and legal aspects as well as warrants room for (and wants to encourage) discussion of challenges and even critical aspects. As for every new technology it requires time to successfully impact current practice of medicine. AI/ML will most likely transform modern medicine and especially innovative fields such as nuclear medicine and hybrid imaging, but despite a potential disruptive impact in the long run this will be rather an evolution over time requiring regular revisitations on its progress. Also—as time told us after the abovementioned comment—nothing happens overnight.

We as the editors believe that exciting times lay ahead for nuclear medicine. Our field needs to rise up to the opportunities, overcome the challenges but most importantly take ownership of driving our field towards the future. We thank all the contributors, reviewers, and sponsors for accompanying us in this journey and profoundly hope that this book will trigger lively discussions and more importantly joint actions!

Toronto, ON, Canada   Patrick Veit-Haibach
Essen, Germany   Ken Herrmann

Contents

Part I

Technology

Role and Influence of Artificial Intelligence in Healthcare, Hybrid Imaging, and Molecular Imaging

Guido A. Davidzon and Benjamin Franc

Contents

Artificial Intelligence (AI) is a broad term commonly used to describe one of the highest growth industries worldwide, which is quickly finding new and exciting applications in healthcare, particularly for image-based diagnostic workup [1–3]. The concept of AI has evolved significantly since early work using model-driven algorithms in the 1940s to its current state where computational power allows observational learning of pattern by a computer algorithm (i.e., machine learning (ML)) from large amounts of now digitally available medical data, precluding the need for a priori knowledge of an underlying process and thus eliminating the requirement for human-driven modeling and feature engineering [1]. ML, a narrower subfield of AI, develops algorithms that learn to perform tasks, make decisions, or predictions automatically from data, rather than having a behavior explicitly programmed. ML can be broadly further subdivided in supervised and unsupervised types of learning. The latter techniques find patterns in data and provide structural learning (e.g., classes within a dataset) with-

G. A. Davidzon (✉) · B. Franc
Division of Nuclear Medicine & Molecular Imaging, Department of Radiology, Stanford University, Stanford, CA, USA
e-mail: gdavidzon@stanford.edu

© The Author(s), under exclusive license to Springer Nature Switzerland AG 2022
P. Veit-Haibach, K. Herrmann (eds.), *Artificial Intelligence/Machine Learning in Nuclear Medicine and Hybrid Imaging*, https://doi.org/10.1007/978-3-031-00119-2_1

out the need for data annotation, making these suitable to learn from large and unlabeled datasets. Clustering analysis and Principal Component Analysis (PCA) are techniques typically used for these tasks. A recent study using the former technique identified four new different clinical phenotypes in septic patients, each with its corresponding host-response pattern and clinical outcome [2].

In contrast, supervised learning techniques may be applied in learning tasks using "cleaned" data. That is data that is organized and provided in the form of input examples (and its features) paired with those examples' specific outputs which constitute the "ground truth" (or labels) to be predicted when building a certain inference model. Supervised learning techniques include regression and classification algorithms such as linear and logistic regression, discriminant analysis, decision tree, random forest, naïve Bayes, support vector machines (SVM), and neural networks. These type of ML models have been evolving for decades and continue to be the most commonly used in healthcare. An early example is *DXplain*, a medical decision support system developed at the Laboratory of Computer Sciences at Massachusetts General Hospital, that takes a set of clinical findings (signs, symptoms, laboratory data) and produces a ranked list of differential diagnoses [3].

Deep Learning (DL) started having an impact in the early 2000s and it took over an additional decade for its use in healthcare. It also encompasses methods in the family of ML, and most frequently referrers to supervised learning using Artificial Neural Networks (ANN), which use multiple layers of features from inputs to progressively extract higher level features in order to predict labeled outputs. Examples of ANN include convoluted neural networks (CNN), deep belief networks (DBN), and recurrent neural networks (RNN). DL may also be used in unsupervised or semi-supervised learning and can become competent in exceedingly complex relationships between features and labels, for which have shown similar or exceeding capabilities to humans in solving problems of computer vision (CV) in medicine [4–6]. Usually the process of preparing datasets with features and labels can be time consuming; however, once readily available, ML algorithms can rapidly be trained and tested.

For instance, during a developing pandemic, when essential swab and serologic testing was lacking in the USA and around the globe, a pretrained ANN showed high accuracy in diagnosing coronavirus disease 2019 (COVID-19) while differentiating this disease from other types of viral or bacterial pneumonias using plain chest X-rays; similar ANN validated chest CT against viral RNA RT-PCR (reverse transcription polymerase chain reaction) test as a sensitive modality for diagnosis of COVID-19 [7–9].

Other computational training tasks use unstructured data to build models that can, for example, diagnose from physician's notes in medical records (a.k.a. as "free text") in combination with the medical literature, using either supervised or unsupervised natural language processing (NLP) learning techniques. Recent examples in this domain have shown that complications from spinal surgery can be screened from operative reports, septic shock, suicide risk can be predicted from clinicians' notes and patients that need follow-up imaging can be detected using previous radiology reports [10–13].

Each of these ML methods is uniquely suited to certain tasks, but their products—models predicting a class or outcome in a narrow specific area of healthcare or medical imaging—are the current essence of AI in medicine.

AI's proposed applications in healthcare are diverse, from hospital finance to diagnostic and therapeutic applications, promising to improve efficiency by decreasing both the time that tasks take and the potential for medical error [14]. A key characteristic of AI's current and proposed applications is expanding what is possible today, not only increasing the speed or accuracy of current processes.

1.1 AI Applications Support the Infrastructure and Interventions of Healthcare, Including Molecular Imaging

At the time of writing this chapter there were 114,002 results for "Artificial Intelligence" in PubMed and, while these entries date back to the year 1951, over fifty percent of the results correspond to the last 7 years. This highlights the importance of time in scientific breakthroughs. While models and theoretical concepts for the now call AI/Deep Learning revolution were first introduced over half-a-century ago by Frank Rosenblatt, a psychologist from Cornell University [15] and Marvin Minsky, a cognitive scientist from MIT [16], it was not until recently that these concepts were perfected and implemented at scale in various industries (including more recently healthcare) by computer and data scientists due to more recent explosive growth in the global digital datasphere and computational power.

1.1.1   Drug Development

In drug development AI models predict the chemical and pharmaceutical properties of small-molecule candidates for drug design and development, new applications of existing drugs, and new patients who can benefit from drugs, predict bioactivity and identify patient characteristics for clinical trials [17–20]. Moreover, AI in combination with sources of large amounts of data in the biosciences has been used to build in silico models of disease processes, such as cancer, to enable computer-aided design and testing of potential therapeutic compounds [21]. In the realm of infection, an approach using ML known as computational phenotyping, was capable to predict antibiotic resistance phenotypes in various bacterial pathogens and another showed it could facilitate rapid drug development against SARS coronavirus 2 (SARS-CoV-2) the causative organism in COVID-19 [22, 23].

1.1.2   Clinical Workflow

In clinical medicine, some of the tasks most amenable to being performed by a computer, as well as some that can only be performed with levels of computational ability beyond the human brain, reside in the clinical workflow itself. By streamlining patient experience and clinical operations, and improving patient flow through key points in

the clinical experience including admissions, discharges, and ICU transfers, AI has the potential to significantly improve the efficiency of clinical care [24]. AI also extends the capability of clinical care implementation, for example, through AI's incorporation into robotic surgical guidance systems [25, 26]. During the COVID-19 pandemic, AI has also been proposed as a real-time forecasting tool [27], and for early infection identification, monitoring, surveillance, and prevention as well as mitigation of the impact to healthcare indirectly related to COVID-19 [28].

AI is now imbedded in various day-to-day operations of many imaging departments including scheduling, image acquisition, dose reduction, image reconstruction and post-processing, prioritization for reporting, classification of findings for reporting, and the reporting task itself [1]. Beyond plugging AI into various pieces of the existing workflow, eventually molecular imaging workflows will need to be redesigned to take full advantage of AI, for example through merging data sources into a data model to enable easier data exploration and visualization [29].

1.2   AI's Clinical Applications with a Focus on Molecular Imaging

From a clinical perspective, models developed using modern DL methods can, in certain circumstances, be generalized across diseases and imaging modalities and are typically less susceptible to errors in predictions secondary to noise. The interactions of various systems within a disease as well as complex dependencies of disease states on each other can be better understood with AI through DL because of its ability to aggregate multiple data streams from imaging, laboratory, genomics, proteomics, pathology, as well as data from the electronic medical record, social networks, wearable sensors, and other data sources to create integrated diagnostic systems [30]. One could envision multimodality DL modeling approaches integrating multiple data streams not only to compute disease prognosis but in every step of the diagnostic imaging workflow to involve both upstream and downstream applica-

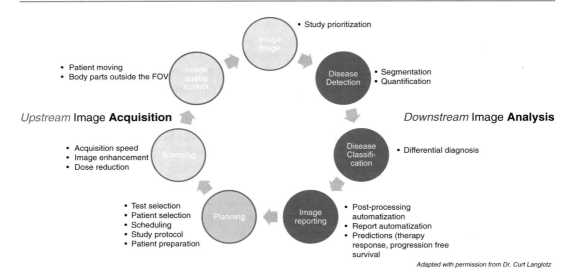

Fig. 1.1 Schematic representation of potentially useful AI applications along the image life cycle including potential applications in the upstream (planning through image quality control) and downstream (triage through image reporting) domains. Adapted with permission from Dr. Curt Langlotz

tions. Such instances could include: *planning* (e.g., patient selection and scheduling based on a patient's disease profile, previous and future interactions with the healthcare system) to *scanning* (e.g., reducing diagnostic study radiation dose and bettering image quality), to *reading* (e.g., automated detection and classification of pathologies), and *reporting* (e.g., automating reports with reproducible measurements, automating prediction of clinical outcomes) (Fig. 1.1).

1.2.1 Understanding Disease

More and more, the concept that diseases are a manifestation of interconnected organ systems is gaining traction. Understanding these systems and their sequalae of signs and symptoms is an area where combined molecular and anatomic imaging modalities can contribute. However, the connections within and between these systems is highly complex and models built on AI can help in pattern elucidation. For example, areas of the brain associated with specific cognitive changes typical of genetic disorders affecting the brain primarily or secondarily have been identified using machine learning approaches [31, 32]. In their study of the

ability of ^{18}F FDG PET to predict neuropsychological performance (NPP) in patients with neurofibromatosis Type 1 (NF 1), Schutze and colleagues built on the anatomical findings of MRI studies of NF 1, concluding that the accuracy in predicting NPP based on PET suggested an underlying metabolic pattern of cognitive function [32].

1.2.2 Diagnosis

AI is used in a plethora of diagnostic tasks using data from traditional and untraditional sources. In primary care, patients report their symptoms and concerns to chatbots that then route their care to the appropriate channel for further diagnosis or treatment [33]. Difficult diagnoses are aided by piecing together symptoms of the patient with those of millions of other patients for diagnosis [34]. Given its particularly complicated origins including genetic and environmental factors interacting with the immune system and other normal tissues in the body, cancer diagnosis is another area where AI is helping in diagnostic tasks using data from general health screening and diagnostic tests, including blood testing, imaging, and pathology [35]. In addition to the field of cancer, numerous AI applications have been developed in neurology and cardiology [36, 37].

In diagnostic imaging tasks, methods of using computational analysis to aid in the detection of lesions have evolved from early work in temporal subtraction methods and artificial neural networks performed in the 1960s–1980s to sophisticated DL methodologies of today [38, 39]. AI can recognize specific diagnoses on imaging, such as pathologic bacteria on microscopy of blood samples or findings on a radiograph [40].

In cancer detection and diagnosis, AI can facilitate the workflow efficiency and accuracy of imaging clinician expertise through precise determination of tumor volume and its change over time and tracking of multiple lesions [30]. Automated PET segmentation of nodules based on neural networks trained in the spatial and wavelet domains have been shown to be reproducible, volumetrically accurate, and demonstrate lower absolute relative error when compared to other automated techniques [41]. Other ML approaches have been useful in dealing with segmentation of larger and more complicated tumors of the head and neck, particularly in the setting of heterogeneous radiopharmaceutical uptake, in segmenting brain tumors and classifying brain scans [42–44]. In evaluating measures that are not typically detectable by an imaging physician, AI can help further guide additional testing and patient management [45].

The greatest strength of AI may be its ability to integrate far more factors than are possible for a single physician. For example, by analyzing images in tandem with blood and other laboratory testing, genomics, and unstructured data from patient medical records, AI algorithms are being used to make diagnoses in a more wholistic manner, decreasing the physician's difficulty of integrating disparate results from numerous tests and the medical history [46]. This approach is known as multimodality deep learning. A recent study using this approach showed that combining clinical, pathological, and imaging information increased the predictive power of clinical outcomes in glioblastoma multiforme, where survival is poor and ranges from one to two years in most patients [47]. Another recent promising methodol-

ogy in this domain could be useful for pancancer prognosis prediction using clinical data, mRNA expression data, microRNA expression data, and whole slide histopathology images [48].

1.2.3   Radiologic-Pathology Correlation

The power of AI over the experience of any single imaging physician or pathologist is the ability to cross-reference imaging or other data from individual tumors to databases of limitless cases for comparison, rather than limiting comparison to those cases seen over the physician's career [30]. AI solutions for pathology have been shown to make diagnoses over tenfold faster than pathologists; while having obvious direct clinical applications, AI-based pathology has shown high value in applications in the pharmaceutical industry [49].

1.2.4   Characterization

Beyond connecting lesions on imaging with specific pathologic correlations, AI can assist with other areas of classification as well. For example, in neurology, Parkinson's Disease severity can be classified with 99mTc-TRODAT-1 SPECT Imaging based on support vector machine models [50]. Several applications of AI have been published in the cancer field including detection, characterization, and monitoring response to treatment of various cancer types [30]. In the realm of hybrid imaging molecular imaging modalities such as PET or SPECT provide molecular characterization of lesions possibly seen on companion anatomic imaging, such as CT. Increasingly, work is focusing on predicting the data that would be produced by the functional modality using the traditional anatomic modality in combination with artificial intelligence. For example, uptake of ^{68}Ga DOTATATE on PET has been used to label bone metastases as active on PET-CT, with subsequent development of AI models to predict activity using only radiomic data from the CT portion of the study [51]. This new paradigm may enable a greater global reach of the benefits of molecular imaging, allowing even those geographies that lack molecular imaging systems the ability to better characterize lesions using staple and inexpensive modalities.

AI has been key in the proliferation of the field of radiomics. Radiomic approaches aim to identify imaging phenotypes specific to diseases that can be used in their diagnosis, characterization, and treatment management, approaches that some have coined as "radiomic biopsy." These imaging phenotypes can be defined by characteristics of the images measured or observed by an imaging specialist or features extracted based upon pre-defined statistical imaging features, of which over 5000 have been described. Such radiomic features can identify key components of tumor phenotype for multiple lesions at multiple time points over the course of treatment, potentially allowing enhanced patient stratification, prognostication, and treatment monitoring for targeted therapies, although care must be taken in evaluating the generalizability of the results of these approaches [52]. Radiogenomics, the translation of intratumoral phenotypic features to genotypes, has been most explored in cancer imaging. Making these types of correlations requires the development of new methodologies to summarize phenotypes of large heterogenous populations of cells within a single tumor and look for underlying genotypic similarities [53].

1.2.5   Treatment Planning

In the realm of treatment, AI has become a pillar of the concept of personalized healthcare whereby machine-based learning based on numerous and seemingly endless sources of medical data is anticipated to identify insights into patterns of disease and prognosis [54, 55]. Models predicting response based upon any given choice of therapy would greatly inform choices of drug therapy made by patients and their physicians.

In the delivery of radiation, AI has enabled dose distribution prediction for intensity-modulated treatment planning based on patient-specific geometry and prescription dose on CT of cancers of the head and neck [56, 57]. Similarly, AI models can predict radiation dose to normal

organs for preemptive adjustment of technique [58]. Ideally, these types of techniques will also inform therapies based on radiopharmaceuticals as the field of theranostics grows.

In treatments involving radiation, AI has the potential to improve safety and quality. For example, in the realm of radiation oncology, DL with convolutional neural networks has been used to identify radiotherapy treatment delivery errors using patient-specific gamma images [59]. However, AI can't be treated as a black box whose output should be trusted at face value, particularly when this output directly affects therapy. Rather, the fields of molecular theranostics and radiation therapy must recognize the fallibility of any technology that is misused with potentially significant consequences and that the workforce, including physicians, technologists, and radiation physicists, must become more conversant in various AI approaches and algorithm development [60].

1.2.6   Prediction of Response to Treatment

Many current pharmacologic therapies and radiotherapy approaches rely on indirect actions on disease, requiring the decoding of complicated molecular inter-relationships to define response to therapy, a task that is suited for AI. Such predictive models may require input of clinical factors; for example, one study using pretherapeutic clinical parameters to predict the outcome of ^{90}Y radioembolization in patients with intrahepatic tumors [61]. Alternatively, models may focus on predictions made solely upon imaging, such as the prediction of radioresistant primary nasopharyngeal cancers from CT, MR, and PET imaging prior to IMRT using radiomics analysis combined with machine learning to identify the most predictive features [62]. Finally, models may rely on a combination of predictors, such as a study by Jin et al. investigating the ability to predict treatment response based on a machine learning model combining computed tomography (CT) radiomic features and dosimetric parameters for patients with esophageal cancer (EC) who underwent concurrent chemoradiation (CRT) [63].

1.2.7   Overall Prognosis

Evaluations of overall prognosis can be helpful to guide therapeutic choices in highly aggressive diseases or diseases that have a more chronic course with multiple therapeutic options. Just as in the case of models to predict response to therapy, overall prognostic models may incorporate clinical information, imaging data, or a spectrum of data from in vivo molecular imaging to ex vivo tissue analysis and patient characteristics.

For example, the ability to train neural network models on data from a single low-cost, widely available test such as bone scan to predict prognosis in patients with metastatic prostate cancer or breast cancer enables the development of a widely applicable prognostic model [64] By comparison, models developed from studies such as one using a combination of highly specialized inputs including ^{11}C methionine (^{11}C MET) PET, tumor grade, histology, and isocitrate dehydrogenase 1 R132H mutational status to predict survival in glioma patients may only be applied under very specialized circumstances [65].

1.2.8   Reporting

The ability to provide a *timely*, *accurate* and *actionable* imaging report is paramount to ensure providing quality of care and better clinical outcomes. It is known that medical image reporting errors are not rare [66, 67]. A plausible explanation for this may be the increasing number and complexity of clinical imaging studies with lagging in training of radiologist specialists, rendering attending radiologists overburdened. Hence, solutions to augment imaging specialists improve and expedite clinical reporting could be helpful (Fig. 1.2). Already an AI framework that could provide considerable benefits for patient safety and quality of care for busy emergency and trauma imaging services that press radiologists to meet the demand of increased imaging volume and provide accurate reports has been proposed [68]. Similarly, another AI framework could potentially increase threefold the measurements of target lesions in oncologic scans and provided faster notification of

actionable findings to referring clinicians [69]. Likewise, a recent study by Rao and colleagues demonstrated an AI tool that can serve as peer reviewer to augment radiologists diagnosing intracranial hemorrhage and reducing error rates [70].

Finally, healthcare records, imaging, medical decision-making, and treatment data are now continuously recorded within the boundaries of healthcare systems in siloed fashion. In part due to this, most of current machine learning efforts in healthcare, including those in hybrid imaging and molecular imaging, are unfortunately only based on data from single institutions. AI and machine learning are inherently statistical methodologies, and as such, they benefit the most from large and heterogenous datasets, ideally from multiple institutions. Never before has the failure to build robust data-sharing systems for large-scale and near real-time analysis in healthcare has been more evident than with the outbreak of COVID-19 pandemic. Nevertheless, an international shared data model exist for information from intensive care units (ICUs): MIMIC database is such model, it is publicly available, deidentified, and widely used by investigators and engineers around the world, helping to drive research in clinical informatics, epidemiology, and machine learning [71]. Efforts like this that can enable global researchers generate AI applications that empower imaging specialists and other healthcare workers to make data-driven decisions, are sadly lacking in the hybrid and molecular imaging community. MIMIC or other established models that enable medical data sharing between institutions may serve as direction for the molecular imaging and other medical communities yet, while such endeavor could boost the task of modeling using retrospective medical data, prospective multicenter validation of developed ML models should be warrant before and during clinical deployment.

1.3   Conclusion

With all these abilities, the boundary between the job of AI and the role of the human imaging specialist will be debated. While some prognosticate an era of medical specialists like radiologists and

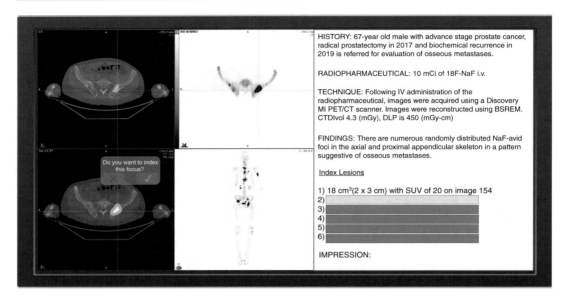

Fig. 1.2 This screen displays a mockup depicting an AI automated clinical reporting workstation. On the left hand side an 18F-NaF PET/CT is displayed. Here, the back-end generates VOIs in overlapping PET/CT images. The AI system detected and segmented lesions and prompts a clinical reader to accept or deny the addition of these to the clinical report (right hand side)

pathologists being augmented by large-scale computation from AI-based applications, others foresee a future where traditional imaging physicians and pathologists cease to have a role, replaced by a physician "information specialist" trained less-so in radiology/pathology and more-so in the data sciences, statistics, and parallel fields that serve as information sources, such as genomics and proteomics [72]. Beyond its influence on medical diagnosis and therapy, AI will have effects throughout the healthcare continuum, including keeping people healthy [73]. As the role and influence of AI in healthcare continues to evolve, real and potential benefits become certain, and so far suggest AI will not replace radiologists and physicians, but radiologists and physicians who use AI will replace those who don't [74].

References

1. Nensa F, Demircioglu A, Rischpler C. Artificial intelligence in nuclear medicine. J Nucl Med. 2019;60(2):29S–37S.
2. Seymour CW, et al. Derivation, validation, and potential treatment implications of novel clinical phenotypes for sepsis. JAMA. 2019;321(20):2003–17.
3. Barnett GO, et al. DXplain. An evolving diagnostic decision-support system. JAMA. 1987;258(1):67–74.
4. Jiang F, et al. Artificial intelligence in healthcare: past, present and future. Stroke Vasc Neurol. 2017;2(4):230–43.
5. Esteva A, et al. Dermatologist-level classification of skin cancer with deep neural networks. Nature. 2017;542(7639):115–8.
6. Gulshan V, et al. Development and validation of a deep learning algorithm for detection of diabetic retinopathy in retinal fundus photographs. JAMA. 2016;316(22):2402–10.
7. Hall LO, et al. Finding Covid-19 from chest X-rays using deep learning on a small dataset. arXiv e-prints. 2020. arXiv:2004.02060.
8. Gozes O, et al. Rapid AI development cycle for the coronavirus (COVID-19) pandemic: initial results for automated detection and patient monitoring using deep learning CT image analysis. arXiv e-prints. 2020. arXiv:2003.05037.
9. Ai T, et al. Correlation of chest CT and RT-PCR testing in coronavirus disease 2019 (COVID-19) in China: a report of 1014 cases. Radiology. 2020;2020:200642.
10. Karhade AV, et al. Natural language processing for automated detection of incidental durotomy. Spine J. 2019;20(5):695–700.
11. Vermassen J, et al. Automated screening of natural language in electronic health records for the diagnosis septic shock is feasible and outperforms an approach based on explicit administrative codes. J Crit Care. 2020;56:203–7.

12. Levis M, et al. Natural language processing of clinical mental health notes may add predictive value to existing suicide risk models. Psychol Med. 2020; https://doi.org/10.1017/S0033291720000173.

13. Lou R, et al. Automated detection of radiology reports that require follow-up imaging using natural language processing feature engineering and machine learning classification. J Digit Imaging. 2020;33(1):131–6.

14. Balasubramanian R, Libarikian A, McElhaney D. Insurance 2030 - the impact of AI on the future of insurance. 2018.

15. Rosenblatt F. The perceptron: a probabilistic model for information storage and organization in the brain. Psychol Rev. 1958;65(6):386–408.

16. Minsky M. Steps toward artificial intelligence. Proc IRE. 1961;49(1):8–30.

17. Zhavoronkov A, et al. Deep learning enables rapid identification of potent DDR1 kinase inhibitors. Nat Biotechnol. 2019;37(9):1038–40.

18. Mamoshina P, et al. Machine learning on human muscle transcriptomic data for biomarker discovery and tissue-specific drug target identification. Front Genet. 2018;9:242.

19. Aliper A, et al. Deep learning applications for predicting pharmacological properties of drugs and drug repurposing using transcriptomic data. Mol Pharm. 2016;13(7):2524–30.

20. Fleming N. How artificial intelligence is changing drug discovery. Nature. 2018;557(7707):S55–7.

21. Bhattacharya T, et al. AI meets exascale computing: advancing cancer research with large-scale high performance computing. Front Oncol. 2019;9:984.

22. Drouin A, et al. Predictive computational phenotyping and biomarker discovery using reference-free genome comparisons. BMC Genomics. 2016;17(1):754.

23. Stebbing J, et al. COVID-19: combining antiviral and anti-inflammatory treatments. Lancet Infect Dis. 2020;20(4):400–2.

24. Tsay D, Patterson C. From machine learning to artificial intelligence applications in cardiac care. Circulation. 2018;138(22):2569–75.

25. Max DT. Paging Dr. Robot: a pathbreaking surgeon prefers to do his cutting by remote control. The New Yorker. 2019.

26. Gormley B. Impact of Auris Health's acquisition could be felt across med-tech. In: The wall street journal. New York: Dow Jones & Company; 2020.

27. Hu Z, et al. Artificial intelligence forecasting of Covid-19 in China. arXiv e-prints. 2020. arXiv:2002.07112.

28. Ting DSW, et al. Digital technology and COVID-19. Nat Med. 2020;26(4):459–61.

29. Brodbeck D, et al. Making the radiology workflow visible in order to inform optimization strategies. Stud Health Technol Inform. 2019;259:19–24.

30. Bi WL, et al. Artificial intelligence in cancer imaging: clinical challenges and applications. CA Cancer J Clin. 2019;69(2):127–57.

31. Ding Y, et al. A deep learning model to predict a diagnosis of Alzheimer disease by using (18)F-FDG PET of the brain. Radiology. 2019;290(2):456–64.

32. Schutze M, et al. Use of machine learning to predict cognitive performance based on brain metabolism in Neurofibromatosis type 1. PLoS One. 2018;13(9):e0203520.

33. Winn AN, et al. Association of use of online symptom checkers with patients' plans for seeking care. JAMA Netw Open. 2019;2(12):e1918561.

34. Tomasev N, et al. A clinically applicable approach to continuous prediction of future acute kidney injury. Nature. 2019;572(7767):116–9.

35. Putcha G. Blood-based detection of early-stage colorectal cancer using multiomics and machine learning. In: American Society of Clinical Oncology Gastrointestinal Cancers Symposium. 2020.

36. Bouton CE, et al. Restoring cortical control of functional movement in a human with quadriplegia. Nature. 2016;533(7602):247–50.

37. Mannini A, et al. A machine learning framework for gait classification using inertial sensors: application to elderly, post-stroke and Huntington's disease patients. Sensors. 2016;16(1):134.

38. Shiraishi J, et al. Computer-aided diagnosis and artificial intelligence in clinical imaging. Semin Nucl Med. 2011;41(6):449–62.

39. Shiraishi J, et al. Development of a computer-aided diagnostic scheme for detection of interval changes in successive whole-body bone scans. Med Phys. 2007;34(1):25–36.

40. Smith KP, Kang AD, Kirby JE. Automated interpretation of blood culture gram stains by use of a deep convolutional neural network. J Clin Microbiol. 2018;56(3):e01521.

41. Sharif MS, et al. Artificial neural network-based system for PET volume segmentation. Int J Biomed Imaging. 2010;2010:105610.

42. Belhassen S, Zaidi H. A novel fuzzy C-means algorithm for unsupervised heterogeneous tumor quantification in PET. Med Phys. 2010;37(3):1309–24.

43. Blanc-Durand P, et al. Automatic lesion detection and segmentation of 18F-FET PET in gliomas: a full 3D U-Net convolutional neural network study. PLoS One. 2018;13(4):e0195798.

44. Nobashi T, et al. Performance comparison of individual and ensemble CNN models for the classification of brain 18F-FDG-PET scans. J Digit Imaging. 2020;33(2):447–55.

45. Dagan N, et al. Automated opportunistic osteoporotic fracture risk assessment using computed tomography scans to aid in FRAX underutilization. Nat Med. 2020;26(1):77–82.

46. Kaplan DA. How radiologists are using machine learning. In: Diagnostic imaging. New York: Springer; 2017.

47. Peeken JC, et al. Combining multimodal imaging and treatment features improves machine learning-based prognostic assessment in patients with glioblastoma multiforme. Cancer Med. 2019;8(1):128–36.

48. Cheerla A, Gevaert O. Deep learning with multimodal representation for pancancer prognosis prediction. Bioinformatics. 2019;35(14):i446–54.

49. Pokkalla H, et al. Machine learning models accurately interpret liver histology in patients with nonalcoholic steatohepatitis (NASH). Hepatology. 2019;70(S1):187.

50. Hsu SY, et al. Feasible classified models for Parkinson Disease from 99mTc TRODAT-1 SPECT imaging. Sensors. 2019;19:1740.

51. Acar E, et al. Machine learning for differentiating metastatic and completely responded sclerotic bone lesion in prostate cancer: a retrospective radiomics study. Br J Radiol. 2019;92(1101):20190286.

52. Morin O, et al. A deep look into the future of quantitative imaging in oncology: a statement of working principles and proposal for change. Int J Radiat Oncol Biol Phys. 2018;102(4):1074–82.

53. Chidester B, Do MN, Ma J. Discriminative bag-of-cells for imaging-genomics. Pac Symp Biocomput. 2018;23:319–30.

54. Mamoshina P, et al. Blood biochemistry analysis to detect smoking status and quantify accelerated aging in smokers. Sci Rep. 2019;9(1):142.

55. Ahmad MA, et al. Death vs. data science: predicting end of life. In: Association for the advancement of artificial intelligence conference on artificial intelligence.

56. Fan J, et al. Automatic treatment planning based on three-dimensional dose distribution predicted from deep learning technique. Med Phys. 2019;46(1):370–81.

57. Chen X, et al. A feasibility study on an automated method to generate patient-specific dose distributions for radiotherapy using deep learning. Med Phys. 2019;46(1):56–64.

58. Avanzo M, et al. Prediction of skin dose in low-kV intraoperative radiotherapy using machine learning models trained on results of in vivo dosimetry. Med Phys. 2019;46(3):1447–54.

59. Nyflot MJ, et al. Deep learning for patient-specific quality assurance: identifying errors in radiotherapy delivery by radiomic analysis of gamma images with convolutional neural networks. Med Phys. 2019;46(2):456–64.

60. Kearney V, et al. The application of artificial intelligence in the IMRT planning process for head and neck cancer. Oral Oncol. 2018;87:111–6.

61. Ingrisch M, et al. Prediction of (90)Y radioembolization outcome from pretherapeutic factors with random survival forests. J Nucl Med. 2018;59(5):769–73.

62. Li S, et al. Use of radiomics combined with machine learning method in the recurrence patterns after intensity-modulated radiotherapy for nasopharyngeal carcinoma: a preliminary study. Front Oncol. 2018;8:648.

63. Jin X, et al. Prediction of response after chemoradiation for esophageal cancer using a combination of dosimetry and CT radiomics. Eur Radiol. 2019;29(11):6080–8.

64. Inaki A, et al. Fully automated analysis for bone scintigraphy with artificial neural network: usefulness of bone scan index (BSI) in breast cancer. Ann Nucl Med. 2019;33(10):755–65.

65. Papp L, et al. Glioma survival prediction with combined analysis of in vivo (11)C-MET PET features, ex vivo features, and patient features by supervised machine learning. J Nucl Med. 2018;59(6):892–9.

66. Waite S, et al. Interpretive error in radiology. AJR Am J Roentgenol. 2017;208(4):739–49.

67. Sokolovskaya E, et al. The effect of faster reporting speed for imaging studies on the number of misses and interpretation errors: a pilot study. J Am Coll Radiol. 2015;12(7):683–8.

68. Jalal S, et al. Exploring the role of artificial intelligence in an emergency and trauma radiology department. Can Assoc Radiol J. 2020;72(1):167–74.

69. Do HM, et al. Augmented radiologist workflow improves report value and saves time: a potential model for implementation of artificial intelligence. Acad Radiol. 2020;27(1):96–105.

70. Rao B, et al. Utility of artificial intelligence tool as a prospective radiology peer reviewer - detection of unreported intracranial hemorrhage. Acad Radiol. 2020;28(1):85–93.

71. Cosgriff CVE, Celi LA. Data sharing in the era of COVID-19. Lancet Digital Health. 2020;2(5):E224.

72. Jha S, Topol EJ. Adapting to artificial intelligence: radiologists and pathologists as information specialists. JAMA. 2016;316(22):2353–4.

73. Duncan DE. Can AI keep you healthy. In: MIT technology review. Boston: MIT; 2017.

74. Cl L. Will artificial intelligence replace radiologists? Radiology. 2019;1(3):e190058.

Introduction to Machine Learning: Definitions and Hybrid Imaging Applications

2

Jens Kleesiek

Contents

2.1 Introduction

In everyday life, the terms machine learning (ML) and artificial intelligence (AI) have become indispensable. All conceivable domains are pre-destined to be optimized and enhanced by techniques summarized by these expressions. This especially holds true for the medical domain, which in turn has various subdisciplines and spe-cialties that are affected to varying degrees by the hope and hype associated with these methods.

ML and AI algorithms, although often tailored to specific tasks and data types, come in different flavors, but usually follow a generic principle. They can be understood as a function mapping that relates an input to an output. At their core, an objective is optimized during training to opti-mally establish this mapping, i.e., to generalize well for unseen data.

Within the vast field of precision (personal-ized) medicine, many approaches are grounded in imaging. These comprise, but are not limited to, the discovery of imaging biomarkers and the establishment of correlations between imaging phenotype, genotype, or clinical outcome

J. Kleesiek (✉)
Institute for AI in Medicine (IKIM), University Hospital Essen, Essen, Germany

German Cancer Consortium (DKTK), Essen, Germany
e-mail: jens.kleesiek@uk-essen.de

parameters for improved disease and therapy monitoring. So far, most of these applications have been demonstrated for radiological images. Technically, these methods can also be applied in the same manner to nuclear and hybrid imaging use cases. Yet, due to particular differences in what can be measured as well as in the acquisition and processing of the images, there are other applications unique to the field of nuclear imaging that can be enhanced by AI. As always, domain knowledge is important for devising novel applications that truly lead to a clinical impact.

2.2   History and Basic Definitions

The term artificial intelligence dates back to the 1950s where it was coined by John McCarthy. The general opinion is that the date of founding for AI as a research field was established in a summer conference at Dartmouth in 1956, bringing together some of the brightest minds of that time. Two years later, Frank Rosenblatt presented the perceptron, the first artificial neural network (ANN). Altered variants of these artificial neurons still serve as building blocks of modern architectures and applications. Less than two decades and many research projects later, the initial hype was followed by the first AI-Winter, presumably triggered by a book published by Marvin Minsky and Seymour Papert revealing limitations of the perceptron. The field recovered due to knowledge representations that thrived in the form of expert systems being utilized for decision-making. Yet, it was hit by the second AI-Winter started in the late 1980s, not meeting the ambitious expectations once again. This second trough of disillusionment[1] ended in 1997 with the famous chess game in which IBMs Deep Blue defeated the reigning world champion Garry Kasparov. Since then, the field prospered and was

propelled forward by several remarkable milestones. In 2012, a convolutional neural network (CNN) termed AlexNet won the ImageNet visual recognition challenge by a large margin. The authors stated that the depth of the model, i.e., the number of layers of the artificial neural network, was one of the primary reasons for its performance [1]. Although the term deep learning (DL) was coined earlier [2], this key event pushed deep learning to the mainstream. Training of deep models is made feasibly by utilizing graphical processing units (GPUs) that have and still are pushing the limits for fast matrix multiplications, the very same requirements dominating within the computer gaming industry. Increasing volumes of data available for training and novel network architectures, intelligently designed for certain tasks, are additional components for the ongoing success story. Since 2016, the error rate for image classification on ImageNet data is considerably better than the reported human error rate of 5.1% [3].

Artificial intelligence often refers to the ability of a machine to display intelligent human behavior. However, this is not a rigorous disambiguation as there is no distinct definition for human intelligence either. The movement toward a general artificial intelligence of machines, i.e., the ability to solve arbitrary problems, is often referred to as strong AI. Yet, the vast majority of, if not all, AI-driven applications to this date are weak or narrow AI systems, tuned for a specific task, e.g., the detection of a tumor lesion within a medical image. The machine detects this pattern, and even might do this better and more consistently than any human physician, but it does not understand the content nor the implications it might have for a patient.

It is worth mentioning that, nonetheless, many algorithms can be utilized as general-purpose tools. The very same network architecture that was used for the detection of tumor lesion can be trained with data from a different domain and is then, for instance, able to detect pedestrians in a street scene. In turn, this means that we can

---

[1] Segment of the hype-cycle established by Gartner consultant Jackie Fenn.

expect many promising algorithms established within the computer vision community to be transferred to the hybrid imaging field.

2.3 Learning Paradigms

Machine learning is a subfield of AI subsuming various techniques for building mathematical models using data. Instead of explicitly programming the computer how to perform a task or solve a problem, the methods are designed to discover relationships or semantic meaning within the data, e.g., learning a mapping between input and output or generative models of the data.

Different learning approaches can be distinguished. In *supervised learning*, the input data x and associated labeled output data y are available. Together they are called training data. Supervised learning algorithms learn, using n input and output pairs (x_n, y_n), to predict an output label y for a new input x, unseen during training. Sometimes it is described as learning with a teacher. Supervised learning algorithms are often used for classification or regression and usually display a better performance in comparison to other approaches. The drawback is that a lot of training data is needed to obtain good models, and even if this data is available, annotating this data can be quite laborious and thus is expensive w.r.t. time and money. Due to these reasons, *weakly supervised learning* relies on training labels that are either noisy or imperfect but cheaper to obtain.

In *classification* algorithms, the output is restricted to a limited set of categories. Input data is categorized to belong to a predefined class, for instance, to label a region with elevated SUV_{max} to be either physiological or pathological uptake. In turn, the output of a *regression* algorithm is a numerical value, e.g., a floating-point number that corresponds to an SUV for a given voxel.

In *unsupervised learning*, only input data without labels or other output values is available. The goal is to discover structures and relationships within data. A famous example is clustering analysis that groups, usually high dimensional data, based on a similarity measure. Other approaches are entitled autoencoders. In this set of methods, the input data serves at the same time as the output. During training, a compression or representation is learned that encodes the data. There are other approaches, all have in common, that at some point meaning needs to be attributed to structures discovered in the data. This step usually is a task reserved for humans.

In *self-supervised learning*, the data itself provides the supervision. There are different approaches in imaging applications where this paradigm has been successfully applied. Procedures include randomly sampling two patches from an image and letting the network learn to predict their relative position, using a monochrome version of the images for predicting pixel color or making a jigsaw puzzle from the image and learning to reassemble the original image. These tricks enable the learning of a semantic representation of the data that can be exploited in downstream tasks, e.g., classification. We are not aware that self-supervised approaches have been utilized in the hybrid imaging community, yet. This could be due to the fact that normally substantial amounts of data are needed, and often supervised approaches perform better.

Semi-supervised learning is a mixture of supervised and unsupervised methods. Often a small part of the data is properly annotated, whereas the rest of the training data lack labels. This combination can often boost performance in comparison to only utilizing either labeled or unlabeled data during training.

Another important approach to deal with scarcely available data is referred to as *transfer learning*. In this setting, data is trained on available data from a different but to some extent related problem, and the model is then fine-tuned on less data stemming from the actual problem at hand. An example would be the classification of radiological images utilizing a model pretrained for a classification task on the aforementioned

ImageNet data. The problems share the same natural imaging statistics, i.e., the images are composed of textures and edges. Thus, if these statistics are already learned, only higher level meanings need to be established for the medical imaging data. In *multi-task learning*, several tasks are solved at once, again being distinct tasks that do share commonalities. It has been demonstrated that this can be beneficial to training separate models for each task, presumably by improving learning efficiency.

Reinforcement learning (RL) is yet another learning paradigm [4]. In this family of algorithms, learning incorporates an interaction with a real or simulated environment. Usually, the task comprises a policy and a value function. The policy function determines an action and the value function, the expected reward for this action. Next to robotics tasks, RL has been used in the past for solving imaging applications such as filtering [5], segmentation [6–10], feature extraction [11–13], and others. A very famous example that combines RL with DL is Google's AlphaGo [14]. In the ancient and very complex board game Go, the proposed algorithm was able to defeat a world champion and is presumably the strongest player in history. When thinking out of the box, detecting a tumor lesion within a PET scan can also be reformulated in terms of a game: scrolling through the stack of images in the least amount of time, while integrating clinical and historic information, to predict the treatment (action) that will yield the highest reward (value), i.e., overall survival time for the individual patient. Again, the very same algorithms that mastered Go could be employed to solve this task in precision oncology. However, for the Go game, data can be simulated, whereas for the medical example, we would need disease histories from millions of patients.

2.4 General Concepts of Machine Learning Methods

Despite sharing commonalities, there are different ways to categorize ML methods. One way is to distinguish between discriminative and generative models. Discriminative models aim at determining a decision boundary. This boundary can be either linear or nonlinear (Fig. 2.1a). In probabilistic terms, this means that a conditional probability distribution $p(y|x)$ is learned that allows to assign a class label y for a given data point x. In contrast, in generative models, the joint probability distribution $p(x,y)$ is sought, explicitly modeling the actual distribution of each class y. Next to transforming the joint probability into a conditional probability using Bayes' rule, this allows to actually generate data from the model by sampling from the distributions, hence the name. Looking for a higher accuracy, discriminative models are often the preferred choice.

Many ML algorithms are parameterized. For instance, parameters that are adjusted during learning are the weights of the neural network or the coefficients of a regression model. In addition, there are also hyperparameters. These hyperparameters are manually set by the user prior to starting the learning algorithm and include, e.g., the number of training steps and the learning rate.

A general approach often found, and one of the most fundamental components of ML algorithms, is that during learning, an objective function, a.k.a. loss, error, or cost function, is optimized. Often this is accomplished using gradient descent, comprising a variety of iterative algorithms, or combinatorial approaches. This is necessary, because, as in real-world problems, an analytical solution usually cannot be found. Dozens of objective functions are available, and developing the right one for a given problem is an important part of designing an algorithm. A popular error is the mean squared error (MSE) that computes the average squared difference between the predicted and true values. For an image, this would result in comparing each pixel value of the predicted to the real image by summing over all squared differences normalized by the total number of pixels. In imaging applications, other loss functions have been described, e.g., the perceptual loss [15]. This loss aims at capturing higher level differences between images, like content or style. The advantage of such a loss is immedi-

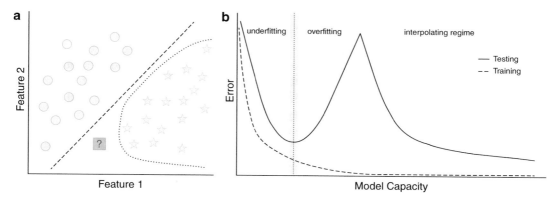

Fig. 2.1 (**a**) Two-dimensional toy problem. Features 1 and 2, e.g., weight and height, characterize the instances of the two different classes, represented by blue circles and green stars. The dashed line shows a linear and the dotted line a nonlinear decision boundary. The decision boundary is learned by the ML model. For instance, if the model is too powerful or non-representative training data was used, overfitting might occur, i.e., it does not generalize well on unseen data. Depending on the type of model used, a different classification might result for an unknown data point (question mark in red box). Overfitting can be prevented by regularization. (**b**) Bias-Variance trade-off for training ML models. The classical goal is to find the sweet spot that balances under- and overfitting (dotted vertical line within blue shading), as the models tend to perform worse on unseen test data (solid line) even though the training error (dashed line) further decreases. A recent publication proposed the existence of an interpolating regime: very powerful models, like neural networks, can be trained to interpolate the training data, classically considered as overfitting, and nevertheless display an improved performance on unseen data

ately apparent, as similar looking images, for instance, identical images that are only shifted by a few pixels, would yield a higher MSE in comparison to the perceptual error.

During the, often iterative, training procedure, the parameters of the model are adjusted so that the total error is minimized. Together with this procedure, several additional concepts are important. One of these is the bias-variance trade-off that is useful in understanding the different types of error sources affecting the model quality. A high bias leads to underfitting, not capturing the relationship present in the data. This might be due to choosing the wrong learning algorithm or model capacity for the problem. On the other hand, a high variance is given when the model captures noise in the training data or the algorithm is trained with nonrepresentative data. It causes overfitting to the training data, and the model usually displays poor generalizability. Apart from bias and variance, the irreducible error, inherent to the problem itself, contributes to the total expected model error. The classical goal is to find the sweet spot that balances under- and overfitting. However, a recent publication suggests that this view might need to be extended

[16]. Empirical evidence exists that very powerful models, like neural networks, can be trained to interpolate (and extrapolate from) the training data, classically considered as overfitting, and nevertheless display improved performance on unseen data (Fig. 2.1b).

A way to control overfitting is regularization. Regularization can be described as reducing the variance of the model, without substantially increasing its bias. This can be realized by introducing constraints on the model parameters, e.g., that they do not become too large (L2-norm, ridge regression) or a sparse solution is preferred (L1-norm, Lasso). It restrains the model from becoming too flexible and, thus, prevents fitting the data exactly. For neural networks, techniques like dropout are used to prevent overfitting. In this procedure, neurons are randomly disabled (dropped out) during training, reducing the effect of specific neurons (and their weights) on the overall output of the network.

Another way of addressing overfitting is cross-validation (CV). In cross-validation, the data is split into different folds of training and validation data. The model is trained and evaluated on each of these splits, identifying the model with a parameter set that probably works best for new data not being part of the CV procedure, e.g., which on average worked best on the validation sets.

The available data should be split into training, validation, and test sets.[2] The training data is used during training, the validation data to evaluate the model during learning (serving as a proxy for test data) and the test data should only be touched at the very end for producing the final results. This allocation of the data can be quite challenging, especially if only few data is available as it is quite often the case in the medical imaging field. Therefore, when reading publications on AI applications, attention should be paid if the division of the data in these three groups has been carried out or if CV has been conducted.

To assess the performance of a classification algorithm, quite often the area under the curve (AUC) of the receiver operator characteristics (ROC) is reported. The value scales between 0.0 and 1.0, the higher the AUC the better the model. The ROC curve is obtained by plotting the true-positive rate (sensitivity) versus the false-positive rate (1.0, specificity). Dozens of performance measures exist for assessing segmentations in images [17], and novel metrics are proposed constantly. A popular measure is the DICE score that geometrically describes the area of the overlap of two segmentations divided by the total size of the two areas. For regression problems, other metrics exist. Quite often, these or similar objective functions, like MSE or the perceptual loss, can be found in medical imaging. They encode the difference between two images with a single number. It always should be kept in mind that these numbers might not reflect the human impression, e.g., when visually comparing images, and thus, the result should not be evaluated purely based on them. Instead, looking at the data and the actual results of an algorithm is of utmost importance (Fig. 2.2). If perfect metrics for assessing the results existed, they could be utilized as objective functions, and even better results could be achieved by the learning algorithm. Further, it

has been pointed out that the ranking of algorithms, as seen in biomedical imaging competitions, should be interpreted with care, and reproducibility is often not possible due to missing information [18]. Thus, comparing two algorithms designed for solving an identical task is far from trivial.

2.5 Classical Machine Learning Approaches

Despite a noticeable shift to DL methods within the last years, several classical machine learning methods are frequently used. Especially, within radiomics applications, they are still the predominant approach for relating imaging features to genetic or clinical results. Next to simple regression analysis, decision trees and support vector machines are often encountered for classification as well as regression tasks. But there are plenty of other approaches beyond the scope of this manuscript, e.g., Bayesian networks and genetic algorithms.

A *decision tree* is a very common and powerful data structure in computer science. It is built up out of layers of nodes and edges. There is a single root at the top and at the end of the edges of the last layer are the leaf nodes that contain the results. Based on an input to the root node, the tree is traversed according to decision rules encoded in the nodes, e.g., if the SUV_{max} is larger than 10.0, take the left edge otherwise the right edge to the succeeding node. Decision trees are easy to understand and train, and they are also computationally efficient. Fortunately, the rules for building up the tree can be learned from data and do not have to be set manually. A *random forest* consists of many individual decision trees that are combined to form an ensemble. When building up the forest, each individual tree is built by randomly sampling with replacement from the training data, resulting in different trees. Further, random subsets of features are chosen, enforcing an even greater variation among the trees in the model. Each individual decision tree in the random forest results in a class prediction and the class with the most votes wins—note the analogy

---

[2]In some sources, the meaning of test and validation set is reversed. But usually it can be deduced in context.

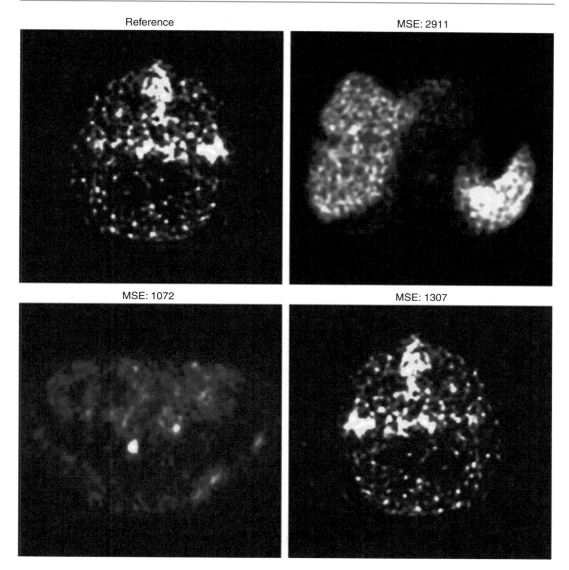

Fig. 2.2 MSE between different PET images. In comparison to the reference image (head, upper left), the MSE is smaller for the pelvis region (lower left) than for the vertically mirrored but otherwise identical head image (lower right). Largest MSE results from comparing the reference to an upper abdominal PET slice (upper right). This illustrates the importance of choosing an appropriate loss function for the learning algorithm that, for instance, incorporates information about the context and not only raw pixel values

to crowd intelligence. By combining simple classifiers, i.e., individual trees, the decision boundary can become substantially more complex. Methods following this idea are subsumed as *ensemble methods*.

For quite some time, *support vector machines* (SVMs) were among the most popular algorithms in the field. They often lead to a very good performance on reasonably sized data sets. However, as they are computationally expensive, they do not scale well with the number of training examples. SVMs are synonymously called maximum margin classifiers or kernel methods. Taking these three names together yields a very good description for the method. It is possible to transform any data (or features extracted thereof), so that the underlying classes can be separated with a linear decision boundary (Fig. 2.1a). This transformation can be performed by using any positive definite function as a kernel. During training, the optimal decision boundary is found, i.e., the line separating the classes which results in the maximum margin between the data points on either side of it. The data points that lie closest to the decision boundary are called support vectors. They are actually the most important points for our classification, as they are the ones where errors might occur and also because they are the only data points we need for defining the decision boundary. All other data points are not needed to perform the classification and can be discarded.

2.6 Artificial Neural Networks

The term deep learning summarizes a group of models utilizing artificial neural networks (ANNs) at their core. Especially, since 2012, they gained more and more importance and nowadays comprise a significant share of the employed machine learning methods. One major reason for this success is grounded in the way they work. In

contrast to classical ML approaches, where features are handcrafted, i.e., chosen by humans, the ANNs learn to extract features that are relevant for solving a given task. In fact, this can be confirmed visually and relates to the hierarchical structure of the networks (Fig. 2.3a). Within the lower layers, neurons are tuned during the training process to detect fundamental properties, like edges and their orientation, that are combined to more complex features in the top layers, e.g., detecting a nose, an eye, or an entire face [20]. Due to the resemblance to biological visual systems, this explains why networks can be pre-trained on photos from a different domain (see above), which share the same low-level image features, and, for instance, then can be adapted to perform well on medical images. The deep layered architecture makes them very powerful and allows to unravel hidden high dimensional relationships that are too complex for humans to discover [21, 22]. However, this usually comes at the cost of requiring substantial training data.

ANNs are built up out of several components. There are connections linking neurons, i.e., the output of a neuron serves as the input to a single or multiple subsequent neurons. The individual

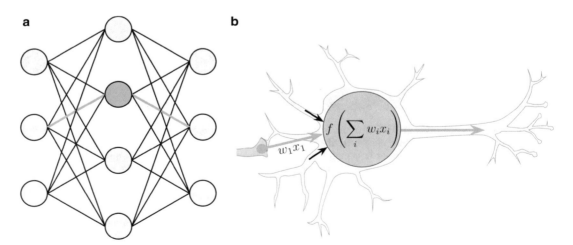

Fig. 2.3 (**a**) Simple ANN. Its hierarchical structure is composed of three layers of neurons schematically represented by nodes arranged in vertical columns. Input layer (left, 3 neurons), hidden layer (middle, 4 neurons), and output layer (right, 3 neurons). The number of hidden layers refers to the depth in DL models. (**b**) Drawing of a single artificial neuron overlayed on its biological role

model. The activation of the neuron is calculated by a weighted sum of the incoming connections from upstream neurons. This sum is transformed using an activation function f and passed on to the neurons of the next layer. During training, the weights w are adjusted using backpropagation. Image taken from [19]

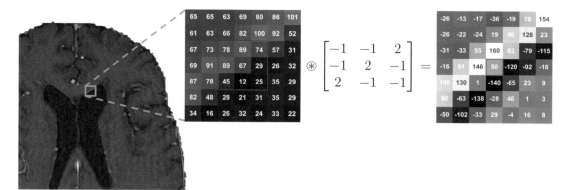

Fig. 2.4 Convolution leading to edge detection. An enlarged section of a brain MRI scan shows gray values of individual pixels (left matrix). Convolution with a filter for diagonal edges (middle matrix) results in an activation map. The filter response, i.e., the detection of an edge is seen as the result of the convolution operation (right matrix). As an example, the value 50 is highlighted, which is the sum of the multiplication of the red marked values with the filter. During CNN training, weights are learned that compose different filters. Image taken from [19]

neurons (units) (Fig. 2.3b) combine their inputs as a weighted sum. The result is transformed by an activation function introducing nonlinearities. Activation functions represent an abstraction of the dependency of a biological neuron's spiking frequency on its synaptic input currents and are also called squashing or transfer functions, because they "squash" the input by transformation into a predefined value range. Activation functions have been the focus of intensive research as they can significantly influence the result of the computation. Hence, dozens of variants are described in literature.

In the end, a mapping between an input and output is learned by a neural network. It has been stated that in theory arbitrary functions can be approximated by feed-forward networks that have at least one hidden layer [23]. In feed-forward networks, the connections between neurons do not form cycles. In contrast, recurrent neural networks do display those cycles, leading to a form of internal memory. This is very useful for sequence learning, e.g., needed for speech processing, and, thus, explains why these models are especially successful in this domain.

During training, the weights of the neural network are optimized. Initially, random values are assigned. Propagating an input through the network results in a series of transformations, initially generating a random output. In supervised learning, the correct output is known, and the error between the current and desired output can be computed. The derivative of the error function (see above) can be calculated, and by using the chain rule, the weights of individual neurons can be updated proportionally to their total error contribution. This mechanism is called backpropagation as the error is propagated back through the network. This is done with thousands of training examples until the weights of the network have converged to produce a minimal error.

Backpropagation is the key principle of most deep learning algorithms and is also used for the training of convolutional neural networks (CNNs). Especially, in the field of image processing, CNNs are the top dog. In order to understand why this is the case, one must first consider what a computer "sees." The individual pixels of an image correspond to gray values[3] that can be displayed in a matrix (Fig. 2.4). For example, a gray scale image of size 256×256 would result in $256 \times 256 = 65,563$ neurons connected via weights to a single neuron in the first hidden layer of a fully connected ANN. Clearly, this does not scale. This is one manifestation of the curse of dimensionality [24], as deep architectures with real color photos or radiological images would result in

---

[3]In the case of color images there are channels added for each color component leading to a 3-D matrix.

billions of weights (parameters) rendering the problem intractable or susceptible to overfitting. For this purpose, in CNNs, neurons are only connected to a small region of the preceding layer. This is achieved by introducing convolutional layers. A convolution operation involves small matrices, called filters, which are shifted over the image. The values are multiplied and added together. For each of these operations, a numerical value is computed. Taken together, these values correspond to new "images" (one for each filter), referred to as activation maps. Each pixel value in these maps represents the filter response for a spatial location within the image of the previous layer. Combined they serve as input for the next layer and so forth. As the network learns, it creates better and better filters. The numerical values of the filters thus correspond to the weights that are optimized during training. Filters are said to be activated when they "recognize" a feature, e.g., an edge (Fig. 2.4).

Dozens of different architectures have been proposed and successfully employed for biomedical imaging tasks [25–28]. Most of them use convolutional layers, sometimes even exclusively (fully convolutional). A very popular variant, especially for medical image segmentation, is the U-Net [29, 30]. It has a u-shaped architecture, consisting of a contracting part (encoder), where spatial information is reduced while feature information is increased, followed by an expanding part (decoder). Crucially, resolution is increased again by simultaneously incorporating high-resolution features directly from the contracting path. This allows to preserve the structural integrity of the image leading to superior results. Examples where this architecture has been used and additional imaging applications are introduced below.

Another family of very powerful methods is called generative adversarial networks (GANs) [28]. As the name implies, it consists of two competing networks: one network, the generator, is trained to generate images indistinguishable from real images, whereas a second network, the discriminator, is trained to distinguish real from fake images. During training, the two adversaries compete and improve until they reach an equilib-rium—the generator is able to produce realistically looking images and the discriminators performance is at chance level as it is not able to tell generated from real images apart. Despite being difficult to train, they have proven to be very powerful, e.g., for transforming one image into another, e.g., an MRI scan into a CT image (see below). In contrast to hand-specified losses, e.g., the MSE, the generator will be driven to learn the full distribution of the original data, instead of summary statistics, such as the mean, which usually results in significantly more realistic samples.

2.7   Radiomics and Radiogenomics

Radiomics describes the quantitative evaluation of imaging markers in radiological data and their correlation to clinical assessment, molecular data or genetic information. Radiomics is an artificial word formed by combining *radiology* and *omics*. Originally, the term radiogenomics was introduced in radiooncology for investigating the radiation response of cells based on their genetic profile [31]. Meanwhile, the term radiogenomics is often used synonymously with radiomics, when establishing a connection between the (imaging) phenotype and the genotype.

A radiomics analysis comprises several steps (radiomics pipeline), including data acquisition and preprocessing, image segmentation followed by the computation and selection of imaging markers. These markers are used for the development of the radiomics model by relating them to desired target parameters—up until now most commonly by employing classical machine learning approaches (see above). The identified imaging markers are referred to as the radiomics signature.

There are several categories of the radiomics features, including shape features, first-order, second-order, and higher-order statistics, resulting in hundreds of features that can be computed for a region of interest (ROI). An example for first-order statistics would be the mean of the Hounsfield units for a delineated area within a

CT scan or the SUV_{max} within a PET scan. For instance, second-order statistics relate to texture features capturing the heterogeneity of a ROI. It should be stressed, that these are usually pre-defined handcrafted features, originating from classical computer vision approaches, and the advantage of DL methods for automatically learning relevant features is not part of the canonical radiomics cascade. Nevertheless, recent publications do take modern DL approaches into account (e.g., [32, 33]). Also, for the automatic segmentation of the ROIs, modern AI algorithms are increasingly being utilized.

All steps of the pipeline are susceptible to errors and must be carried out carefully. Data acquisition and preprocessing can devastatingly influence the results, as image characteristics directly impact the feature computation. In the past, different equations have been employed for feature computations, e.g., with or without normalization. To tackle this source of variation, standardization attempts by the image biomarker standardization initiative (ISBI) and Quantitative Imaging Biomarkers Alliance (QIBA) have been put forward [34–36].

Radiomics studies often display an imbalance between patients included (N) and features examined (P), impeding the establishment of statistically sound claims. Increased false-positive rates have been reported in these "large-p-small-n" scenarios [37]. In a recent review, the majority of studies included less than 100 patients [38]. As the feature space grows exponentially with the number of features included, powerful ML models tend to adapt very strongly to the few existing points in this high-dimensional space and thus do not generalize well (see overfitting above). Further observed failure points for reproducibility include inadequate corrections for multiple testing as well as an improper separation of data into training, validation, and test set (see above).

In oncological studies, the genetic heterogeneity of tumor tissue also should be paid attention to. The biopsy contains only a sample of the tumor and already a neighboring site within the same lesion, not even to consider a metastasis at a different location, might have a deviating genomic profile. This needs to be considered when mapping the radiomics features for a given ROI to the genomic target parameters.

In the last years, the radiomics-related publications increased constantly and are considered as a valuable component for achieving the goal of precision medicine. It has been conjectured that the quantitative analysis of imaging features generates more and better information than the assessment of images by a physician alone [39]. Of course, the underlying principles and processes of the radiomics pipeline are very general. They can be directly applied to any kind of medical images, e.g., stemming from pathology or nuclear medicine. For example, it has been demonstrated that radiomics features extracted from multiparametric PET/MRI images can be used to classify gliomas as well as to predict their mutational status [40].

2.8 Imaging Applications

In the previous part, the groundwork for understanding AI methods has been established. This section will look at ML imaging applications that have been proposed for hybrid imaging tasks. Broadly, two major categories can be distinguished: (1) image acquisition and processing and (2) clinical applications. Within this chapter, we focus on the first set of applications; the clinical applications will be presented in detail in the second part of the book.

In addition to methods for segmentation of PET images and the improved quantification of SUV-related parameters, e.g. [41], ML methods for faster image acquisition, dose reduction, and the synthesis of PET contrasts from other modalities have been proposed. It has been demonstrated that CNNs can learn image reconstruction based on PET sinogram raw data [42]. This inverse problem has also been addressed by an approach coined DeepPET, leading up to a drastic reconstruction speedup in comparison to iterative techniques [43]. Next to this potential speedup for PET image reconstruction, there is also ongoing work for improving the acquisition times of MR images starting with undersampled k-space data [42, 44]. Interestingly, Facebook AI Research is one of the major partners of the fastMRI challenge that addresses this problem [45].

To obtain a quantitative signal, attenuation correction (AC) is carried out during PET image reconstruction. In PET/CT, the CT data can be directly used for this purpose. However, as most MR images do not correlate with tissue density, the AC of PET/MRI examinations is a major challenge. It has been shown that next to classical approaches, e.g., atlas-based, this challenge can also be solved with ML approaches. For instance, DL neuronal networks allow to transform MRI scans into synthetic CT images [46–49]. This is often done with GANs and called image synthesis. Sometimes, the resulting synthetic CT images consist of only a few classes, e.g., bone, air, and soft tissue, that are nonetheless sufficient for a good attenuation correction. It even has been claimed that some of these methods achieve better results than the currently available commercial solutions [46, 48].

The use of MR or CT images for AC might lead to disadvantages in case of an incorrect co-registration of the hybrid image data, for example, if the patient moves during the acquisition. For this reason, DL approaches have also been proposed for generating synthetic CT images from nonattenuation corrected (NAC) PET data and to use them in a subsequent step for AC of the original data [50, 51]. Of course, this suggests that this can also be realized in a single step by transforming an NAC PET directly into its AC counterpart as shown by Shiri et al. [52]. The applications that use only NAC PET data as input are limited to tracers that are taken up in the entire body (e.g., FDG), since otherwise not enough morphological information would be available as input for the ANN.

Due to detector characteristics and image reconstruction effects, PET images often display a suboptimal signal-to-noise ratio (SNR) [53]. Most classical approaches denoise the image data at the expense of the local or temporal resolution resulting in a decreased image contrast [54]. Again, ML methods have been proposed for denoising PET images. One way to achieve this goal is to add artificial noise to existing high-resolution data. In turn, these noisy images and

the denoised original scans can be utilized as training in- and output pairs for the learning algorithm. Thereby, the method learns to remove the artificially added noise component. Within this scope, it has been demonstrated that the integration of anatomical information, i.e., CT or MRI scans, has a favorable effect on the final result [53, 55].

Low tracer doses also lead to a decreased SNR. Similar to denoising an image, as described above, the image quality can be increased by learning to transform low-dose images into standard dose images using deep neural networks. However, deliberately decreasing the radiation exposure is a desired effect as it potentially leads to additional PET applications for which a beneficial risk–benefit ratio currently might not be given. Additionally, it reduces the costs and duration of an examination. It has been demonstrated that a standard dose PET can be predicted from the combination of low-dose PET and T1-weighted MR images [56, 57]. Also Chen and colleagues demonstrated that 100-fold dose reduced amyloid (18F-florbetaben) PET images together with T1-, T2-, and FLAIR-weighted MRI images can be used to predict standard dose images [58]. The quality of the synthesized images was assessed by specialists to be only slightly worse in comparison to the ground truth data. In addition, a quantitative comparison yielded that the amyloid status reached an accuracy of almost 90% and that it was similar to the intra-rater reproducibility determined with full-dose images. They also demonstrated that the usage of hybrid images, i.e., the integration of the structural MRI data, leads to an added value for the prediction. Nevertheless, recent work suggests that by utilizing a GAN, a similar performance can be achieved even when omitting MR images and solely relying on low-dose PET scans as input for the neural network [59]. It should be noted that for all methods presented above, low-dose scans were artificially generated from full-dose scans and the clinical verification with actual low-dose image data is still pending. In addition, prospective studies are needed to evaluate if in AI-generated full-dose PET images information is lost or artifacts are introduced that could unfavorably influence the reading of the image.

The logical next step after reducing the dose is to artificially generate PET images from other imaging modalities without the application of any tracer substance. Although this might not be deemed possible as molecular and functional information from PET scans should not be captured in anatomical images, initial publications explore this as well as other tasks. For multiparametric MR images, it has been demonstrated that, using a DL architecture, the gadolinium contrast enhancement of brain tumors can be predicted solely based on the pre-contrast scans [21]. It has also been shown that it is possible to reliably predict some fluorescent labels from unlabeled transmitted-light microscopy images [22]. During reading of morphological scans, specialists often have a strong suspicion about how certain lesions will behave in PET scans. Thus, it could be possible that ML methods are able to identify phenotypic "traits" in images that are indicative of tracer uptake. This notion is also supported by a recent study that investigated CNNs in predicting the 68Ga-PSMA-PET lymph node status from the lymph node appearance and its surrounding in CT images alone [60]. The results were susceptible to the composition of the training set but, nevertheless, yielded a classification accuracy higher than radiologists. When examining the regions in the images that were pivotal to the decision of the best performing neural network, the authors found that the anatomical location in combination with the appearance of the lymph node were the key factors.

2.9 Conclusions and Perspectives

This chapter gave an overview of machine learning and its application to hybrid imaging, emphasizing data acquisition and image processing. Combining low-dose AI-enhanced imaging with faster acquisition times of PET as well as MRI scans will lead to shorter and safer examinations for the benefit of patients. Large-scale prospective multicenter studies are needed for the critical evaluation of these novel techniques. It still needs to be established if, given the clinic context in addition to an AI enhanced image, the same conclusion for diagnosis and therapy can be drawn. Furthermore, boundary conditions and application areas for ML algorithms need to be specified more thoroughly for real clinical applications. Entire ML subfields have evolved that investigate the explainability and out-of-distribution conditions of algorithms. The first subject aims at developing methods that make the decision plausible for the physician, whereas the second examines what data statistics are mandatory for an algorithm to deliver reliable results for unseen data. This stresses also the need for the incorporation of representative training data w.r.t to the target application when training an algorithm. Luckily, an increasing number of publications provide code and sometimes also data, allowing for reproducibility of the results. This will accelerate the progress within this exciting field and also open up the possibilities for novel applications. Among other, dual-tracer applications will probably benefit from the recent developments in machine learning and open up yet another area of active research in the near future, e.g., disentangling the signal from the individual tracers.

Acknowledgments The author would like to thank Kai Ueltzhöffer, Jacob Murray, and Christian Strack for their advice and comments on this manuscript.

References

1. Krizhevsky A, Sutskever I, Hinton GE. ImageNet classification with deep convolutional neural networks. In: Pereira F, CJC B, Bottou L, Weinberger KQ, editors. Advances in neural information processing systems. Red Hook: Curran Associates, Inc. p. 1097–105.
2. Dechter R. Learning while searching in constraint-satisfaction-problems. In: Proceedings of the fifth AAAI national conference on artificial intelligence. Palo Alto: AAAI Press; 1986. p. 178–83.
3. Dodge S, Karam L. A study and comparison of human and deep learning recognition performance under visual distortions. ArXiv170502498 Cs. 2017. Available from http://arxiv.org/abs/1705.02498
4. Sutton RS, Barto AG. Reinforcement learning: an introduction. Cambridge: MIT Press; 1998.

5. Taylor GW. A reinforcement learning framework for parameter control in computer vision applications. In: First Canadian conference on computer and robot vision, 2004 proceedings. 2004, pp. 496–503.

6. Peng J, Bhanu B. Closed-loop object recognition using reinforcement learning. IEEE Trans Pattern Anal Mach Intell. 1998;20(2):139–54.

7. Sahba F, Tizhoosh HR, Salama MM. Application of opposition-based reinforcement learning in image segmentation. In: 2007 IEEE symposium on computational intelligence in image and signal processing. 2007, pp. 246–251.

8. Sahba F, Tizhoosh HR, Salama MM. Application of reinforcement learning for segmentation of transrectal ultrasound images. BMC Med Imaging. 2008;8(1):8.

9. Shokri M, Tizhoosh HR. A reinforcement agent for threshold fusion. Appl Soft Comput. 2008;8(1):174–81.

10. Ghajari S, Naghibi Sistani MB. Improving the quality of image segmentation in ultrasound images using reinforcement learning. Commun Adv Comput Sci Appl. 2017;2017(1):33–40.

11. Jodogne S, Piater JH. Interactive selection of visual features through reinforcement learning. In: Bramer M, Coenen F, Allen T, editors. Research and development in intelligent systems XXI. London: Springer; 2005. p. 285–98.

12. Piñol M, Sappa AD, Toledo R. Multi-table reinforcement learning for visual object recognition. In: Kumar SS, editor. Proceedings of the fourth international conference on signal and image processing 2012 (ICSIP 2012). New Delhi: Springer; 2013. p. 469–79.

13. Liu D-R, Li H-L, Wang D. Feature selection and feature learning for high-dimensional batch reinforcement learning: a survey. Int J Autom Comput. 2015;12(3):229–42.

14. Silver D, Schrittwieser J, Simonyan K, Antonoglou I, Huang A, Guez A, et al. Mastering the game of Go without human knowledge. Nature. 2017;550(7676):354–9.

15. Johnson J, Alahi A, Fei-Fei L. Perceptual losses for real-time style transfer and super-resolution. ArXiv160308155 Cs. 2016. Available from http://arxiv.org/abs/1603.08155

16. Belkin M, Hsu D, Ma S, Mandal S. Reconciling modern machine-learning practice and the classical bias–variance trade-off. Proc Natl Acad Sci. 2019;116(32):15849–54.

17. Taha AA, Hanbury A. Metrics for evaluating 3D medical image segmentation: analysis, selection, and tool. BMC Med Imaging. 2015;15(1):29.

18. Maier-Hein L, Eisenmann M, Reinke A, Onogur S, Stankovic M, Scholz P, et al. Why rankings of biomedical image analysis competitions should be interpreted with care. Nat Commun. 2018;9(1):1–13.

19. Kleesiek J, Murray JM, Strack C, Kaissis G, Braren R. Wie funktioniert maschinelles Lernen? Radiology. 2020;60(1):24–31.

20. Jones N. Computer science: the learning machines. Nat News. 2014;505(7482):146.

21. Kleesiek J, Morshuis JN, Isensee F, Deike-Hofmann K, Paech D, Kickingereder P, et al. Can virtual contrast enhancement in brain MRI replace gadolinium? A feasibility study. Investig Radiol. 2019;54(10):653–60.

22. Christiansen EM, Yang SJ, Ando DM, Javaherian A, Skibinski G, Lipnick S, et al. In silico labeling: predicting fluorescent labels in unlabeled images. Cell. 2018;173(3):792–803.

23. Leshno M, Lin VY, Pinkus A, Schocken S. Multilayer feedforward networks with a nonpolynomial activation function can approximate any function. Neural Netw. 1993;6(6):861–7.

24. Bellman RE. Dynamic programming. Mineola: Dover Publications, Inc.; 2003.

25. Simonyan K, Zisserman A. Very deep convolutional networks for large-scale image recognition. ArXiv14091556 Cs. 2015. Available from http://arxiv.org/abs/1409.1556

26. He K, Zhang X, Ren S, Sun J. Deep residual learning for image recognition. ArXiv151203385 Cs. 2015. Available from http://arxiv.org/abs/1512.03385

27. Huang G, Liu Z, van der Maaten L, Weinberger KQ. Densely connected convolutional networks. ArXiv160806993 Cs. 2018. Available from http://arxiv.org/abs/1608.06993

28. Goodfellow IJ, Pouget-Abadie J, Mirza M, Xu B, Warde-Farley D, Ozair S, et al. Generative adversarial networks. ArXiv14062661 Cs Stat [Internet]. 2014. Available from http://arxiv.org/abs/1406.2661

29. Ronneberger O, Fischer P, Brox T. U-Net: convolutional networks for biomedical image segmentation. ArXiv150504597 Cs. 2015. Available from: http://arxiv.org/abs/1505.04597

30. Isensee F, Kickingereder P, Wick W, Bendszus M, Maier-Hein KH. No New-Net. ArXiv180910483 Cs. 2018. Available from http://arxiv.org/abs/1809.10483

31. Andreassen CN, Schack LMH, Laursen LV, Alsner J. Radiogenomics – current status, challenges and future directions. Cancer Lett. 2016;382(1):127–36.

32. Xu Y, Hosny A, Zeleznik R, Parmar C, Coroller T, Franco I, et al. Deep learning predicts lung cancer treatment response from serial medical imaging. Clin Cancer Res. 2019;25(11):3266–75.

33. Lou B, Doken S, Zhuang T, Wingerter D, Gidwani M, Mistry N, et al. An image-based deep learning framework for individualising radiotherapy dose: a retrospective analysis of outcome prediction. Lancet Digit Health. 2019;1(3):136–47.

34. Kinahan PE, Perlman ES, Sunderland JJ, Subramaniam R, Wollenweber SD, Turkington TG, et al. The QIBA profile for FDG PET/CT as an imaging biomarker measuring response to cancer therapy. Radiology. 2020;294(3):647–57.

35. Sullivan DC, Obuchowski NA, Kessler LG, Raunig DL, Gatsonis C, Huang EP, et al. Metrology standards for quantitative imaging biomarkers. Radiology. 2015;277(3):813–25.

36. Zwanenburg A, Vallières M, Abdalah MA, Aerts HJ, Andrearczyk V, Apte A, et al. The image biomarker standardization initiative: standardized quantitative

radiomics for high-throughput image-based pheno-typing. Radiology. 2020;295(2):328–38.

37. Park JE, Park SY, Kim HJ, Kim HS. Reproducibility and generalizability in radiomics modeling: possible strategies in radiologic and statistical perspectives. Korean J Radiol. 2019;20(7):1124–37.

38. Bodalal Z, Trebeschi S, Nguyen-Kim TDL, Schats W, Beets-Tan R. Radiogenomics: bridging imaging and genomics. Abdom Radiol. 2019;44(6):1960–84.

39. Lambin P, Rios-Velazquez E, Leijenaar R, Carvalho S, van Stiphout RG, Granton P, et al. Radiomics: extracting more information from medical images using advanced feature analysis. Eur J Cancer. 2012;48(4):441–6.

40. Haubold J, Demircioglu A, Gratz M, Glas M, Wrede K, Sure U, et al. Non-invasive tumor decoding and phenotyping of cerebral gliomas utilizing multiparametric 18F-FET PET-MRI and MR fingerprinting. Eur J Nucl Med Mol Imaging. 2020;47(6):1435–45.

41. Seifert R, Herrmann K, Kleesiek J, Schafers MA, Shah V, Xu Z, et al. Semi-automatically quantified tumor volume using Ga-68-PSMA-11-PET as biomarker for survival in patients with advanced prostate cancer. J Nucl Med. 2020;61(12):1786–92.

42. Zhu B, Liu JZ, Cauley SF, Rosen BR, Rosen MS. Image reconstruction by domain-transform manifold learning. Nature. 2018;555(7697):487–92.

43. Häggström I, Schmidtlein CR, Campanella G, Fuchs TJ. DeepPET: a deep encoder-decoder network for directly solving the PET image reconstruction inverse problem. Med Image Anal. 2019;54:253–62.

44. Eo T, Jun Y, Kim T, Jang J, Lee H-J, Hwang D. KIKI-net: cross-domain convolutional neural networks for reconstructing undersampled magnetic resonance images. Magn Reson Med. 2018;80(5):2188–201.

45. Knoll F, Zbontar J, Sriram A, Muckley MJ, Bruno M, Defazio A, et al. fastMRI: a Publicly available raw k-Space and DICOM dataset of knee images for accelerated MR image reconstruction using machine learning. Radiol Artif Intell. 2020;2(1):e190007.

46. Bradshaw TJ, Zhao G, Jang H, Liu F, McMillan AB. Feasibility of deep learning–based PET/MR attenuation correction in the pelvis using only diagnostic MR images. Tomography. 2018;4(3):138–47.

47. Kläser K, Varsavsky T, Markiewicz P, Vercauteren T, Atkinson D, Thielemans K, et al. Improved MR to CT synthesis for PET/MR attenuation correction using imitation learning. In: Burgos N, Gooya A, Svoboda D, editors. Simulation and synthesis in medical imaging. Cham: Springer International Publishing; 2019. p. 13–21.

48. Ladefoged CN, Marner L, Hindsholm A, Law I, Højgaard L, Andersen FL. Deep learning based attenuation correction of PET/MRI in pediatric brain tumor patients: evaluation in a clinical setting. Front Neurosci. 2019;12:01005.

49. Liu F, Jang H, Kijowski R, Bradshaw T, McMillan AB. Deep learning MR imaging–based attenuation correction for PET/MR imaging. Radiology. 2017;286(2):676–84.

50. Dong X, Wang T, Lei Y, Higgins K, Liu T, Curran WJ, et al. Synthetic CT generation from non-attenuation corrected PET images for whole-body PET imaging. Phys Med Biol. 2019;64(21):215016.

51. Liu F, Jang H, Kijowski R, Zhao G, Bradshaw T, McMillan AB. A deep learning approach for 18F-FDG PET attenuation correction. EJNMMI Phys. 2018;5(1):24.

52. Shiri I, Ghafarian P, Geramifar P, Leung KH-Y, Ghelichoghli M, Oveisi M, et al. Direct attenuation correction of brain PET images using only emission data via a deep convolutional encoder-decoder (Deep-DAC). Eur Radiol. 2019;29(12):6867–79.

53. Liu C-C, Qi J. Higher SNR PET image prediction using a deep learning model and MRI image. Phys Med Biol. 2019;64(11):115004.

54. Klyuzhin IS, Cheng J-C, Bevington C, Sossi V. Use of a tracer-specific deep artificial neural net to denoise dynamic PET images. IEEE Trans Med Imaging. 2019;1:1.

55. Cui J, Gong K, Guo N, Wu C, Meng X, Kim K, et al. PET image denoising using unsupervised deep learning. Eur J Nucl Med Mol Imaging. 2019;46(13):2780–9.

56. Wang Y, Zhou L, Wang L, Yu B, Zu C, Lalush DS, et al. Locality adaptive multi-modality GANs for high-quality PET image synthesis. In: Frangi AF, Schnabel JA, Davatzikos C, Alberola-López C, Fichtinger G, editors. Medical image computing and computer assisted intervention – MICCAI 2018. Cham: Springer International Publishing; 2018. p. 329–37.

57. Xiang L, Qiao Y, Nie D, An L, Lin W, Wang Q, et al. Deep auto-context convolutional neural networks for standard-dose PET image estimation from low-dose PET/MRI. Neurocomputing. 2017;267:406–16.

58. Chen KT, Gong E, de Carvalho Macruz FB, Xu J, Boumis A, Khalighi M, et al. Ultra–low-dose 18F-florbetaben amyloid PET imaging using deep learning with multi-contrast MRI inputs. Radiology. 2018;290(3):649–56.

59. Ouyang J, Chen KT, Gong E, Pauly J, Zaharchuk G. Ultra-low-dose PET reconstruction using generative adversarial network with feature matching and task-specific perceptual loss. Med Phys. 2019;46(8):3555–64.

60. Hartenstein A, Lübbe F, Baur ADJ, Rudolph MM, Furth C, Brenner W, et al. Prostate cancer nodal staging: using deep learning to predict 68 Ga-PSMA-positivity from CT imaging alone. Sci Rep. 2020;10(1):1–11.

Radiomics in Nuclear Medicine, Robustness, Reproducibility, and Standardization

3

Reza Reiazi

Contents

The original version of this chapter was revised. A correction to this chapter can be found at https://doi.org/10.1007/978-3-031-00119-2_16

R. Reiazi (✉)
Princess Margaret Bioinformatics and Computational Genomics Laboratory, University Health Network, Toronto, ON, Canada
e-mail: Reza.Reiazi@uhnresearch.ca

3.1 Introduction

Quantitative information is the main form of gathering information in digital imaging systems that follows by transforming to qualitative and sensible information for the human eye, but this process may lead to missing some worth data which could help us to complete clinical evaluations [1]. Usage of images biomarkers is the principal issue in the field of radiomics that can provide useful information, absolutely noninvasively, about the behavior and characteristics of suspected tissue and lesion in the body [2]. Radiomics tries to access those forms of quantitative information of medical images that are hidden from the physician's eyes and eventually help them to improve their prognosis and diagnosis tasks. Repeatability and reproducibility are the two main characteristics of radiomic features that are necessary for clinical trial applications [1]. The objective of this chapter is an evaluation of the influence of nuclear medicine imaging parameter changes on radiomic features variability extracted from these images. Also, try to bring a comparison between the recent article's results and a demonstration of the most robust and sensitive features from these researches (Table 3.1).

3.2   Robustness of Radiomic Features

Like other new methodologies difficulty and limitations along with usefulness are inevitable, likewise, sensitivity and difference potentiality to imaging parameters are the most important limitations of the application of radiomic features [14]. However, repeatability and reproducibility both refer to robustness of features, there are some differences though. When the same features from the same subject, situations, and imaging parameters are extracted, these are repeatable features and, if the same features from different parameters and situations are extracted, these are reproducible features [15]. These two properties of radiomic features are such obstacles that limit application and generalization of them to the broad manner in medicine [1]. Researches dedicated to assessing these characteristics can open new bright paths for radiomics employment in precision medicine and clinics as well [7, 16]. The main factors that have a significant impact on radiomic features consist of image acquisition parameters, image reconstruction methodologies, and settings, contouring and delineation processes, image processing and feature extraction parameters, etc. [14, 17].

3.3   Image Acquisition

Image acquisition parameters such as tracer uptake time or level, scan mode, number of views, view matrix size, attenuation correction, type of scanner, etc. can be a source of variation in radiomics features [13, 17]. Decreasing the level of injected lead to a lower dose receiving by the patient. This is important especially for pediatrics nuclear imaging as high organ sensitivity of this group. Some recent studies have shown that keeping tumor diagnostic power with a diminishing volume of tracer could be done simultaneously [2].

Branchini et al. in their research have shown that robust features can be extracted from pediatrics PET/MRI scans even with lower tracer volume. In this study features from shape and intensity families had an acceptable range of stability (ICC > 0.9) [2]. Another study that assessed the impact of acquisition parameter consisting of the number of views, view matrix size, with or without attenuation correction, on radiomic features variability, demonstrated that DE(GLDM), RLNUN, SRE, RP(GLRLM), ZE(GLSZM) and IDMN, IDN, IMC2(GLCM) have significant stability (Table 3.2). Also, it can be recognized from this article that matrix size and number of views are two factors that have the most effect on radiomic biomarkers [13].

3.4   Image Reconstruction

Another source of variation in radiomic features is reconstruction parameters that its effect has studied and proven by multiple assessments [3, 5, 6, 8, 13]. Edalat-javid et al. in their research about the influence of reconstruction parameters on radiomic features extracted from SPECT scans, illustrated that FWHM of Gaussian filter has maximum effect on features between other parameters they studied. Besides, in their study, some of the most robust features for instance: RLNUN, SRE, RP(GLRLM), and most sensitive features like SDLGLE, LDLGLE, DV (GLDM) have reported [13]. The stability of features included in GLRLM and GLSZM families is proven by multiple studies that have evaluated the variability of PET/CT radiomic features [3, 5, 6, 8, 13]. Among these features, RP and SRE from GLRLM represented maximum stability.

Table 3.1 Identification of multiple variation sources evaluated by lectures and comparing of robustness and sensitivity of extracted features

	Author	Source of variation	Most robust features	Most sensitive features	Most affecting source
1	Gallivanone et al. [3]	1. Segmentation method 2. Lesion uniformity 3. Reconstruction parameter	To recon: 1. GLRLM 2. GLSZM 3. Morphological features — To seg: 1. Contrast (GLCM) 2. Dissimilarity (GLCM) 3. HGRE (GLRLM) 4. SRHGE (GLRLM) 5. HGZE (GLSZM)	To recon: 1. Intensity histogram — To seg: 1. Morphological 2. Intensity histogram	Segmentation method
2	Papp et al. [4]	1. Extraction parameters Voxel size, bin size, lesion volume change	1. Information correlation (GLCM) 2. Compactness, volume and Spheric dice coefficient (shape features)	1. Contrast and difference variance (GLCM) 2. Contrast (NGTDM)	Lesion volume change
3	Pfaehler et al. [5]	1. Discretization method 2. Noise 3. Recon method 4. Underlying data	1. GLSZM 2. GLRLM 3. GLCM		Discretization Sphere size Activity uptake
4	Pfaehler et al. [6]	Reconstruction method	1. LocINT	1. NGLDM	FBN discretization
5	Yang et al. [7]	Contouring	1. GLNDM (for 3,264,128 discretization) 2. GLCOM (for 256 discretization)	Most of #GLSZM features	Low discretization schemes
6	Shiri et al. [8]	Reconstruction settings	1. Entropy, homogeneity, dissimilarity, correlation (GLCM) 2. SRE, LRE, RLV, RP(GLRLM) 3. SZE, IV, ZP (GLSZM) 4. Entropy, homogeneity, dissimilarity (NGLCM) 5. SUVmean, entropy, SULpeak and 16 other features (intensity and SUV) 6. SNE, NNU, SM, entropy (NGLD) 7. Homogeneity (TFC) 8. Entropy, homogeneity, intensity, IDMcglcm, CE (GLCM-coding)	1. NGTDM 2. TS	Matrix size

(continued)

Table 3.1 (continued)

	Author	Source of variation	Most robust features		Most sensitive features		Most affecting source
7	Belli et al. [9]	Delineation (manual, semi-automatic, fully automatic)	1. First order SUV families 2. Co-occurrence matrix (higher-order)		VA and ISZ families		Automated (>50%)
8	Lv et al. [10]	Extraction parameters	1. GLRLM		1. GLSZM		
9	Catherine Guezennec [11]	1. Three contouring methods 2. Two observers	For observers 1. Homogeneity 2. Correlation 3. Entropy	For contouring methods 1. Busyness	For observers 1. Busyness	For contouring methods Homogeneity, correlation, entropy, and LZLGE	Contouring methods
10	Branchini et al. [2]	1. Statistics count reduction 2. Discretization method	1. GLCM		1. GLRLM		Discretization method
11	Vuong et al. [12]	Segmentation methods	Shape and intensity features		Wavelet features		Threshold-based segmentation
12	Edalat-Javid et al. [13]	Image acquisition and reconstruction settings	1. DE from GLDM 2. RLNUN and SRE and RP from GLRLM 3. ZE from GLSZM 4. IDMN and IDN, IMC2 from GLCM		1. SDLGLE, LDLGLE, and DV from GLDM 2. SALGLE, LALGLE and LGLZE from GLSZM		1. Matrix size 2. Number of views 3. FWHM of the Gaussian filter

Suv standard uptake value, *VA* voxel-alignment, *ISZ* intensity-size zone

Table 3.2 Abbreviations

Gray-level co-occurrence matrices (GLCM or GLCOM)	Inverse difference moment (IDMcglcm)
	Code entropy (CE)
	Inverse difference moment Normalized (IDMN)
	Inverse difference normalized (IDN)
	Informal measure of correlation (IMC)
Gray level run length matrix (GLRLM)	High gray-level run emphasis (HGRE)
	Short run high gray-level emphasis (SRHGE)
	Short run emphasis (SRE)
	Long run emphasis (LRE)
	Run-length variability (RLV)
	Run percentage (RP)
	Run length non-uniformity Normalized (RLNUN)
Gray-level size zone matrices (GLSZM)	High gray-level zone emphasis (HGZE)
	Short-zone emphasis (SZE)
	Intensity variability (IV)
	Zone percentage (ZP)
	Zone Entropy (ZE)
	Small area low gray level emphasis (SALGLE)
	Large area low gray level emphasis (LALGLE)
	Low gray level zone emphasis (LGLZE)
Neighborhood gray-level dependence matrix (NGLDM)	
Gray-level neighborhood difference matrices (GLNDM)	
Neighboring gray level dependence (NGLD)	Small number emphasis (SNE)
	Number non-uniformity (NNU)
	Second moment (SM)
Texture feature coding (TFC)	
Texture spectrum (TS)	
Long-zone low gray-level emphasis (LZLGE)	

Table 3.2 (continued)

Gray level dependence matrix (GLDM)	Dependence entropy (DE)
	Small dependence low gray level Emphasis (SDLGLE)
	Large dependence low gray level emphasis (LDLGLE)
	Dependence variance (DV)
Normalized gray-level co-occurrence (NGLCM)	

3.5 Segmentation

Radiomic features are extracted from VOI regions. Contouring or delineation are the names of precise recognition VOI on the images, that can perform manually, automatically, and semi-automatically [17]. Comparing all three methods is done by Belli et al. in 2018 in which a semi-automatic contouring method named PET/Edge represented best repeatability (DICE > 0.95) [9]. The impact of applying different segmentation methods on image features alteration is proven as well. For example, in a study in 2018 it has illustrated that between parameters influencing PET imaging features which have studied, segmentation methods had the most effect on radiomic features variability [3].

3.6 Image Processing

Another step of radiomics workflow (after image acquisition) is image processing consisting of discretization methods, normalizations, interpolations, noise filtering, etc. that always affect the radiomics features [17, 18]. Papp et al. in their research about the effects of extraction parameters changes on radiomic features variability, demonstrated that lesion volume alterations have a larger effect on features in comparison with voxel and bin size [4]. A study concerning the consequence of matrix constructions on radiomic features has indicated that most GLRLM features are independent of matrix parameters meaning there is high stability [10].

3.7   Discretization

Discretization is a process done before feature calculation for some reasons such as noise decreasing, intensity range limiting, and generally to diminish texture matrix dispersal [2]. Among different discretization methods including Max–LIoyd discretization, histogram equalization, fixed bin size (FBS), fixed bin number (FBN), etc. the two last methods are most applicable in radiomics researches [17]. The impact of bin number and bin width, two main parameters related to FBN and FBS respectively, on features variation has proven by multiple studies. Indeed larger influence of FBN and much more repeatable features of FBS have reported too [2, 5].

3.8   Software

It has been seen in some quantitative researches, radiomics papers particularly, the use of home-made software to calculate and extract features. These such works seem to be in contrast to provide a general pipeline for radiomics applications [19]. So it has recommended that to improve and progress in radiomics research and make it closer to clinical reliability, it's necessary to follow IBSI laws and policies [17]. Foy et al. in the assessment of variability of radiomic features against different software implemented, assessed four radiomic packages which two of them were home-made software employed. In this study only a few first- and second-order features were used, they observed that the values calculated by four packages have significant differences so the use of reliable packages for radiomics researches has recommended [20].

3.9   Pitfalls

The last step of radiomics workflow is the creation of models and algorithms for prognostic and diagnostic support tasks. The objective is to achieve such a model which is most relevant to reality. For this purpose, first, we need high-quality and reliable data to construct models and after that examination and performance tests of models should be done to evaluate the function and also differentiate authentic and actual results from false ones. Among multiple pitfalls existing in model creation, overfitting, the condition in which the model performance is pretty good for training data but disappointing for real situations, is a common problem that has been mentioned by plenty of papers [1, 14, 15]. Lack of external validation, class imbalance, incorrect model calibration, use of nonrobust image biomarkers, incomplete reporting, etc. are other mentioned pitfalls that should be considered [17].

3.10   Standardization

Reproducibility of radiomic features and also difference in methodologies to achieve these features are the crucial challenges in the radiomics field [21, 22]. Uncertainty in feature reproducibility is the factor that directly impacts on the translation of these features to clinical area [22, 23]. So, ascertain the reliable and stable features in order to interpretations and also establish a uniform workflow for radiomic features achievement so that it would be followed by all researches in this field are two ineluctable requisites for future of the radiomics [21]. There has been trying recently to develop a defined framework and features nomenclature by the image biomarker standardization initiative (IBSI) researchers in order to integrate the routes and outcomes in future researches [24].

3.11   Discussion

Stability of radiomic features is the recent and critical issue in translating these features for prognostic and diagnostic context. For this purpose, the objective of this chapter was an assessment of the robustness and repeatability of radiomic quantities against imaging parameter changes. Medical imaging has great potential to provide a wide range of information about the internal construction and function of the body completely noninvasively, so it's necessary to accelerate researches in this area. Along with offering new methods and procedures in this field, the reliability and dependability of these methods are also important as practical application is the goal. In this review, searching main keywords including repeatability, reproducibility, robustness, stability, radiomic features, nuclear medicine, etc. tries to collect all recent researches directly relevant to the variability of radiomic features against imaging parameters changes. The priority of the last three-year articles was one of the reasons that limited the number of articles.

In addition to imaging parameter changes, inter-patient and inter-scanner repeatability need to be evaluated too, so the need for a general procedure for the execution of this kind of researches is seriously vital. One of the existing problems in the field of radiomics researches is the extended range of research methodologies. For example, although the use of retrospective data is prevalent for many studies, implementing multiple kinds of phantoms including digital phantom, anthropomorphic phantom, software simulated phantom, etc. is another source of data. Moreover, various ways to feature extraction and feature robustness analysis can aggravate the condition. This dispersion of operation pathes can lead to the accumulation of a large volume of new and raw data which without any reliability characteristics are not applicable and maybe cause to the confusion of newcomers to this branch of science. So it seems necessary to present a coherent and integrated methodology to achieve meaningful results.

3.12 Conclusion

Radiomics is a developing field of research that connects imaging technology and statistical analysis to achieve more information that may be hidden or unclear for the human eye. Repeatability and reproducibility of radiomic features are the most recent issues that got more attention due to the tendency of employing radiomics in clinics [1]. Variability of features caused by imaging parameter changes is mentioned in several arti-

cles and it is exactly why clinicians can't benefit from radiomics abilities. To identify what parameter can alter radiomic features we have to investigate the influence of each parameter to the attainment of an optimized set of radiomics features. In this chapter we reviewed some relevant papers that assessed the robustness and stability of radiomic features along with different changes in imaging parameters like image acquisition, segmentation, image reconstruction, etc. also by comparing the response of extracted features to parameter changing, the most robust and sensitive features highlighted. Acquiring robust and reproducible features need homogenous use of influencing parameters (scan protocols) which have optimized to radiomics usage. More researches and endeavors are necessary to take this field into its appropriate place of science.

References

1. Park JE, Park SY, Kim HJ, Kim HS. Reproducibility and generalizability in radiomics modeling: possible strategies in radiologic and statistical perspectives. Korean J Radiol. 2019;20(7):1124–37.
2. Branchini M, Zorz A, Zucchetta P, Bettinelli A, De Monte F, Cecchin D, et al. Impact of acquisition count statistics reduction and SUV discretization on PET radiomic features in pediatric 18F-FDG-PET/MRI examinations. Phys Med. 2019;59:117–26.
3. Gallivanone F, Interlenghi M, D'Ambrosio D, Trifirò G, Castiglioni I. Parameters influencing PET imaging features: a phantom study with irregular and heterogeneous synthetic lesions. Contrast media. Mol Imaging. 2018;2018:5324517.
4. Papp L, Rausch I, Grahovac M, Hacker M, Beyer T. Optimized feature extraction for radiomics analysis of (18)F-FDG PET imaging. J Nucl Med. 2019;60(6):864–72.
5. Pfaehler E, Beukinga RJ, de Jong JR, Slart RHJA, Slump CH, Dierckx RAJO, et al. Repeatability of 18F-FDG PET radiomic features: a phantom study to explore sensitivity to image reconstruction settings, noise, and delineation method. Med Phys. 2019;46(2):665–78.
6. Pfaehler E, van Sluis J, Merema BBJ, van Ooijen P, Berendsen RCM, van Velden FHP, et al. Experimental multicenter and multivendor evaluation of the performance of PET radiomic features using 3-dimensionally printed phantom inserts. J Nucl Med. 2020;61(3):469–76.
7. Yang F, Simpson G, Young L, Ford J, Dogan N, Wang L. Impact of contouring variability on oncological

PET radiomics features in the lung. Sci Rep. 2020;10(1):369.

8. Shiri I, Rahmim A, Ghaffarian P, Geramifar P, Abdollahi H, Bitarafan-Rajabi A. The impact of image reconstruction settings on 18F-FDG PET radiomic features: multi-scanner phantom and patient studies. Eur Radiol. 2017;27(11):4498–509.

9. Belli ML, Mori M, Broggi S, Cattaneo GM, Bettinardi V, Dell'Oca I, et al. Quantifying the robustness of [¹⁸F]FDG-PET/CT radiomic features with respect to tumor delineation in head and neck and pancreatic cancer patients. Phys Med. 2018;49:105–11.

10. Lv W, Yuan Q, Wang Q, Ma J, Jiang J, Yang W, et al. Robustness versus disease differentiation when varying parameter settings in radiomics features: application to nasopharyngeal PET/CT. Eur Radiol. 2018;28(8):3245–54.

11. Guezennec C, Bourhis D, Orlhac F, Robin P, Corre J-B, Delcroix O, et al. Inter-observer and segmentation method variability of textural analysis in pretherapeutic FDG PET/CT in head and neck cancer. PLoS ONE. 2019;14(3):e0214299.

12. Vuong D, Tanadini-Lang S, Huellner MW, Veit-Haibach P, Unkelbach J, Andratschke N, et al. Interchangeability of radiomic features between [18F]-FDG PET/CT and [18F]-FDG PET/MR. Med Phys. 2019;46(4):1677–85.

13. Edalat-Javid M, Shiri I, Hajianfar G, Abdollahi H, Arabi H, Oveisi N, et al. Cardiac SPECT radiomic features repeatability and reproducibility: a multiscanner phantom study. J Nucl Cardiol. 2020;28(6):2730–44.

14. Mayerhoefer ME, Materka A, Langs G, Haggstrom I, Szczypinski P, Gibbs P, et al. Introduction to radiomics. J Nucl Med. 2020;61(4):488–95.

15. Traverso A, Wee L, Dekker A, Gillies R. Repeatability and reproducibility of radiomic features: a systematic review. Int J Radiat Oncol Biol Phys. 2018;102(4):1143–58.

16. Kuhl CK, Truhn D. The long route to standardized radiomics: unraveling the knot from the end. Radiology. 2020;295(2):339–41.

17. Zwanenburg A. Radiomics in nuclear medicine: robustness, reproducibility, standardization, and how to avoid data analysis traps and replication crisis. Eur J Nucl Med Mol Imaging. 2019;46(13):2638–55.

18. Ibrahim A, Vallières M, Woodruff H, Primakov S, Beheshti M, Keek S, et al. Radiomics analysis for clinical decision support in nuclear medicine. Semin Nucl Med. 2019;49(5):438–49.

19. Reuzé S, Schernberg A, Orlhac F, Sun R, Chargari C, Dercle L, et al. Radiomics in nuclear medicine applied to radiation therapy: methods, pitfalls, and challenges. Int J Radiat Oncol Biol Phys. 2018;102(4):1117–42.

20. Foy JJ, Robinson KR, Li H, Giger ML, Al-Hallaq H, Armato SG. Variation in algorithm implementation across radiomics software. J Med Imaging. 2018;5(4):044505.

21. Zwanenburg A, Vallières M, Abdalah MA, Aerts HJ, Andrearczyk V, Apte A, et al. The image biomarker standardization initiative: standardized quantitative radiomics for high-throughput image-based phenotyping. Radiology. 2020;295(2):328–38.

22. Welch ML, McIntosh C, Haibe-Kains B, Milosevic MF, Wee L, Dekker A, et al. Vulnerabilities of radiomic signature development: the need for safeguards. Radiother Oncol. 2019;130:2–9.

23. McNitt-Gray M, Napel S, Jaggi A, Mattonen S, Hadjiiski L, Muzi M, et al. Standardization in quantitative imaging: a multicenter comparison of radiomic features from different software packages on digital reference objects and patient data sets. Tomography. 2020;6(2):118.

24. Hagiwara A, Fujita S, Ohno Y, Aoki S. Variability and standardization of quantitative imaging: monoparametric to multiparametric quantification, radiomics, and artificial intelligence. Investig Radiol. 2020;55(9):601.

Evolution of AI in Medical Imaging

4

Josh Schaefferkoetter

Contents

In the field of medical imaging, the application of computer vision to solve radiologic problems has been proposed since the mid-twentieth century [1]. As computers became more prevalent and imaging became digitized, the infrastructure was in place upon which to build sophisticated analysis pipelines to be used in routine workflow—this workflow has included, and will certainly continue to include, different applications of artificial intelligence. Today, AI is fundamental in many facets of everyday life, from semantic searches on the internet to facial and voice recognition in mobile devices, and it has made remarkable progress in recent years. There are various potential applications of AI in medicine, and AI has already impacted radiology in some regards, introducing quantification into a space which was historically based purely on subjectivity [2, 3]. This however is just the beginning—it is widely recognized that medical imaging is one of the many fields in which advanced AI will cause a complete paradigm shift. Molecular imaging in particular is an especially likely candidate to benefit, and it is in a position which would allow it to readily integrate this technology.

Molecular imaging technologies have continually improved year over year. MRI developments include higher field strength magnets,

J. Schaefferkoetter (✉)
Siemens Medical Solutions USA, Inc.,
Knoxville, TN, USA
e-mail: joshua.schaefferkoetter@siemens-healthineers.com

improved RF coil arrays increasing acquisition SNR, and a growing catalog of pulse sequences for various applications. Single photon emission computed tomography (SPECT) systems routinely employ advanced correction techniques now producing quantitative images, and modern positron emission tomography (PET) scanners are using smaller crystals leading to better spatial resolution, with detection systems approaching timing resolution close to 200 ps. All of these modalities have realized concurrent progress in data processing as well, including sophisticated reconstruction and motion correction techniques. These advances have yielded extraordinary levels of image quality, but point is approaching where it is becoming less clear how these improvements are practically realized in terms of clinical outcomes. For instance, producing images with superfine resolution for routine examinations might not significantly impact diagnostic reliability, staging, or treatment planning. In fact, the additional time taken for the data acquisition and radiologist interpretation would potentially have adverse effects on the clinical workflow. Furthermore, in recent years, the amount of medical imaging data has grown exponentially, and this has already increased the pressure on radiologists to maintain accuracy at higher throughput. While novel imaging innovations will continue to have impact on patient care and be welcomed by the medical community, it is likely that technological developments in the near future will focus on increasing efficiency, reliably standardizing care, and improving patient safety.

Artificial intelligence, by definition, is the branch of computer science, developing computer algorithms to perform jobs normally requiring human intelligence. Machine learning (ML) is a subgroup of AI connoting any algorithm which improves through experience. There are many different schemes, ranging in complexity from simple regression models and component analyses to more complex methods like random forests and support vector machines. However, most of the remarkable successes and resulting excitement of recent times belong to the class of ML known as deep learning (DL). State-of-the-art results have been achieved in the fields of object detection, classification, image segmentation, speech recognition, and image generation—in fact, DL models have matched and even surpassed human performance in certain tasks [4–6]. It is impossible to ignore that these tasks are ubiquitous components in many aspects of radiology, and novel applications for DL are immediately identified. Indeed, there are many areas of active research in medicine and remarkable successes have been reported. Most reviews or general overviews of DL in medicine cite the growing number of related publications on PubMed, and at the time of this writing, the search phrase "deep learning" returned 5315 results for 2019. This is up from 3004 in the previous year, and for 2020, there are already 3994 results in the first 6 months. This trend is certainly a testament to the applicability and success of DL in medicine.

It is difficult to understand the evolution and future direction of AI without a basic understanding of the recent advances in AI techniques. This section gives an abbreviated overview, detailing a few specific examples. It cannot possibly cover all aspects but will instead focus on DL, since it is, without question, the dominant trend and direction of recent AI research; it has demonstrated promising improvements even over other traditional ML approaches. Almost all DL techniques are based on artificial neural networks (ANNs) comprising layers of numerical weights and "activation" nodes. More specifically, each node within a layer generally consists of a linear operation involving the summed product of its weights and input (the outputs of the previous layer), followed by a nonlinear operation, e.g., sigmoid, hyperbolic tangent, rectified linear—there may be thousands of nodes in a given layer. By stacking many of these layers, through densely interconnected nodes, one can effectively piecewise construct complex functions which are able to be shaped throughout many degrees of freedom. In this sense, a network can be shaped to "learn" mapping functions between different domains. Unlike most other ML approaches, DL does not require inputs which explicitly define the discriminating features of the population; through training, it inherently learns the features which best represent the data for the current task. This data-driven approach allows DL applications to characterize more abstract features and makes these systems more generalizable, but it is predicated on the availability of large amounts of training data to enable accurate characterizations of the sample populations.

Convolutional neural networks (CNNs) are an extension of neural networks, designed to handle data with higher dimensionality, usually in 2D or 3D, and so are well suited for image-based tasks. In conventional ANNs, the weights at each layer have a single, unique value for every combination of nodes of its layer and the nodes of the previous layer, and so the corresponding total number of weights at each layer is the product of these numbers. For CNNs, instead of a single value, there is a matrix of values, which can be thought of as a weighted filter; the size of the matrices is relatively small. The filters are passed over the layer input data like a convolution kernel, resulting in output feature maps of the same dimensionality as the input. This approach exploits the spatial dependencies within the data and makes the network invariant to input translations, while at the same time significantly reducing the total number of network parameters. For example, say we have a single 2D input image with pixel dimensions 100×100, and this feeds a layer with 128 channels. A conventional ANN would handle each of the 10,000 input pixels independently, and so the total number of parameters would be 1,280,000 for that single layer. For a CNN, this corresponding layer would handle the whole image as a single, multidimensional input—with a filter size 3×3, the total number of layer parameters would then only be 1152 ($1 \times 3 \times 3 \times 128$). This scheme is not only more efficient but potentially allows the same network to handle inputs of arbitrary sizes. For these reasons, CNNs are currently the AI technique of choice for image analyses and computer vision tasks.

Various CNN architectures are currently used—a few are explicitly mentioned here, but many of the basic concepts are common with many other networks. The convolution layers typically have filters with sizes between 3 and 5 pixels (for each dimension), and most networks also have multiple resolution downsampling (or encoding) layers. Many of the early uses for CNNs were focused on classification tasks and used a nonconvolutional, densely connected layer at the last layer to sort the output in scalar class probabilities [7]. Fully convolution networks (FCNs), however, do not contain any densely connected layers and preserve the input dimensionality throughout the network—this architecture is better suited to certain analysis tasks, i.e., when requiring a dense prediction map over all pixels [8]. The U-Net architecture has become widely used in image analyses [9] and uses a dedicated encoding and decoding path to produce outputs of the same size as the inputs. A major contribution of U-Net was the introduction of skip connections between the encoding and decoding paths at each resolution level in order to preserve spatial detail throughout the network—this feature makes this architecture popular for medical image segmentation tasks. Another useful architecture is ResNet, which is built on residual blocks containing multiple convolution layers, with the block input directly connected to its output [10]. This direct connection results in an alternate identity path, and so each convolutional block needs only to learn the pixel residuals and is pre-conditioned to learn mappings which are close to identity; the ResNet architecture has facilitated training stability in some of the deepest networks. The last relevant architecture is called Inception [11]. It contains blocks of multiple streams, each with different numbers of convolutions, under the premise that explicit filter sizes need not be defined since the image is now analyzed at multiple scales at the same level, i.e., taking the network wider rather than deeper. There is also a powerful extension of this called Inception-ResNet, which as the name implies, uses Inception blocks, rather than blocks of single-convolution streams, to calculate the block residuals.

Alongside the evolution of network architectures were concurrent advances in network training approaches. In the context of ML, training refers to the minimization of an objective loss metric corresponding to a certain task, i.e., some measure of distance between the network output and target value. In more basic terms, this means the values of the network weight parameters are gradually modified so that the desired outputs are obtained. This is usually accomplished by back-propagating the derivative of the loss through the network. Backpropagation is a computationally efficient method, combining simple mathematical operations, to generate a gradient of partial derivatives comprising the influences on the loss of every parameter in the network. After a complete backpropagation cycle, each network parameter is updated according to a predefined schedule in the direction which minimizes the loss. This process is repeated for many, sometimes millions, of iterations until acceptable performance is achieved.

In general, there are two fundamental approaches to training ML systems, supervised and unsupervised. Under supervised approaches, the input data have corresponding labels, and gradient backpropagation begins with a loss calculation over every output element of the network. For example, a CNN designed for classification might predict the correct class for a given input image by finding the maximum of the discrete probabilities calculated over all possible classes—during training, it would compare this prediction to the correct label and backpropagate its error differentials. In a simple classification task, each possible class might be represented as a single node in the output layer. This concept is readily extended to FCNs, in which a classification framework might be used for organ segmentation, for example. In this situation, the loss would be calculated over each pixel, giving the likelihood that it belongs to a given tissue class. Supervised methods provide a direct objective but require manual data labeling or annotating, which is a laborious task and is often the main challenge given the large scale of data typically needed for training. Unsupervised methods, on the other hand, do not require labeled data and instead rely on the algorithm itself to extract the discriminating features within different sample populations to minimize the loss for the task at hand. There are several methods for unsupervised network training, but one approach stands out for its range of applicability and remarkable recent results, and it is designed for image-based tasks performed by CNNs. Generative adversarial networks (GANs), introduced in 2014, comprise a system of two networks [12]. The first is the primary network, the generator, which for simplicity, can be regarded no differently than the networks discussed above—its job is to perform the desired task. However, instead of defining the training loss directly at its top layer with labels, the generator's output is fed into the second network, the discriminator, and the job of this network is to distinguish the generator's outputs from a corresponding set of real samples. During training, the discriminator learns the features that are common to the real and generated populations as a whole and uses this information to discriminate between the two sample sets. However, this same information can also be backpropagated to the generator and used to improve its own output. In this way, the two networks are adversaries in that they are each constantly trying to outperform the other, but at the same time, both the networks can simultaneously improve together. Deep learning systems built on the GAN framework have been tailored for specific applications in a wide range of fields and have demonstrated state-of-the-art performance, especially for image generation, translation, and transformation tasks.

Artificial intelligence has already established applications in the medical field. Novel investigations however, particularly those based on DL, are yielding especially impressive results, and these provide a glimpse of the direction of AI and hint at its potential future role in molecular imaging. The following sections provide an abbreviated outline of its historical and current uses and also highlight some areas of emerging research.

4.1 Disease Characterization

Characterization is a general term implying the segmentation, diagnosis, and staging of disease. These tasks are achieved by identifying and measuring the imaged properties of a pathologic abnormality. A radiologist performing these analyses is therefore required to process large amounts of data for each examination, and he or she must then distill it down into a manageable, and much smaller, number of qualitative features, e.g., size, shape, heterogeneity, to serve as the basis for the final interpretation. Inevitably, some radiological information is lost throughout this process. Furthermore, every physician is different, and there will be unavoidable variability among human observers. Artificial intelligence can help to automate this procedure. It has the capacity to consider large numbers of quantitative features, potentially orders of magnitude greater than a human, and it could perform the task in a fraction of the time in a reproducible way. For example, benign and malignant pulmonary nodules have similar appearances, and hence, the status of malignancy in the lungs is difficult to assess. AI can account for many features simultaneously and automatically determine those which are most relevant to the current case. The relevant features could be treated as imaging biomarkers to be used in the malignancy prediction, along with other clinical endpoints like risk assessment and prognosis [13].

The idea to use AI for disease characterization and diagnosis dates back to the mid-twentieth century [14–17]. Many of these studies focused on the improved interpretation of electrocardiograms by computers [18–21] since these data are particularly suitable for computer analyses. Other related work included the differential diagnosis of hematological diseases [22], automatic biochemical analysis of bodily substances [23], and sclerosis prediction in the coronary arteries [24]. These efforts mostly comprised smaller pilot studies and reported some success. Although larger-scale, definitive experiments were not performed during this time, these efforts led to the general belief that automatic diagnoses by computers were not just feasible, but necessary as part of a comprehensive medical data control system [25–27]. These early studies fostered an optimistic outlook for the potential of machine-assisted diagnosis and led to many advancements in computer-aided diagnostic (CAD) programs.

Dedicated CAD programs have early roots [28], but researchers only started large-scale development toward practical solutions in the 1980s. Significant effort was made in the research

arena, but the benefits to the real clinical applications fell short [29], and it was not until 1998 that the FDA approved its use in screening and diagnostic mammography, as well as in plain chest radiography and CT imaging. Today, several systems are in clinical use with screening mammograms [30]. They are typically recommended to serve as a second opinion, complementing the initial radiologist assessment [31], and these led to the development of similar systems for other imaging modalities, including ultrasonography and MRI [32].

These conventional CAD systems generally consist of two components: detection of suspicious lesions and reduction of the false positive findings. The detection system is based on radiologist-defined criteria like tumor volume, shape, texture, etc. which are translated into a pattern-recognition problem where the most robust features are fed into an algorithm to highlight suspicious objects in the image [33]. The false-positive reduction part is also based on traditional ML, but can pose a bigger challenge to these algorithms. Even with sophisticated programs, the general performance of current CAD systems is not good, and this limits their extensive clinical use. Several trials have concluded that these systems, at best, deliver no benefit [34, 35]. It is more concerning though that these systems were actually found to reduce radiological accuracy in some cases [36], leading to higher recall and biopsy rates [37, 38].

Conventional CAD systems are built on rigid ML algorithms, mostly relying on expert knowledge, established a priori, for engineering features to be extracted from regions of interest. In contrast, new programs built on DL algorithms offer potential advantages regarding the degrees of freedom and level of abstraction in which the detection and classification tasks are defined. Furthermore, the performance of conventional CAD systems is notoriously sensitive to image noise and selected scanning protocol, and DL has demonstrated flexibility with regard to these parameters [39].

Largely due to the advances in computer hardware and processing technology, DL applications have emerged only recently for CAD systems—perhaps the earliest use in radiology was first reported in 1990, when a group at the University of Chicago developed an ANN for improving differential diagnosis of interstitial lung diseases using clinical and radiographic information. They claimed that the decision performance of the neural network was comparable to that of the chest radiologists and even superior to that of the senior radiology residents [40]. This led to several subsequent studies at that institution investigating neural network-aided diagnoses of lung disease [41–43]. The first object detection system using CNNs was proposed a few years later in 1995 at Georgetown University Medical Center, using a CNN with four layers to detect nodules in X-ray images [44].

Since then, DL-based CAD systems have been developed for the identification, detection, diagnosis, and risk analysis of various pathologies. Breast cancer, for example, was an obvious target since there was a historical precedent, and recent studies have demonstrated promising results regarding the performance of these next-generation systems in detecting and staging the diseases [45, 46]. In particular, it was reported that the automatic feature exploration and higher noise tolerance of DL-based CAD systems were responsible for the performance gains, which were quantified using different metrics, including sensitivity, specificity, and receiver operating characteristic analyses [47]. Lung cancer detection and screening is another attractive application, and several studies have evaluated the implementation of DL-based CAD systems for this purpose [48, 49]. These have also shown potential to effectively predict lung cancer and classify pulmonary nodules [47, 50]. In dermatology, deep convolutional networks have been used to classify skin lesions according to malignancy [51]. This large study found that AI achieved equivalent performance to all tested experts on two separate classification tasks, and further, it suggested that smartphone cameras could be used in conjunction with this technology to provide low-cost access to vital diagnoses. Other groups have also investigated DL with multi-modal imaging data. One notable study used PET and computed tomography (CT) data together in order to reduce false-positive results

in lung lesion detections [52]. Simultaneous PET/CT data have also been used to classify lymph node metastases; a recent work found that this approach yielded higher sensitivities than radiologists [53]. Studies are consistently showing that the detection performance of AI in dedicated tasks is rivaling that of physicians [54], and recent interest in pursuing large-scale CAD solutions suggests the future for developing robust, high-performance systems based on deep learning [55].

Deep learning has also demonstrated success for using radiological information, not just for disease detection and characterization, but for predicting patient diagnosis and prognosis. Early works in this area included survival predictions in patients with lung adenocarcinoma [56] and high-grade gliomas [57]. More recently, DL algorithms have been developed to predict the risk of lung cancer from a patient's current and prior CT volumes [58]. This work achieved a state-of-the-art predictive performance on thousands of national lung cancer screening trial cases and independent clinical validation sets. This work also noted that its AI-based model reduced many risks associated with conventional low-dose CT screening, including false positives, overdiagnoses, and radiation exposure. The computer-aided detection and diagnosis of Alzheimer's disease (AD) is another area of active DL research. SPECT and PET are both used by physicians to image the metabolism, protein aggregation, or amyloid deposition associated with AD, and a few studies have investigated DL-based CAD systems for early AD diagnoses. The flexibility of DL allows brain data from multiple modalities to be assessed together [59–61]. Two notable recent works even used 3D CNNs to classify patients having AD [62, 63]. In other functional neurological studies, Parkinson's disease has been automatically diagnosed in dopamine active transporter SPECT scans, achieving sensitivities around 95% [64, 65]. Other work has been performed with PET/CT and PET/MR data, and the inclusion of multimodal inputs, exploiting functional and structural information, has the potential to further improve the performance of AI-based disease characterization.

4.2 Segmentation

Segmentation is an important component of medical image analyses—indeed, many of the aforementioned applications regarding the characterization of disease may be predicated on accurate delineations of organs, tissue or pathologic region of interest. It can often be a tedious and arduous task, and techniques to reliably speed the process would be welcomed by medical practitioners. Automatic segmentation methods using computer vision date back to the 1980s [66], with continual improvement over the following decades. Early approaches were based on clustering to isolate areas of similar intensities or region growing algorithms which spatially expanded regions around a user-selected seed point until homogeneity dropped below a certain criterion [67]. The next-generation algorithms used statistical learning and optimization to improve accuracy. One such approach is the watershed algorithm, in which image values are used to construct topology-like maps [68]. More advanced systems were able to use previous knowledge to construct a probability map to inform the segmentations. This approach is analogous to Bayesian inference, and the use of prior information lends itself, for example, to situations where objects are ill-defined in terms pixel intensities. The use of probability maps has proven especially helpful for oncologic segmentation within patient populations, since they contain information regarding the expected location of tumors [69]. Other segmentation systems based on prior knowledge-based probability maps have also been applied to radiotherapy planning in head and neck CT images [70] and segmenting gliomas in brain MRIs [71].

These past techniques have realized some success in the clinical workflow, but the algorithms are somewhat inflexible and were designed for specific tasks. Segmentation programs built on DL technology will significantly outperform their predecessors, and for these applications, fully convolutional networks are well suited. A major step toward semantic segmentation by FCNs was reported by UC Berkeley in 2015 [8]. This group first constructed FCNs by "decapitat-ing" the fully connected layers from conventional CNNs, and replacing them with new layers to expand the resolution. This resulted in a network which produced an output having the same dimensions as its input, and by fine-tuning only the new layers, the parameters of the original layers which had already been trained on millions of images for classification tasks were not affected. The result was a network which was able to exploit the feature extraction mechanisms of the original network and apply this information to a dense prediction matrix. These researchers achieved impressive results, effectively using an FCN to segment detailed regions based on multi-class probabilities predicted for every discrete pixel [72]. Although this work focused only on natural images, the concept is readily extended to medical images.

Substantial attention has been paid to CNNs to resolve the challenges associated with medical imaging segmentation. Many techniques have been evaluated for various applications—a few specific examples include the automatic segmentation of lungs [73], biological cells and membranes [74, 75], tibial cartilage [76], bone tissue [77], brain structures [78], prostate [79], and tumors [80–83]. An important contribution came in 2015 with the introduction of the U-Net architecture and skip connections [9]. U-Net has been the de facto choice for many applications, including segmenting multiple organs on thoracic CT images with 3D data [84] or as incorporated into a GAN framework [85]. This network architecture also led to other derivatives like V-Net, which introduced a novel loss function directly based on the Dice coefficient [86].

Segmentation platforms built on DL offer other general advantages over older AI techniques as well. One study describes that DL methods for brain MRI segmentation completely eliminate the need for image registration required by other approaches like atlas-based methods [87]. It has also been reported that a single DL system is able to perform diverse segmentation tasks, without task-specific training, across multiple modalities and tissue types, including brain MRI, breast MRI, and cardiac CT angiography [88]. Considering this with the fact that current

DL technologies are already equivalent in many regards to radiologists' performance for segmentation [89], it is expected that the presence of DL-based segmentation algorithms in routine clinical tools will increase dramatically in the near future.

4.3 Image Generation/ Reconstruction

Images are fundamental in radiology and diagnostic medicine. It was Wilhelm Roentgen who first discovered X-rays could be used to image bone just prior to the turn of the twentieth century. These early images were created directly, simply by exposing photographic film with the high-energy radiation. Over the next few decades, several other scanners were developed and some became digitized. This included the first positron-annihilation coincident detection system in the 1950s. A simple rectilinear scanner with sodium iodide detectors was designed and built by Gordon Brownell at Massachusetts General Hospital to image tumors in the brain. As imaging technology advanced throughout the century, so did the methods used to process the acquired data and produce the images. Certainly, one of the most groundbreaking inventions was the CT scanner in the 1970s by Sir Godfrey Hounsfield. This achievement ushered in the era of volumetric tomography, i.e., cross-sectional imaging of a 3D body, in the medical setting. The CT scanner acquired X-ray projection data at various angles for sequential axial positions. The projection data were used to reconstruct image slices by filtered back-projection (FBP), a direct reconstruction technique which is still used even today. FBP was used to reconstruct projection data for emission modalities as well like PET and SPECT as they made their way into nuclear medicine departments in the 1980s and 1990s. During this time, MRI systems also became a mainstream diagnostic tool. MR is unique from the others in that its images are generated directly through inverse Fourier transforms of the acquired frequency and phase data. For all imaging modalities, processing methods have made great strides over recent

years, and through many recent advances, the images which are routinely produced in the clinic are of unprecedented quality. Artificial intelligence has the potential to push this even higher.

Until recent times, AI had not realized an overwhelming presence in image reconstruction. Conventional approaches relied on physics and closed-form mathematics to define the acquisition process and translate the data into images. However, recent decades have seen processing schemes which have become less rigid and more adaptive. Although these may not be considered AI, per se, they incorporate some of the same components. For example, direct reconstruction methods like FBP have been replaced by iterative algorithms. The objective of these algorithms is to find the image which is the most likely source of the projections—this framework can account for data which may be incomplete which results in far less image noise. The optimal image may be found by maximizing some likelihood or minimizing some cost measure, a technique which is often used in clustering machine learning algorithms. Also, many MR systems are moving toward compressed sensing to perform routine examinations in fractions of the time. Combining these under sampled data with prior information, images of high fidelity can still be produced.

Deep learning algorithms based on CNNs have incredible potential for applications in image reconstruction and generation. Research in this field is rapidly increasing, with the large majority of work focusing on MRI—only a relatively small subset of studies is mentioned here. A popular area is looking to AI for acceleration of MR imaging through improving compressed sensing techniques [90, 91]. Neural networks have demonstrated the ability to learn spatio-temporal dependencies which enable them to improve the accuracy of reconstructed MR images from highly undersampled complex-valued k-space data. This concept can be applied to dynamic MR imaging and may be especially interesting for cardiac cine protocols [92]. Furthermore, this idea has been extended to various MRI acquisition strategies. Recent algorithms have proved to be flexible for treating the MR reconstruction process as a supervised learning task, mapping the scanner sensors to resultant images [93]. Deep learning has also been used to reduce the gadolinium dose in contrast-enhanced brain MRI by an order of magnitude while preserving the quality of the images [94] and for inferring advanced MRI diffusion parameters from limited data [95]. Quantitative susceptibility mapping, which aims to estimate the magnetic susceptibility of biological tissue, is currently a growing field in MRI research [96, 97]. The estimation of magnetic susceptibility from local magnetic fields is an ill-posed problem, and recent AI methods are being used here as well. One work developed a CNN based on the U-Net architecture which was able to generate high-quality susceptibility maps from single orientation data [98]. MR-fingerprinting (MRF) is another recent technique [99]. The idea is to use a pseudo-randomized acquisition that captures a unique signal from different tissues. These tissue "fingerprints" are then mapped back to standard parameters, T1, T2, proton density, etc. by matching them to a predefined dictionary of predicted signal evolutions. This mapping is a difficult problem and has usually employed a pattern recognition approach—deep learning methodology is now being investigated for this purpose. A four-layer neural network was trained to map the recorded signal magnitudes to their corresponding tissue T1 and T2 values [100]. This group found reconstruction times using this approach were 300–5000 times faster than conventional dictionary-matching techniques in both phantom and human brain studies. Other similar approaches have been used to predict quantitative tissue parameter values from undersampled MRF data [101, 102].

Although MRI has so far realized the largest number of deep learning research efforts, these have potential applications extending to many areas in medical imaging on a more general scale. The last few years have seen impressive results for synthesizing photo-realistic images, especially using GANs [12, 103–105], and these techniques have also been used for biological image synthesis [106, 107]. One recent study designed a system to generate synthetic tumors in otherwise normal brain images [108]. This approach high-

lights a tremendously powerful use for generative networks, namely creating or augmenting training data. This is highly interesting for medical imaging as datasets are often sparse or imbalanced, with few examples of pathological findings. Overcoming this challenge would help alleviate a huge limitation commonly encountered in training deep learning models. This approach has been used for brain tumor segmentation [109], synthesizing realistic prostate lesions [110], augmenting data for improved liver lesion classification [111], and generating synthetic retinal fundus images [112]. GANs have also been used for unsupervised generation of T1-weighted brains [113] and image synthesis for tissue recognition and computer-assisted intervention [114, 115]. Inter-modality translation has even been performed by GANs, transforming MR to CT images [116, 117] and to PET images [118]. This work even showed that generated images can be used in CAD systems for improving the diagnosis of Alzheimer's disease when the patient data are incomplete.

Artificial intelligence has provided a new paradigm for solving inverse problems in medical imaging [119–123]. Furthermore, studies have demonstrated the ability of DL to not only improve existing image reconstructions [124, 125] but also replace the reconstruction altogether, generating images directly from acquisition data [126]. This work found that a deep convolutional encoder–decoder network could be successfully used to generate quantitatively accurate PET images in a fraction of the time taken by conventional reconstruction methods. These works, and others like them, are incredibly encouraging. As a result, they have provoked a new, and necessary, avenue for research focusing solely on the potential pitfalls of DL-based reconstruction, and it has been found that deep learning can often cause unstable reconstruction methods. One recent work reported that these instabilities occur in several forms including: severe reconstruction artifacts caused by small perturbations in both the image or sampling domain; incomplete or incorrect representation of small structural changes, e.g., tumors; and more training samples yielded poorer reconstruction performance for several of the models investigated [127]. Numerical accuracy and stability are essential components of medical image reconstruction, and so the limitations of new technology are important to understand before it can be reliably used in the clinic. It is likely that, in the future, the image reconstruction process will be omitted altogether for certain applications, since a computer can theoretically extract any information contained in an image directly from the acquired data. For now, however, since humans perform the clinical interpretation, medical images need to be generated, and AI will continue to impact this process in unprecedented ways.

4.4   Data Corrections

As alluded to in the previous section, the methods to create medical images must be accurate and stable in order to be reliable—these requirements become even more critical when medical decisions depend on measurements of precisely quantified image values. Hence, the entire reconstruction process may comprise multiple steps to address different aspects. The backprojection algorithm, the cornerstone of tomographic reconstruction, can help to illustrate this. Data that are acquired as projections are mathematically regarded as a set of 1D line integrals, and backprojection seeks to invert this process and transform the sets of projections back to their original 2D form. However, due to the nature of the acquisition, low frequencies have a stronger latent prevalence within the projections than do the higher frequencies. So, to avoid a blurry reconstructed image dominated by low frequencies, the projection data must first be convolved with a ramp filter to boost the high frequencies. Additionally, the cylindrical geometry of the detection system results in nonuniform radial sampling, and this nonuniformity must also be accounted for in the reconstruction. This example demonstrates some of the steps necessary for a correct reconstruction approach, but backprojection is considered a direct method—newer, more sophisticated techniques usually require many additional considerations.

In addition to the corrections needed to compensate for the limitations of the acquisition method, the acquired data themselves may not be of high inherent quality. For PET, the true data come from pure annihilation photons, detected within a small coincidence window. However, the scanner also captures coincident events arising from scattered and random photons which must be corrected. These are not generally abled to be measured directly, so they must be estimated—this is currently accomplished by modeling the underlying physics. Photon scattering and absorption also leads to signal attenuation, and this requires an additional correction, usually based on an accompanying anatomical map. For MRI, the quality of the acquired data depends on the homogeneity of the static magnetic field, linearity of the gradients and stability of the receiver coils. These properties are bound by engineering limitations, and many techniques are routinely used to correct anomalies; for example, shimming is used to adjust the field homogeneity and spherical harmonic polynomial models can be used to characterize high-order gradient nonlinearities. However, sometimes these attempts are insufficient. Additionally, the MR scanner is very sensitive to environmental perturbations, and these can also lead to image noise. Artificial intelligence has proven adept at finding solutions to inference problems and should be able to help with issues related to incomplete or corrupted imaging data—indeed, it has already attained some notable successes.

Deep learning has recently been introduced to image denoising for many applications. In one study, neural networks were specifically developed to learn the implicit brain manifolds in MR images [113]. This group tested their approach by adding various levels of noise to several hundred T1-weighted brain images and reported improved performance over current denoising methods in terms of peak signal-to-noise ratios. Denoising has also been applied to dynamic contrast enhanced MR data, using multiple networks to improve the signal quality, both spatially and temporally [128]. Emission modalities have also been a focus of AI denoising research since they are inherently noisy. For instance, each projection bin of a routine PET acquisition may contain only a few coincident events, introducing uncertainty into the reconstruction. Several works within the last few years have reported success for PET image denoising using both supervised and unsupervised training approaches [129–131]. One notable study incorporated a 2D network pretrained on millions of natural images as a perceptual loss network [132]. This group reported that image resolution and noise properties were improved by optimizing the perceptual loss in this way, rather than simply using a per-pixel supervised loss like L1- or L2-norm. This approach has also been successfully applied for denoising CT images at various noise levels [133]. These reported successes have driven other research to investigate the potential clinical impacts of these methods. One such work reported improvements in physician lesion detectability performance when low-count PET images where denoised by a CNN [134].

Artifacts are another common nuisance in medical images—physiological or random patient motion, metal implants and temporal or spatial aliasing all cause distortions in the reconstructions. Deep learning methods have been used for correcting these. Techniques have been applied to automatically detect and correct patient motion for both MRI [135] and PET [136]. Motion does not only compromise imaging data. It can also affect techniques like MR spectroscopy, and approaches based on DL have been developed to remove ghosting artifacts in these studies [137, 138]. Regardless of their source, artifacts degrade the reconstructed spatial resolution. This of course limits the value of medical images for diagnoses, since good resolution properties are required to extract fine details from small pathological foci.

Improving medical image resolution has been the sole focus of many research efforts. Super-resolution in MRI has been around for over a decade [139]. These approaches enabled the reconstruction of a 3D volume with high isotropic resolution by acquiring the data typically through regular angular sampling about a common frequency encoding axis [140] or through modulation of the longitudinal magnetization to acquire independent k-space data [141]. Studies have reported success for estimating quantitative high-resolution T1 maps from a corresponding set of low-resolution maps [142] and even using conventional machine learning techniques to generate 7T-like MR images from 3T data [143]. Within the last few years, image super-resolution has become an interesting application for DL methods. Novel methods have produced state-of-the-art results for resolution up-sampling in natural images [144], and applications specific to MRI followed closely. Deep convolutional networks have constructed super-resolution brain [145] and musculoskeletal [146] images. These networks have also been adapted to generate super-resolution images from another modality [147].

The transformational mapping between multiple image domains is yet another exciting application for DL [148]. Due in part to recent advances in unsupervised training methods [149], this concept has found applications in medical research. Deep convolutional networks have been developed for transforming Flair to T1 MRI [150], CT to PET [151], and T1 MRI to CT [117]. Clinical interpretations and therapy planning based on images synthesized from another, unrelated modality could have far-reaching effects in the future of diagnostic and therapeutic medicine; this should be approached cautiously though, as synthesized images may contain incorrect pathological information and could lead to critical errors [150]. Notwithstanding this, image transformation based on DL may have the immediate potential to be a valuable tool for some technical problems. One popular current focus is related to PET/MR systems, transforming MR data to CT for PET attenuation correction. In order to produce quantitative images, photon attenuation must be corrected in all PET scans. This can be accurately estimated when an anatomical correlate of quantified attenuation values is available for directly generating a correction map, as it is with PET/CT. For PET/MR, however, this problem is more complicated since MR data do not contain information regarding photon scattering and absorption. Transforming MR images into quantified CT data has been implemented by several groups with promising results [152–154].

Furthermore, the PET/MR attenuation correction problem has also been addressed by omitting the CT transformation step altogether, using a CNN to estimate the correction map directly from the attenuated PET data themselves [155].

4.5   Image Registration

Once accurate medical images are produced, the image data must be translated into information which can be used for clinical patient management by a physician. In certain situations, the information obtained from multiple images read concurrently may be of much greater value than that obtained from reading them independently. The frequency of these situations dramatically increased at the turn of the twenty-first century for multimodal imaging with the invention of the PET/CT [156]. Multimodality imaging brought a new perspective into the field of clinical imaging. In this case, the combination of functional information with anatomical and morphological information provided an advanced medical tool, and countless studies over the past two decades have unequivocally established its diagnostic value. Other situations in which multiple images may be analyzed simultaneously include dynamic acquisitions, longitudinal comparisons or multiparametric MRI. In each of these cases, it is helpful, or even necessary, for the images to be spatially matched. For this reason, image registration is a constant focus of research, and techniques continue to evolve.

There are many potential sources of misregistration between two images of the same object, but assuming the differences are only spatially variant, one space can be mapped to the other through linear and nonlinear transformations. It is then the job of the registration algorithm to find the optimal transformation. For rigid structures, e.g., the head, linear transformations comprising global translations and rotations may be sufficient for coregistration. However, most other natural movement contains local, elastic deformations, and more complex methods are additionally needed to characterize and compensate for it. This is conventionally handled by project-ing one image onto a grid, which is then deformed in a way which increases some joint similarity measure. Many different similarity metrics have been proposed and investigated, but common ones include correlation (for single-modality data) or mutual information (for multimodal data). The optimization algorithm typically combines these approaches within some convergence framework to try and maximize the relative similarity.

The registration problem comprises a challenging combination of many factors; decisions regarding the spatial transformations, similarity metrics, optimization strategies and numerical framework all play important roles in the performance. Machine learning techniques have been applied successfully for some specific applications in the past. However, as with other traditional ML techniques, these algorithms require explicitly handcrafting the features and have limited flexibility. In many cases, they are unable to meet the accuracy requirements of high-resolution medical imaging [157–160]. Recently, DL methods have been applied to image registration in order to improve accuracy and speed [161]. Image registration depends fundamentally on the identification of relevant information in the images, and this is a strength of deep neural networks. Convolution stacked auto-encoder networks, for example, have demonstrated the ability to identify intrinsic features in image patches [162], and CNNs have been developed for regressing the transformation parameters of the registration for multimodal data [163]. The flexibility of DL makes it well suited to address applications involving deformable registrations [162, 164]. Many groups have reported recent successes for specific tasks including elastic registration between 3D MRI and transrectal ultrasound for guiding prostate biopsy [165], deformable brain MRI registration [166], unsupervised CNN-based deformable registration for CT and MRI [167–169], and DL-based 2D/3D registration for registration of preoperative 3D data and intraoperative 2D X-ray images in image-guided therapy [170].

As diagnostic medicine continues to evolve, more complementary and multiparametric tissue information will be acquired in space and time—accurate image registration will become increasingly critical. Methods based on AI have shown impressive results and will undoubtedly play important roles in the automated clinical workflow, enabling quantitative comparisons at multiple timepoints and across different imaging modalities.

4.6 Radiology Reporting

The underlying goal of any medical imaging examination is a noninvasive survey of pathological information. Regardless of the imaging modality, the radiologic data must be read and translated into reports which are able to be used toward guiding patient management—these reports lie at the intersection of radiology and multiple downstream clinical subspecialties. These reports are sensitive to errors in the previous steps of the imaging pipeline, and so great care must be taken to clearly and accurately outline the relevant findings. This makes it an arduous and time-consuming task. Furthermore, subjectivity and inter-reader variability may introduce communication inconsistencies between radiology and other physicians. AI presents an attractive option for increasing speed and improving standardization of radiology reports.

Artificial intelligence algorithms for voice recognition and text generation were first proposed nearly two decades ago [171], and today, they are used routinely for radiologic reporting. Since then, machine learning techniques have made great strides in natural language processing, and now several vendors have developed powerful tools capable of speech-to-text translation, along with compatible hardware, e.g., dictation microphones [172]. These solutions have proven themselves invaluable for automatic transcription without the need for typing dictation content from radiologists, substantially reducing report generation times and improving clinical workflow.

Radiologic tools driven by deep learning algorithms have the potential to further streamline this process. Recently, DL has been used to automatically produce captions for natural photographic images [173], and this has led to many studies investigating potential applications for generating textual descriptions for medical images [174–181] and also for identifying findings in radiology reports [182–184]. Such AI tools could also replace the conventional qualitative nature of radiologic reporting with a more interactive quantitative one, and this approach has been shown to improve collaboration between radiology and oncology [185]. For example, it is plausible to expect that in the future, an AI-powered platform would be able to identify and diagnose pathological abnormalities and annotate them in a textual format that included quantified information about size, location, and probability of malignancy with associated confidence levels. These data would reduce subjective bias in decisions regarding patient management. Additionally, these well-structured reports would prove very beneficial to population sciences and big data mining initiatives. Another related avenue of DL research is using the generated radiologic reports themselves to annotate and label the imaging data. Medical PACS systems typically store thousands of free-text reports containing valuable information describing the images. Parsing this text and turning it into accurate annotations or labels requires sophisticated text-mining method—this is a field in which DL is currently being applied. Reports with higher degrees of structure more readily lend themselves to this purpose, and there are already some emerging applications. For example, there has been work reporting success leveraging radiologists' BI-RADS categorizations for training deep neural networks for characterizing breast lesions [174]. Considering the point that labeled data can be used to improve classification accuracy, one study was motivated by the fact that large amounts of annotated data might be unobtainable. This work proposed to create semantic description labels for the data, using both images and textual reports [186]. This group reported that semantic information can increase classification accuracy for different pathologies in medical images. Advanced AI algorithms are also being applied in other ways to improve efficiency in radiology practice. Convolutional neural networks can be used to determine scanning protocols from short text classification [187] and to improve time-sensitive decisions by prioritizing urgent cases [188]. One of the most interesting recent endeavors, however, addressed the challenges summarizing and representing patient data from electronic health records [189]. This work presented a novel unsupervised DL method for constructing general-purpose patient representations. This value of such data would be huge, since it could then potentially facilitate clinical predictive modeling on a large scale.

The applications mentioned above involved, to some degree, image interpretations based on human perception. Years of collecting data in routine clinical practice have produced an incredibly rich resource of quantified radiological data along with the associated clinical outcomes. These data are being leveraged to refine the field of radiomics. Radiomics in medicine refers to the high-throughput extraction of large amounts of features from medical images [190]. Radiomic analyses, sometimes involving high order statistics, can be used to identify patterns related to disease characteristics—patterns which may be undetectable by a traditional observer. Radiomics emerged from the field of oncology with the hypothesis that imaged tumors may reveal distinctive features pertaining to the disease which can be useful for predicting prognoses and planning personalized therapy [191, 192]. Early work in radiomics involved analyzing large sets of images and building correlations among various predefined features characterizing, for example, tumor morphology, intensity, and texture. Following this, many efforts have successfully applied radiomic evaluations for assisting clinical decision-making in oncology. For example, radiomics has been used to predict metastatic patterns in lung adenocarcinoma [193] as well as disease recurrence [194] and prognoses [195]. Recently, deep learning has been applied in this space [161]. As with many other examples presented in this chapter, DL poses advantages over traditional methods for automatically extracting the relevant features, while simultaneously providing information regarding their clinical relevance. Deep learning and radiomics are two rapidly evolving technologies, and their symbiosis will likely lead to a single unified framework to support clinical decisions—this has the potential to completely transform the field of precision medicine [13].

4.7 Conclusion

Fundamentally, medical images are generated in order to be presented to physicians for evaluation—optimizing the appearance of images for human viewers almost always includes simplification and down-sampling of the raw data. Quantitative approaches like radiomics represent a step toward automatic image interpretation using the latent information embedded in the images, and following this evolutionary track, it is expected in the future that the presence of automated, AI-driven analyses in routine clinical workflow will continue to increase. In this paradigm, processed medical images may become altogether unnecessary for certain indications. This would avoid the loss of information inherent in the creation of images, leading to reproducible analyses which were faster and more accurate.

In conclusion, AI has made great advances, especially recently, but it is not expected that it will outperform humans for general clinical planning and patient management in the near future. Instead, both will improve together. Although AI is currently able to provide advantages for specific quantitative tasks, medical decisions cannot be strictly regarded as such. They are based on knowledge obtained through life experience and philosophy. To incorporate these characteristics into an AI program, one would be faced with many challenges including data collection and algorithm development [29]. Considering this, it is likely that the trend in AI will move toward advanced unsupervised learning approaches, allowing the immense amounts of readily-available, unlabeled data to be utilized. In any case, the synergy between AI and physicians will certainly grow and continue to be mutually beneficial within the field of medical imaging, leading to unprecedented levels of precision and quality in patient care.

References

1. Ledley RS, Lusted LB. Reasoning foundations of medical diagnosis. Science. 1959;130(3366):9–21.
2. Haug PJ. Uses of diagnostic expert systems in clinical care. In: Proceedings of the annual symposium on computer application in medical care. Bethesda: American Medical Informatics Association; 1993.
3. Ambinder EP. A history of the shift toward full computerization of medicine. J Oncol Pract. 2005;1(2):54.
4. Krizhevsky A, Sutskever I, Hinton GE. Imagenet classification with deep convolutional neural networks. Adv Neural Inf Proces Syst. 2012;25:1097–105.
5. He K, et al. Delving deep into rectifiers: surpassing human-level performance on imagenet classification. In: Proceedings of the IEEE international conference on computer vision. New York: IEEE; 2015.
6. Silver D, et al. Mastering the game of Go with deep neural networks and tree search. Nature. 2016;529(7587):484–9.
7. Simonyan K, Zisserman A. Very deep convolutional networks for large-scale image recognition. arXiv preprint arXiv:1409.1556, 2014.
8. Long J, Shelhamer E, Darrell T. Fully convolutional networks for semantic segmentation. In: Proceedings of the IEEE conference on computer vision and pattern recognition. 2015.
9. Ronneberger O, Fischer P, Brox T. U-net: Convolutional networks for biomedical image segmentation. In: International conference on medical image computing and computer-assisted intervention. New York: Springer; 2015.
10. He K, et al. Deep residual learning for image recognition. In: Proceedings of the IEEE conference on computer vision and pattern recognition. 2016.
11. Szegedy C, et al. Going deeper with convolutions. In: Proceedings of the IEEE conference on computer vision and pattern recognition. 2015.
12. Goodfellow I, et al. Generative adversarial nets. In: Advances in neural information processing systems. 2014.
13. Hosny A, et al. Artificial intelligence in radiology. Nat Rev Cancer. 2018;18(8):500–10.
14. Ledley RS. Using electronic computers in medical diagnosis. IRE Trans Med Electron. 1960;4:274–80.
15. Amosov N, Shkabara E. Experience in determining diagnosis with the aid of diagnostic machines. Eksp Khirurgiia. 1961;6:15–22.
16. Rikli AE, et al. Computer analysis of electrocardiographic measurements. Circulation. 1961;24(3):643–9.
17. Paycha F. Diagnosis with the aid of artificial intelligence: demonstration of the 1st diagnostic machine. Presse Therm Clim. 1968;105(1):22.
18. DeCote R, Horvath WJ. An electronic computer for vector electrocardiography. IRE Trans Med Electron. 1957;1957:31–7.
19. Caceres CA. How can the waveforms of a clinical electrocardiogram be measured automatically by a computer? IRE Trans Biomed Electron. 1962;9(1):21–2.
20. Pipberger HV, Stallmann F. Use of computers in ECG interpretation. Am Heart J. 1962;64:285.
21. Steinberg C, Abraham S, Caceres C. Pattern recognition in the clinical electrocardiogram. IRE Trans Biomed Electron. 1962;9(1):23–30.
22. Lipkin M, Hardy JD. Mechanical correlation of data in differential diagnosis of hematological diseases. J Am Med Assoc. 1958;166(2):113–25.
23. Jonnard R. Random selection system for automatic biochemical analysis-partial functional analysis. IRE Trans Biomed Electron. 1961;8(2):83–98.
24. Moyer D, Talbott G. Instrumentation for the diagnosis of coronary-artery disease. Trans Am Inst Electr Eng. 1962;80(6):717–21.
25. Ledley RS, Lusted LB. Computers in medical data processing. Oper Res. 1960;8(3):299–310.
26. Gillon J. Is automatic diagnosis in the future? Concours Med. 1962;84:3829–33.
27. Schweisheimer W. Can electronic machines facilitate and improve medical diagnosis? Hippokrates. 1962;33:162.
28. Lodwick GS, Keats TE, Dorst JP. The coding of roentgen images for computer analysis as applied to lung cancer. Radiology. 1963;81(2):185–200.
29. Tang X. The role of artificial intelligence in medical imaging research. BJR Open. 2019;2(1):20190031.
30. Champaign JL, Cederbom GJ. Advances in breast cancer detection with screening mammography. Ochsner J. 2000;2(1):33–5.
31. Shiraishi J, et al. Computer-aided diagnosis and artificial intelligence in clinical imaging. In: Seminars in nuclear medicine. London: Elsevier; 2011.
32. Ayer T, et al. Computer-aided diagnostic models in breast cancer screening. Imaging Med. 2010;2(3):313.
33. Nagaraj S, Rao G, Koteswararao K. The role of pattern recognition in computer-aided diagnosis and computer-aided detection in medical imaging: a clinical validation. Int J Comput Appl. 2010;8(5):18–22.
34. Cole EB, et al. Impact of computer-aided detection systems on radiologist accuracy with digital mammography. Am J Roentgenol. 2014;203(4):909–16.
35. Lehman CD, et al. Diagnostic accuracy of digital screening mammography with and without computer-aided detection. JAMA Intern Med. 2015;175(11):1828–37.
36. Fenton JJ, et al. Influence of computer-aided detection on performance of screening mammography. N Engl J Med. 2007;356(14):1399–409.
37. Gilbert FJ, et al. Single reading with computer-aided detection for screening mammography. N Engl J Med. 2008;359(16):1675–84.
38. Oakden-Rayner L. The rebirth of CAD: how is modern AI different from the CAD we know? Oak Brook: Radiological Society of North America; 2019.

39. Lee J-G, et al. Deep learning in medical imaging: general overview. Korean J Radiol. 2017;18(4):570–84.

40. Asada N, et al. Potential usefulness of an artificial neural network for differential diagnosis of interstitial lung diseases: pilot study. Radiology. 1990;177(3):857–60.

41. Lin J-S, et al. Reduction of false positives in lung nodule detection using a two-level neural classification. IEEE Trans Med Imaging. 1996;15(2):206–17.

42. Ashizawa K, et al. Artificial neural networks in chest radiography: application to the differential diagnosis of interstitial lung disease. Acad Radiol. 1999;6(1):2–9.

43. Ashizawa K, et al. Effect of an artificial neural network on radiologists' performance in the differential diagnosis of interstitial lung disease using chest radiographs. AJR Am J Roentgenol. 1999;172(5):1311–5.

44. Lo S-C, et al. Artificial convolution neural network techniques and applications for lung nodule detection. IEEE Trans Med Imaging. 1995;14(4):711–8.

45. Wang D, et al. Deep learning for identifying metastatic breast cancer. arXiv preprint arXiv:1606.05718, 2016.

46. Kallenberg M, et al. Unsupervised deep learning applied to breast density segmentation and mammographic risk scoring. IEEE Trans Med Imaging. 2016;35(5):1322–31.

47. Cheng J-Z, et al. Computer-aided diagnosis with deep learning architecture: applications to breast lesions in US images and pulmonary nodules in CT scans. Sci Rep. 2016;6(1):1–13.

48. Hua K-L, et al. Computer-aided classification of lung nodules on computed tomography images via deep learning technique. Onco Targets Ther. 2015;8:2015–22.

49. Kumar D, Wong A, Clausi DA. Lung nodule classification using deep features in CT images. In: 2015 12th conference on computer and robot vision. New York: IEEE; 2015.

50. Chen J, et al. Use of an artificial neural network to construct a model of predicting deep fungal infection in lung cancer patients. Asian Pac J Cancer Prev. 2015;16(12):5095–9.

51. Esteva A, et al. Dermatologist-level classification of skin cancer with deep neural networks. Nature. 2017;542(7639):115–8.

52. Teramoto A, et al. Automated detection of pulmonary nodules in PET/CT images: ensemble false-positive reduction using a convolutional neural network technique. Med Phys. 2016;43(6): 2821–7.

53. Wang H, et al. Comparison of machine learning methods for classifying mediastinal lymph node metastasis of non-small cell lung cancer from 18 F-FDG PET/CT images. EJNMMI Res. 2017;7(1):11.

54. Chen T, Metaxas D. Medical image computing and computer-assisted intervention—Miccai 2000. Vol. 1935 of lecture notes in computer science. New York: Springer; 2000.

55. Kooi T, et al. Large scale deep learning for computer aided detection of mammographic lesions. Med Image Anal. 2017;35:303–12.

56. Paul R, et al. Deep feature transfer learning in combination with traditional features predicts survival among patients with lung adenocarcinoma. Tomography. 2016;2(4):388.

57. Nie D, et al. 3D deep learning for multi-modal imaging-guided survival time prediction of brain tumor patients. In: International conference on medical image computing and computer-assisted intervention. New York: Springer; 2016.

58. Ardila D, et al. End-to-end lung cancer screening with three-dimensional deep learning on low-dose chest computed tomography. Nat Med. 2019;25(6):954–61.

59. Suk H-I, et al. Hierarchical feature representation and multimodal fusion with deep learning for AD/MCI diagnosis. NeuroImage. 2014;101:569–82.

60. Suk H-I, Shen D. Deep learning-based feature representation for AD/MCI classification. In: International conference on medical image computing and computer-assisted intervention. New York: Springer; 2013.

61. Liu S, et al. Early diagnosis of Alzheimer's disease with deep learning. In: 2014 IEEE 11th international symposium on biomedical imaging (ISBI). New York: IEEE; 2014.

62. Hosseini-Asl E, Gimel'farb G, El-Baz A. Alzheimer's disease diagnostics by a deeply supervised adaptable 3D convolutional network. arXiv preprint arXiv:1607.00556, 2016.

63. Payan A, Montana G. Predicting Alzheimer's disease: a neuroimaging study with 3D convolutional neural networks. arXiv preprint arXiv:1502.02506, 2015.

64. Choi H, et al. Refining diagnosis of Parkinson's disease with deep learning-based interpretation of dopamine transporter imaging. NeuroImage. 2017;16:586–94.

65. Kim DH, Wit H, Thurston M. Artificial intelligence in the diagnosis of Parkinson's disease from ioflupane-123 single-photon emission computed tomography dopamine transporter scans using transfer learning. Nucl Med Commun. 2018;39(10):887–93.

66. Haralick RM, Shapiro LG. Image segmentation techniques. Comput Vis Graph Image Process. 1985;29(1):100–32.

67. Pham DL, Xu C, Prince JL. Current methods in medical image segmentation. Annu Rev Biomed Eng. 2000;2(1):315–37.

68. Grau V, et al. Improved watershed transform for medical image segmentation using prior information. IEEE Trans Med Imaging. 2004;23(4):447–58.

69. Sharma N, Aggarwal LM. Automated medical image segmentation techniques. J Med Phys. 2010;35(1):3.

70. Han X, et al. Atlas-based auto-segmentation of head and neck CT images. In: International conference on medical image computing and computer-assisted intervention. New York: Springer; 2008.

71. Parisot S, et al. A probabilistic atlas of diffuse WHO grade II glioma locations in the brain. PLoS One. 2016;11(1):e0144200.

72. Shelhamer E, Long J, Darrell T. Fully convolutional networks for semantic segmentation. IEEE Trans Pattern Anal Mach Intell. 2017;39(4):640–51.

73. Middleton I, Damper RI. Segmentation of magnetic resonance images using a combination of neural networks and active contour models. Med Eng Phys. 2004;26(1):71–86.

74. Ning F, et al. Toward automatic phenotyping of developing embryos from videos. IEEE Trans Image Process. 2005;14(9):1360–71.

75. Ciresan D, et al. Deep neural networks segment neuronal membranes in electron microscopy images. In: Advances in neural information processing systems. 2012.

76. Prasoon A, et al. Deep feature learning for knee cartilage segmentation using a triplanar convolutional neural network. In: International conference on medical image computing and computer-assisted intervention. 2013. Springer.

77. Cernazanu-Glavan C, Holban S. Segmentation of bone structure in X-ray images using convolutional neural network. Adv Electron Comput Eng. 2013;13(1):87–94.

78. Moeskops P, et al. Automatic segmentation of MR brain images with a convolutional neural network. IEEE Trans Med Imaging. 2016;35(5):1252–61.

79. Zhu Q, et al. Deeply-supervised CNN for prostate segmentation. In: 2017 international joint conference on neural networks (IJCNN). New York: IEEE; 2017.

80. Rastgarpour M, Shanbehzadeh J. Application of ai techniques in medical image segmentation and novel categorization of available methods and in tools. In: Proceedings of the international multiconference of engineers and computer scientists. Princeton: Citeseer; 2011.

81. Pereira S, et al. Brain tumor segmentation using convolutional neural networks in MRI images. IEEE Trans Med Imaging. 2016;35(5):1240–51.

82. Roth HR, et al. Deep learning and its application to medical image segmentation. Med Imaging Technol. 2018;36(2):63–71.

83. Tang X, Wang B, Rong Y. Artificial intelligence will reduce the need for clinical medical physicists. J Appl Clin Med Phys. 2018;19(1):6.

84. Feng X, et al. Deep convolutional neural network for segmentation of thoracic organs-at-risk using cropped 3D images. Med Phys. 2019;46(5):2169–80.

85. Dong X, et al. Automatic multiorgan segmentation in thorax CT images using U-net-GAN. Med Phys. 2019;46(5):2157–68.

86. Milletari F, Navab N, Ahmadi S-A. V-net: fully convolutional neural networks for volumetric medical image segmentation. In: Fourth international conference on 3D Vision (3DV). New York: IEEE; 2016. p. 2016.

87. de Brebisson A, Montana G. Deep neural networks for anatomical brain segmentation. In: Proceedings of the IEEE conference on computer vision and pattern recognition workshops. 2015.

88. Moeskops P, et al. Deep learning for multi-task medical image segmentation in multiple modalities. In: International conference on medical image computing and computer-assisted intervention. New York: Springer; 2016.

89. Ghafoorian M, et al. Location sensitive deep convolutional neural networks for segmentation of white matter hyperintensities. Sci Rep. 2017;7:5110.

90. Sun J, Li H, Xu Z. Deep ADMM-Net for compressive sensing MRI. In: Advances in neural information processing systems. 2016.

91. Wang S, et al. Accelerating magnetic resonance imaging via deep learning. In: 2016 IEEE 13th international symposium on biomedical imaging (ISBI). New York: IEEE; 2016.

92. Qin C, et al. Convolutional recurrent neural networks for dynamic MR image reconstruction. IEEE Trans Med Imaging. 2018;38(1):280–90.

93. Zhu B, et al. Image reconstruction by domain-transform manifold learning. Nature. 2018;555(7697):487–92.

94. Gong E, et al. Deep learning enables reduced gadolinium dose for contrast-enhanced brain MRI. J Magn Reson Imaging. 2018;48(2):330–40.

95. Golkov V, et al. Q-space deep learning: twelve-fold shorter and model-free diffusion MRI scans. IEEE Trans Med Imaging. 2016;35(5):1344–51.

96. Deistung A, et al. Toward in vivo histology: a comparison of quantitative susceptibility mapping (QSM) with magnitude-, phase-, and $R2_*$-imaging at ultra-high magnetic field strength. NeuroImage. 2013;65:299–314.

97. Deistung A, Schweser F, Reichenbach JR. Overview of quantitative susceptibility mapping. NMR Biomed. 2017;30(4):e3569.

98. Yoon J, et al. Quantitative susceptibility mapping using deep neural network: QSMnet. NeuroImage. 2018;179:199–206.

99. Ma D, et al. Magnetic resonance fingerprinting. Nature. 2013;495(7440):187–92.

100. Cohen O, Zhu B, Rosen MS. MR fingerprinting deep reconstruction network (DRONE). Magn Reson Med. 2018;80(3):885–94.

101. Hoppe E, et al. Deep learning for magnetic resonance fingerprinting: a new approach for predicting quantitative parameter values from time series. In: GMDS. 2017.

102. Fang Z, et al. Quantification of relaxation times in MR fingerprinting using deep learning. In: Proceedings of the International Society for Magnetic Resonance in Medicine... Scientific Meeting and Exhibition. International Society for Magnetic Resonance in Medicine. Scientific Meeting and Exhibition. Bethesda: NIH Public Access; 2017.

103. Creswell A, et al. Generative adversarial networks: an overview. IEEE Signal Process Mag. 2018;35(1):53–65.

104. Hong Y, et al. How generative adversarial networks and their variants work: an overview. ACM Comput Surv. 2019;52(1):1–43.

105. Huang H, Yu PS, Wang C. An introduction to image synthesis with generative adversarial nets. arXiv preprint arXiv:1803.04469, 2018.

106. Osokin A, et al. Gans for biological image synthesis. In: Proceedings of the IEEE international conference on computer vision. New York: IEEE; 2017.

107. Antipov G, Baccouche M, Dugelay J-L. Face aging with conditional generative adversarial networks. In: 2017 IEEE international conference on image processing (ICIP). New York: IEEE; 2017.

108. Shin H-C, et al. Medical image synthesis for data augmentation and anonymization using generative adversarial networks. In: International workshop on simulation and synthesis in medical imaging. New York: Springer; 2018.

109. Mok TC, Chung AC. Learning data augmentation for brain tumor segmentation with coarse-to-fine generative adversarial networks. In: International MICCAI brainlesion workshop. New York: Springer; 2018.

110. Kitchen A, Seah J. Deep generative adversarial neural networks for realistic prostate lesion MRI synthesis. arXiv preprint arXiv:1708.00129, 2017.

111. Frid-Adar M, et al. Synthetic data augmentation using GAN for improved liver lesion classification. In: 2018 IEEE 15th international symposium on biomedical imaging (ISBI 2018). New York: IEEE; 2018.

112. Guibas JT, Virdi TS, Li PS. Synthetic medical images from dual generative adversarial networks. arXiv preprint arXiv:1709.01872, 2017.

113. Bermudez C, et al. Learning implicit brain MRI manifolds with deep learning. In: Medical imaging 2018: image processing. Bellingham: International Society for Optics and Photonics. p. 2018.

114. Zhang Q, et al. Medical image synthesis with generative adversarial networks for tissue recognition. In: 2018 IEEE international conference on healthcare informatics (ICHI). New York: IEEE; 2018.

115. Nie D, et al. Medical image synthesis with context-aware generative adversarial networks. In: International conference on medical image computing and computer-assisted intervention. New York: Springer; 2017.

116. Nie D, et al. Estimating CT image from MRI data using 3D fully convolutional networks. In: Deep learning and data labeling for medical applications. New York: Springer; 2016. p. 170–8.

117. Wolterink JM, et al. Deep MR to CT synthesis using unpaired data. In: International workshop on simulation and synthesis in medical imaging. New York: Springer; 2017.

118. Li R, et al. Deep learning based imaging data completion for improved brain disease diagnosis. In: International conference on medical image computing and computer-assisted intervention. New York: Springer; 2014.

119. Strack R. Imaging: AI transforms image reconstruction. Nat Methods. 2018;15(5):309–10.

120. McCann MT, Jin KH, Unser M. Convolutional neural networks for inverse problems in imaging: a review. IEEE Signal Process Mag. 2017;34(6):85–95.

121. Jin KH, et al. Deep convolutional neural network for inverse problems in imaging. IEEE Trans Image Process. 2017;26(9):4509–22.

122. Schlemper J, et al. A deep cascade of convolutional neural networks for MR image reconstruction. In: International conference on information processing in medical imaging. New York: Springer; 2017.

123. Lucas A, et al. Using deep neural networks for inverse problems in imaging: beyond analytical methods. IEEE Signal Process Mag. 2018;35(1):20–36.

124. Kim K, et al. Penalized PET reconstruction using deep learning prior and local linear fitting. IEEE Trans Med Imaging. 2018;37(6):1478–87.

125. Gong K, et al. Iterative PET image reconstruction using convolutional neural network representation. IEEE Trans Med Imaging. 2018;38(3):675–85.

126. Häggström I, et al. DeepPET: a deep encoder–decoder network for directly solving the PET image reconstruction inverse problem. Med Image Anal. 2019;54:253–62.

127. Antun V, et al. On instabilities of deep learning in image reconstruction and the potential costs of AI. Proc Natl Acad Sci. 2020;117(48):30088–95.

128. Benou A, et al. Ensemble of expert deep neural networks for spatio-temporal denoising of contrast-enhanced MRI sequences. Med Image Anal. 2017;42:145–59.

129. Liu C-C, Qi J. Higher SNR PET image prediction using a deep learning model and MRI image. Phys Med Biol. 2019;64(11):115004.

130. Lu W, et al. An investigation of quantitative accuracy for deep learning based denoising in oncological PET. Phys Med Biol. 2019;64(16):165019.

131. Cui J, et al. PET image denoising using unsupervised deep learning. Eur J Nucl Med Mol Imaging. 2019;46(13):2780–9.

132. Gong K, et al. Pet image denoising using a deep neural network through fine tuning. IEEE Trans Radiat Plasma Med Sci. 2018;3(2):153–61.

133. Yang Q, et al. CT image denoising with perceptive deep neural networks. arXiv preprint arXiv:1702.07019, 2017.

134. Schaefferkoetter J, Yan J, Ortega C, et al. Convolutional neural networks for improving image quality with noisy PET data. EJNMMI Res. 2020;10:105. https://doi.org/10.1186/s13550-020-00695-1.

135. Küstner T, et al. Automated reference-free detection of motion artifacts in magnetic resonance images. Medicine. 2018;31(2):243–56.

136. Li T, et al. Motion correction of respiratory-gated PET images using deep learning based image registration framework. Phys Med Biol. 2020;65(15):155003.

137. Gurbani SS, et al. A convolutional neural network to filter artifacts in spectroscopic MRI. Magn Reson Med. 2018;80(5):1765–75.

138. Kyathanahally SP, Döring A, Kreis R. Deep learning approaches for detection and removal of ghosting artifacts in MR spectroscopy. Magn Reson Med. 2018;80(3):851–63.

139. Robinson MD, et al. New applications of super-resolution in medical imaging. Super-Resolut Imaging. 2010;2010:384–412.

140. Shilling RZ, et al. A super-resolution framework for 3-D high-resolution and high-contrast imaging using 2-D multislice MRI. IEEE Trans Med Imaging. 2008;28(5):633–44.

141. Ropele S, et al. Super-resolution MRI using microscopic spatial modulation of magnetization. Magn Reson Med. 2010;64(6):1671–5.

142. Van Steenkiste G, et al. Super-resolution T1 estimation: quantitative high resolution T1 mapping from a set of low resolution T1-weighted images with different slice orientations. Magn Reson Med. 2017;77(5):1818–30.

143. Bahrami K, et al. 7T-guided super-resolution of 3T MRI. Med Phys. 2017;44(5):1661–77.

144. Ledig C, et al. Photo-realistic single image super-resolution using a generative adversarial network. In: Proceedings of the IEEE conference on computer vision and pattern recognition. 2017.

145. Liu C, et al. Fusing multi-scale information in convolution network for MR image super-resolution reconstruction. Biomed Eng Online. 2018;17(1):114.

146. Chaudhari AS, et al. Super-resolution musculoskeletal MRI using deep learning. Magn Reson Med. 2018;80(5):2139–54.

147. Zeng K, et al. Simultaneous single-and multi-contrast super-resolution for brain MRI images based on a convolutional neural network. Comput Biol Med. 2018;99:133–41.

148. Isola P, et al. Image-to-image translation with conditional adversarial networks. In: Proceedings of the IEEE conference on computer vision and pattern recognition. 2017.

149. Zhu J-Y, et al. Unpaired image-to-image translation using cycle-consistent adversarial networks. In: Proceedings of the IEEE international conference on computer vision. 2017.

150. Cohen JP, Luck M, Honari S. Distribution matching losses can hallucinate features in medical image translation. In: International conference on medical image computing and computer-assisted intervention. New York: Springer; 2018.

151. Armanious K, et al. Unsupervised medical image translation using cycle-MedGAN. In: 2019 27th

European signal processing conference (EUSIPCO). New York: IEEE; 2019.

152. Han X. MR-based synthetic CT generation using a deep convolutional neural network method. Med Phys. 2017;44(4):1408–19.

153. Torrado-Carvajal A, et al. Dixon-VIBE deep learning (DIVIDE) pseudo-CT synthesis for pelvis PET/MR attenuation correction. J Nucl Med. 2019;60(3):429–35.

154. Leynes AP, et al. Zero-echo-time and Dixon deep pseudo-CT (ZeDD CT): direct generation of pseudo-CT images for pelvic PET/MRI attenuation correction using deep convolutional neural networks with multiparametric MRI. J Nucl Med. 2018;59(5):852–8.

155. Spuhler KD, et al. Synthesis of patient-specific transmission data for PET attenuation correction for PET/MRI neuroimaging using a convolutional neural network. J Nucl Med. 2019;60(4):555–60.

156. Beyer T, et al. A combined PET/CT scanner for clinical oncology. J Nucl Med. 2000;41(8):1369.

157. Wohlhart P, Lepetit V. Learning descriptors for object recognition and 3d pose estimation. In: Proceedings of the IEEE conference on computer vision and pattern recognition. 2015.

158. Dollár P, Welinder P, Perona P. Cascaded pose regression. In: 2010 IEEE computer society conference on computer vision and pattern recognition. New York: IEEE; 2010.

159. Zach C, Penate-Sanchez A, Pham M-T. A dynamic programming approach for fast and robust object pose recognition from range images. In: Proceedings of the IEEE conference on computer vision and pattern recognition. 2015.

160. Mottaghi R, Xiang Y, Savarese S. A coarse-to-fine model for 3d pose estimation and sub-category recognition. In: Proceedings of the IEEE conference on computer vision and pattern recognition. 2015.

161. Litjens G, et al. A survey on deep learning in medical image analysis. Med Image Anal. 2017;42:60–88.

162. Wu G, et al. Scalable high-performance image registration framework by unsupervised deep feature representations learning. IEEE Trans Biomed Eng. 2015;63(7):1505–16.

163. Sloan JM, Goatman KA, Siebert JP. Learning rigid image registration-utilizing convolutional neural networks for medical image registration. 2018.

164. Yang X, et al. Quicksilver: fast predictive image registration–a deep learning approach. NeuroImage. 2017;158:378–96.

165. Haskins G, et al. Learning deep similarity metric for 3D MR–TRUS image registration. Int J Comput Assist Radiol Surg. 2019;14(3):417–25.

166. Cao X, et al. Deformable image registration using a cue-aware deep regression network. IEEE Trans Biomed Eng. 2018;65(9):1900–11.

167. Shan S, et al. Unsupervised end-to-end learning for deformable medical image registration. arXiv preprint arXiv:1711.08608, 2017.

168. Kearney V, et al. An unsupervised convolutional neural network-based algorithm for deformable image registration. Phys Med Biol. 2018;63(18):185017.

169. de Vos BD, et al. A deep learning framework for unsupervised affine and deformable image registration. Med Image Anal. 2019;52:128–43.

170. Zheng J, et al. Pairwise domain adaptation module for CNN-based 2-D/3-D registration. J Med Imaging. 2018;5(2):021204.

171. Antoniol G, et al. Radiological reporting based on voice recognition. In: International conference on human-computer interaction. New York: Springer; 1993.

172. Liu Y, Wang J. PACS and digital medicine: essential principles and modern practice. Boca Raton: CRC Press; 2010.

173. Karpathy A, Fei-Fei L. Deep visual-semantic alignments for generating image descriptions. In: Proceedings of the IEEE conference on computer vision and pattern recognition. 2015.

174. Kisilev P, et al. Medical image description using multi-task-loss CNN. In: Deep learning and data labeling for medical applications. New York: Springer; 2016. p. 121–9.

175. Shin H-C, et al. Interleaved text/image deep mining on a very large-scale radiology database. In: Proceedings of the IEEE conference on computer vision and pattern recognition. 2015.

176. Shin H-C, et al. Learning to read chest X-rays: recurrent neural cascade model for automated image annotation. In: Proceedings of the IEEE conference on computer vision and pattern recognition. 2016.

177. Wang X., et al. Unsupervised category discovery via looped deep pseudo-task optimization using a large scale radiology image database. arXiv preprint arXiv:1603.07965, 2016.

178. Jing B, Xie P, Xing E. On the automatic generation of medical imaging reports. arXiv preprint arXiv:1711.08195, 2017.

179. Li Y, et al. Hybrid retrieval-generation reinforced agent for medical image report generation. In: Advances in neural information processing systems. 2018.

180. Moradi M, et al. Bimodal network architectures for automatic generation of image annotation from text. In: International conference on medical image computing and computer-assisted intervention. New York: Springer; 2018.

181. Zhang Y, et al. Learning to summarize radiology findings. arXiv preprint arXiv:1809.04698, 2018.

182. Pons E, et al. Natural language processing in radiology: a systematic review. Radiology. 2016;279(2):329–43.

183. Zech J, et al. Natural language–based machine learning models for the annotation of clinical radiology reports. Radiology. 2018;287(2):570–80.

184. Goff DJ, Loehfelm TW. Automated radiology report summarization using an open-source natural language processing pipeline. J Digit Imaging. 2018;31(2):185–92.

185. Folio LR, et al. Quantitative radiology reporting in oncology: survey of oncologists and radiologists. Am J Roentgenol. 2015;205(3):233–43.

186. Schlegl T, et al. Predicting semantic descriptions from medical images with convolutional neural networks. In: International conference on information processing in medical imaging. New York: Springer; 2015.

187. Lee YH. Efficiency improvement in a busy radiology practice: determination of musculoskeletal magnetic resonance imaging protocol using deep-learning convolutional neural networks. J Digit Imaging. 2018;31(5):604–10.

188. Annarumma M, et al. Automated triaging of adult chest radiographs with deep artificial neural networks. Radiology. 2019;291(1):196–202.

189. Miotto R, et al. Deep patient: an unsupervised representation to predict the future of patients from the electronic health records. Sci Rep. 2016;6(1):1–10.

190. Lambin P, et al. Radiomics: extracting more information from medical images using advanced feature analysis. Eur J Cancer. 2012;48(4):441–6.

191. Aerts HJ. The potential of radiomic-based phenotyping in precision medicine: a review. JAMA Oncol. 2016;2(12):1636–42.

192. Kumar V, et al. Radiomics: the process and the challenges. Magn Reson Imaging. 2012;30(9):1234–48.

193. Coroller TP, et al. CT-based radiomic signature predicts distant metastasis in lung adenocarcinoma. Radiother Oncol. 2015;114(3):345–50.

194. Huynh E, et al. Associations of radiomic data extracted from static and respiratory-gated CT scans with disease recurrence in lung cancer patients treated with SBRT. PLoS One. 2017;12(1):e0169172.

195. Parmar C, et al. Machine learning methods for quantitative radiomic biomarkers. Sci Rep. 2015;5:13087.

The Basic Principles of Machine Learning

5

Joshua D. Kaggie, Dimitri A. Kessler,
Chitresh Bhushan, Dawei Gui, and Gaspar Delso

Contents

J. D. Kaggie (✉) · D. A. Kessler
Department of Radiology, University of Cambridge, Cambridge, UK
e-mail: jk636@medschl.cam.ac.uk; dak50@cam.ac.uk

C. Bhushan
GE Research, Niskayuna, NY, USA
e-mail: chitresh.bhushan@ge.com

D. Gui · G. Delso
GE, Waukesha, USA
e-mail: Dawei.Gui@ge.com; GasparDelso@ge.com

5.1 Introduction

Medical imaging encompasses a broad range of methods from the more established to the new (Fig. 5.1). The X-ray radiograph, which is the backbone of computed tomography (CT) imaging, has existed for over a hundred years. Positron emission tomography (PET) and magnetic resonance imaging (MRI) had their earliest clinical developments in the late 1970s. These modalities, among many others, remain subjects of wide research and continue to make strides within

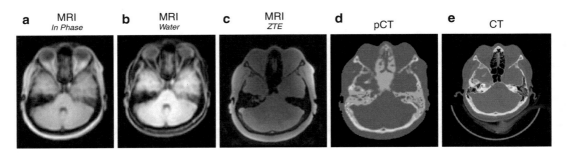

Fig. 5.1 Images of a head using (**a**–**c**) three MRI methods, (**d**) a pseudo-CT image derived from the MRI data using machine learning, and (**e**) a CT image

these fields as new techniques continue to improve them. The preponderance of medical imaging has led to an explosion of data, which in medical settings is then be used by a radiologist to determine whether there are significant diseases. Instead of relying on human observation, this data is increasingly analyzed with machine algorithms. Mathematics is at the heart of the many machine algorithms designed to help in the clinical interpretation of underlying biology.

If you are in medicine, you cannot escape encountering "machine learning" (ML), which is a subset of "artificial intelligence" (AI). "Machine learning" encompasses a wide range of techniques, from the more basic linear regression to combinations of deep neural networks. New methods are frequently developed, and so it is very easy to lose sight of significant developments. It helps to know that at the heart of machine learning are fundamental mathematical principles, which can help with understanding the underlying principles of future methods. It also helps to know a few broad techniques that fall into several major categories.

The reality is that diseases and treatments that can be collected on large scales will likely be replaced by ML methods throughout the next decades. Even with common diseases, simultaneous occurrence of several diseases along with patient's demographics, environment, and treatment history can result in exponential numbers of possibilities. This leads to low numbers of data points with specific/similar inputs. The significant number of rare diseases that exist will not be replaced easily by ML without substantial advancements in ML techniques, due to their low

numbers. ML is unlikely to completely replace routine care in these scenarios, but can greatly help in enriching the overall understanding of diseases and treatments by revealing new relationships between diseases, demographics, treatment outcomes, or other factors. ML within medicine will provide insights into human biology that will feed future clinical advancements.

5.1.1   The Task of ML

Machine learning has been successfully applied to an increasing number of tasks. The success of ML is near inescapable. ML has been successful in computer vision, speech recognition, image and audio generation, drug design, and natural language processing. However, none of these successes are considered a "general AI". A generalized ML algorithm that can be used without user input and can give you an appropriate output is considered a "general AI." Oftentimes, general AI is brought up when discussing the promises and fears of ML, which is confused with routine ML techniques. "ML" is the preferred term within scientific practice to avoid the confusion of the term AI. To perform ML, you will need a question, a computer, an algorithm or model, and data to interpret.

5.1.1.1 A Question
The overall goal of ML in medicine is the specific tasks of predicting and treating disease. ML is being increasingly used wherever computer processing can be involved with the acquisition or analysis of any dataset. ML relies on having a

question to answer, knowledge to gain, or process to improve. There are several questions in medicine that can be tackled with ML, such as: does the person have any disease? If yes, what is the disease? How far along is it? Where is it located? Can it be treated? Can imaging be used in conjunction with any other data to diagnose the disease? In order to have a useful measurement, it is necessary to have a question or hypothesis.

5.1.1.2 A Computer

To perform ML, you will need hardware and software that can perform this task (Fig. 5.2). The hardware will consist of a computer made of a "central processing unit" (CPU) and memory. CPUs are incredibly versatile and can handle nearly all computing tasks. Your home computer will likely contain 2–16 CPUs for its daily computational tasks, whether that is browsing the internet or advanced

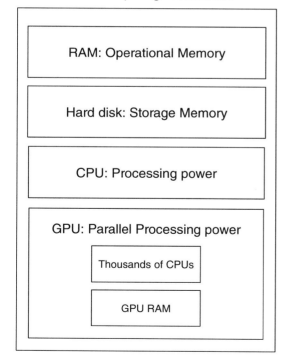

Basic Computing Architecture

Fig. 5.2 An image showing four components that are present in modern computers: RAM, hard disks, CPUs, and a GPU. These four parameters determine the speed that a computer can perform ML, although the data size and algorithm are also important!

image processing. The combination of thousands of low-powered CPUs for parallel computing are commonly used in "graphics processing units" (GPUs), which combines CPUs to optimize calculations for graphical displays and intensive ML tasks. GPUs can contain thousands of CPUs, called 'cores', although these cores will individually be much slower than the CPUs in your home computer. The advantage of the GPU is that it performs highly parallel computations, which allows it to outperform a CPU when many similar computations can be performed at the same time, or parallelized. Within your home, you may have a GPU that could perform ML; however, many of the tasks require higher quality GPUs that can cost thousands of dollars. In order to access high performance GPUs, there are many online websites that offer free trials to quality GPUs. High performance computing centers exist at many universities and offer purchasable time with the possibility of thousands of CPUs and hundreds of GPUs for parallel computing. There are also "tensor processing units" (TPUs), which are a proprietary form of CPUs/GPUs dedicated to ML that use lower numerical precision to enable faster processing.

5.1.1.3 An Algorithm or Model

An ML algorithm or model is the sequence of well-defined instructions, implemented in a computer, to solve a question. Typically, these algorithms are specific to a class of similar questions. Within medical imaging, ML algorithms dominate with solutions of the following three classes of questions: (1) radiomics, e.g., texture analysis, (2) automated segmentation, and (3) disease prediction. These algorithms do not encompass all imaging applications, which can include the optimization of data acquisition routines or the reconstruction of data.

ML algorithms learn or fit a mathematical "model" to solve a question using prior knowledge and observed data, which creates "training data." ML models are generally flexible enough to allow learning a specific solution to a specific question by changing the training data. Perhaps surprisingly, the same ML algorithms can be used to learn models for the (a) segmentation of brain tissues in MRI images and the (b) segmentation of liver lesions in CT images, just by changing the training data!

A significant amount of computer code with different ML algorithm implementations are readily available online for the intrepid researchers who are willing to explore them. There are increasingly more free tools available for individuals to use with their own datasets. ML methods become increasingly impressive, with recent demonstrations that ML can predict what a person may be looking at (after very significant pretraining!). At present, there are no ML algorithm or ML models that enables generalized intelligence ("general AI"), so we work with very specific tasks, data, and models. Not all diseases will be detectable with ML methods, as even ML is subject to the sensitivity and specificity of physical systems. The more specific the data, the more specific the technique can be used.

5.1.1.4 Data to Interpret

ML is specific to the datasets used in training, and thus requires curation of the data to perform a specific task. Data curation remains a limiting factor, as the majority of medicinal techniques require human involvement in order to establish efficacy, and few locations are willing to accept the additional risk when an ML method may misdiagnose a patient. In practice, a large amount of time for machine learning is spent in the preparation of datasets, such as curating or labeling them, and analyzing whether the outputs are meaningful.

There are two axioms presented when discussing ML: "garbage in, garbage out" and "more data is always better." The following question arises: what are the optimal numbers within a dataset to learn and then verify the task at hand? Unfortunately, there is no simple answer to the data amount. This depends largely on the quality of data and the strength of the relationship between the model and observed parameters. Sufficient dataset diversity is a requirement, but too much data diversity will waste resources on unimportant leads. A dataset with large variability in its files/parameters and with fewer individuals will require more resources than a dataset with small files/parameters and more individuals. The stronger the relationship between the input and output, the sooner any model will converge. Datasets where strong correlations exist, such as the segmentation of large features like an entire lung or brain volume, may be trainable on tens of subjects, and tested on tens of other subjects. Datasets with weak correlations may require thousands of subjects or more, if they are even possible to train well.

There are several questions to ask when considering the data: is the data balanced between training types? Are the labels noisy enough to model real-world environments, but not too noisy to be useless? Are all of the interesting values represented? Is the data structured appropriately, such as in a file format type (video, images, XML, etc.), where ML can be performed? Does the data need labels/supervision, and are there sufficient labels? Are the labels accurate? Is the data biased, and can we overcome these biases?

5.1.2 Supervised Learning

Successful ML models in medicine use datasets based on the inputs of an experienced clinician providing outlines or disease scores. These models are trained with very specific questions in mind, often on "labeled" datasets to enable "supervised" learning. Labeling a dataset refers to providing a structured raw dataset, such as images that may have a type of disease present, and a label specific to each image, such as whether that image has the disease present. Supervised learning happens when both the raw data and labels are presented in a structured format. To draw parallels with fitting the curve of a line, raw data is often referred to as "x." The goal of the algorithm would be to identify the curve or formula that best fits the labels "y" corresponding to those "x" data points. After performing supervised learning, a machine learning program will create an output of predicted "y" values, which are then tested against the observed or measured "y" values, which are labels derived from an experienced reader.

5.1.3 Unsupervised Learning

"Unsupervised learning" does not rely on having labels from a trained clinician. Unsupervised learning finds correlations within datasets to automatically categorize the data. As an example of unsupervised learning, imagine that you had two apple and three bananas (Fig. 5.3). You might automatically categorize them, as a human, into two groups: apples versus bananas. Perhaps you did this based on their color or shape. An algorithm that does this automatic categorization is referred to as an unsupervised learning algorithm. There are many ways to categorize these two apples and three bananas. Perhaps we classify or separate these fruits based on their weight, then we might find that the clusters contain a mixture of apples and bananas if we had a wide range of weights within a single fruit category. There may be an algorithm that leads to an intuitive result, such as the "yellowness" of the bananas becoming a distinguishing quantifiable metric. The clustering or separation of these characteristics as chosen by an algorithm may not be as intuitive as one chosen by a human observer. It may be possible to find an algorithm that relies on the same characteristics that a human will choose, or it may be that a computer finds a result that is unfathomable. Regardless of the result, the question remains, "will this algorithm help us understand or treat a disease?" Even unsupervised learning does not occur in a vacuum, so eventually must be tied into other analysis regarding its utility.

5.1.4 Radiomics and Texture Analysis

While a human is able to automatically classify the properties of an image, this classification is often subjective. Texture analysis attempts to make this classification numerical or objective by creating mathematical descriptions of "image features" (Fig. 5.4). An image feature is any mathematical description of the image, which could be as simple as the number of red pixels (or when discussed in 3D, voxels) in an image of an apple, the mean intensity of these pixels, or standard deviation. There is information encoded in space, such as whether red pixels in an image are close together might indicate the presence of an apple, whereas random, scattered pixels may indicate noise.

Mean, variance (and standard deviation), kurtosis, and skew are commonly used features, also referred to as 1D histogram measurements, and do not account for spatial variations. Two-dimensional histograms account for intensity similarities within a mask and are based on work from Haralick et al. who described "gray-level co-occurrence matrices" (GLCMs) [1]. GLCMs are then further processed or transformed into other, more descriptive measurements, many of which are derived from physics equations, such as "entropy" and "energy." Other texture measurements can also be measured, such as gradient measurements, which can also be described as "total variation" [2, 3]. There are many different possible mathematical features, with many of them overlapping each other. Convolutional neu-

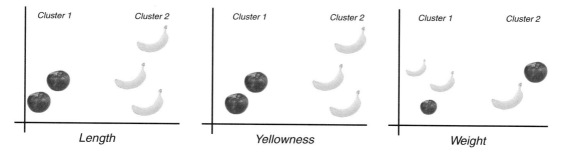

Fig. 5.3 Three plots showing quantifications of apples and bananas based on length, color ("yellowness"), and weight. Depending on the quantification method used, the classification can result in several clusters that can distinguish the apples and bananas or can make them indistinguishable

Fig. 5.4 A 4 × 4 image of white and black block tiles. This image can be used to create quantities that can describe any number of feature dynamics

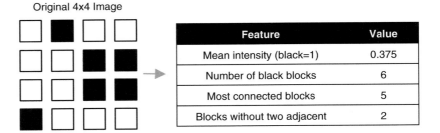

Feature	Value
Mean intensity (black=1)	0.375
Number of black blocks	6
Most connected blocks	5
Blocks without two adjacent	2

ral networks allow learning very complex, task-specific textures that can be used to recognize faces [4] and numbers [5], and segment structures in different types of bio-medical images [6, 7].

Texture measurements can have a confusing relationship with shape and volume. While some textures are shape dependent, others are not. A simple total volume or length may be more important than other texture features because large diseased areas often represent comorbidities. Due to this dependency, many different image combinations are possible. Should you use an arbitrary region outline to extract features of your image that could vary over different disease shapes and sizes, or a rigid shape (such as a square)? Outlining a disease specifically will highlight disease specific features but will result in irregular shapes that are less repeatable than conforming to drawing a rigid shape based on anatomical landmarks; the precise outline required depends on context.

5.1.5 Feature Reduction

One of the difficulties of texture analysis, and in general ML, is that the number of descriptions can quickly outpace the data present. Let us take five different fruits: an apple, orange, banana, cherry, and pear. There are 5! = 120 different orders in which we can arrange these in a line, which is much more than the number of fruit themselves. However, it may be that one of those specific orders is the key to unlocking a mystery. Those 120 orders are not all of the possible representations of those 5 fruits, because we could place the fruits into 5 boxes instead of 1, or 4, 3 or 2. Images have much more than five features, often using pixel dimensions of $256 \times 256 = 65,536$

pixels, before even considering the many layouts possible or 3D layers!

This proliferation of dimensionality obscures the interpretation of the results, making it difficult to understand why an algorithm has reached a certain conclusion. The goal of ML research should be to find new mechanisms underlying the causes of diseases, which will aid future assessments (whether in the physical or computational spaces). Not all data is necessary—it does not *normally* make sense to look for disease correlations within the brain to a predominantly kidney disease. In order to make sense of much of the data, we can perform "ablation" to determine whether these features are primary measurements within our tests. "Ablation" is the removal of a portion of the ML pipeline to see whether the same results are obtained, whether that's removing data, features, or a portion of the ML network. For example, an ablation study might be to randomly remove half of the image features to see whether the same results can be obtained [8, 9].

Large numbers of features are more difficult to train and require more data. Two methods to reduce the number of features are called principal component analysis (PCA) and singular value decomposition (SVD). These are unsupervised algorithms that reduce the number of features by combining them into new features based on linear relationship calculations. By reducing the number of features used before further calculations, ML methods can train more quickly and with reduced dataset sizes. PCA and SVD can be considered to be the same thing for all practical purposes, although PCA can differ in its operational order. These create a reduced set of features based on their linear correlations, calculated based on a linear algebra technique called eigenvalue decomposition.

Feature selection can be performed by the recursive elimination of features (feature ablation) to determine whether an output remains significant. Feature selection can be prior to analysis as well. For example, features can be removed that have strong linear correlations to each other, presupposing that they do not contain new information. This is not strictly true as a quadratic curve could be based off of a linear curve and will not have a strong linear correlation, but would be caused by exactly the same information. Another selection method retains features that have the highest variances, based on the assumption that independent relationships will have high variances - but this could also could be the result of noise. Recursive elimination is the most likely to find significant results, but it is also the most likely to find insignificant results at the same time due to the wide range of repeated tests, which is why linear- or variance-based feature removals are used.

5.1.6   Scaling and Normalization

For a large majority of ML methods, the models are improved when the data is standardized—which means to adjust the scale of the input features. We can show how this relates to features in the five fruit example. If we have measurements of the fruits based on their weights and longest lengths, then we want our output to be consistent regardless of the input. That is, regardless of whether we obtain the weights of the fruits in grams, kilograms, or pounds, we would like the end result to be the same. Furthermore, if we have calculated the features at very different scales, like the weight in milligrams, which would give features in hundreds of thousands, and length in kilometers, which would give features at decimal places, then we may get a nonoptimal outputs. Standardization is necessary partially because a majority of ML methods are built on linear regression, discussed more in depth later.

This normalization process can occur for texture features prior to analysis or for features within neural networks or for outputs between neural network layers (discussed later). Feature

normalization is not always ideal because it can reduce the quantitative nature of outputs; however, rescaling features is often necessary to obtain a meaningful result. For example, if I have two processes, one which results in 1000 ± 100 and another which results in 0.0010 ± 0.0001, then the effect of the one with higher scale may be overestimated during any optimization process. Rescaling also normally results in faster fitting.

A (non-fruit) example might be one below. Let us say we have the feature inputs, x, and the outputs, y, as listed:

Texture (x_1)	Shape (x_2)	eGFR (x_3)	Gender (x_4)	Disease score (y)	Disease (y_{binary})
0.7	1000	65	M (0)	4	Yes (1)
0.1	3000	15	F (1)	5	Yes (1)
0.5	500	110	M (0)	0	No (0)
0.9	7000	80	M (0)	3	Yes (1)
0.5	2500	120	F (1)	1	No (0)

A common standardization method of the input features, x_n, is to subtract all features by their mean and then divide those outputs by their overall standard deviation per each feature or per column. This will normally result in better outputs. This would result in a table as such:

Texture (x_1)	Shape (x_2)	eGFR (x_3)	Gender (x_4)	Disease score (y)	Disease (y_{binary})
0.6	−0.8	−0.3	−0.8	4	Yes (1)
−1.6	0.1	−1.6	1.2	5	Yes (1)
−0.2	−1.0	0.9	−0.8	0	No (0)
1.4	1.8	0.1	−0.8	3	Yes (1)
−0.2	−0.1	1.1	1.2	1	No (0)

5.1.7   Training, Validation, and Testing

A well-known issue when testing statistical problems is called the "multiple comparisons problem." If there are five random measurements of any kind, and a dice is thrown five 50 times, then there will be strong linear correlations between the initial set of random measurements and roughly 10 of these dice rolls, despite having no meaningful linking relationship. These correlations are called false positives or type I errors if there is no underlying causation. ML normally uses too many features or variables while ignoring multiple testing corrections (such as Bonferroni corrections). The high dimensionality of the problems would result in small statistical significance if such corrections were to be used in many of these tests. To work around this limitation and ensure reliable measurements, datasets are often broken up into *"Training," "Validation,"* and *"Testing"* datasets.

The *training* dataset is used while developing an algorithm. The *validation* set is used after an ideal algorithm has been developed to measure initial results on an independent set, which will result in lower scores than a training set. The *testing* set is meant to be a completely independent set of data that has not been tested previously, such that the training and validation would not bias its scores. The test set is considered *measured* or *observed* values. In practice, many datasets have been obtained from online databases that have been tested previously, so there is ambiguity in whether a test set is *"validation"* or *"testing"* set within literature.

These datasets might be split up equally into thirds, or into 30/20/30 splits, or even into 80/20 splits, depending on the data quality and type. For large databases, a full train-validation-test split is possible for sufficient training to obtain high scores (of any metric), while for smaller databases, such as in the case of rare diseases, an 80/20 split is required. It is also possible to do five 80/20 splits, with the 20% of the split coming from the five different portions of the data, and to repeat the training/testing five times, if the dataset numbers are very low [10].

5.2   Linear Regression

While it may seem backwards to begin with linear regression, it is helpful to understand before delving deeper into ML methods. Since the importance of textures can be separated via linear regression and since linear regression is a fundamental component of the majority of neurons in neural networks, having a solid framework of linear regression can help inform a more intuitive understanding of ML structures. Linear regression can be used as its own ML method. The principles demonstrated while performing a simple linear regression are applicable in more advanced machine learning topics.

5.2.1   Under- and Overfitting

Imagine that two points on a line are known exactly: at $x = 1$, $y = 2$, and at $x = 5$, $y = 10$. It is easy to see that the equation for this line would be $y = 2*x$. We have two variables, x and y, which are unknown. We have two points of (x,y): $(1,2)$ and $(5,10)$. If we know those two points exactly and that the model to be fit is a line, then we can fit the curve exactly.

Now imagine that our model is not a line but that it is a second-degree polynomial: $y = ax^2 + bx + c$. This could be the case because we have nonlinear relationships within our dataset. We may not even know what this model is, which does not necessarily have to be a second-degree polynomial but could be any number of other curves. We stick with the second-degree polynomial in this hypothetical example to give an intuitive feel for fitting. Let us assume that we only have those original two points [(1,5) and (2,10)]. The second-degree curve that fits this curve could be $y = -5x^2 + 20x - 10$. It could also be $y = -10x^2 + 35x - 20$. Or any number of solutions that exist. We could continue to extend the parameters with higher orders of polynomials, where even more possibilities exist. For a noiseless problem, we would want the same number of input datasets to match the number of variables to be predicted. In the real world, data collection processes are messy, so we normally require significantly more datasets to average noise out, even for predicting simple linear relationships.

Underfitting occurs when the data follows a more complicated relationship than the final model requires. Underfitting usually results in poor predictions because it does not model all of the complex relationships within the data.

Overfitting is when the data follows a simpler relationship than the final model requires. Many ML tasks will have many more variables predicted than inputs, which is overfitting. Overfitting is unavoidable because we are attempting to predict multiparametric, nonlinear relationships, such as the shape of a liver within images. The cost of overfitting is that it requires a larger number of datasets to have good predictability, it requires more advanced computational equipment (and power!), and it precludes the understanding of underlying models and mechanisms, which should be the goal of every researcher. However, an overfitted model is far from useless—if an overfitted model can be used for future predictions with statistical significance, naively as a lookup table using a very large dataset, then it may point to the existence of a simpler, underlying model or mechanism.

The goals of researchers vary: for some, finding small relationships in large datasets is important where effects are hidden; for others, finding strong relationships in small datasets is important, as that demonstrates very significant effects. Scientific progression relies on both types. Within the ML applications presented hereafter, we primarily focus on the use of large datasets, but note that small datasets require more specific models and stronger correlations to demonstrate efficacy, whether with ML or classical statistics.

In a very strict sense, many ML applications perform "overfitting," as the amount of data present is limited by the number of patients that it is far lower than the number of variable parameters (Fig. 5.5). The number of variable parameters in a typical deep learning model can include 30+ layers of parameters with tens to hundreds of parameters per layer. In this context, both "underfitting" and "overfitting" are when the model cannot be generalized to a group beyond the individuals included in the study, because the model is either not trained on enough data ("overfitting") or does not have enough parameters ("underfitting"). ML generally focuses on future predictions based on past data, whereas medicinal research focuses on better patient treatments or finding new underlying causes of disease progression, which require sensitive techniques and meaningful statistical methods to avoid biases.

5.2.2 Linear Regression Mathematics

This section is included as an easy reference for those who may be required to perform these calculations. It can be skipped for those not wishing to delve deeper into the mathematics.

Linear regression tries to predict a linear relationship between a set of variables and an output. We are most familiar with linear regression in the form of

$$y = f_{m,b}(x) = mx + b$$

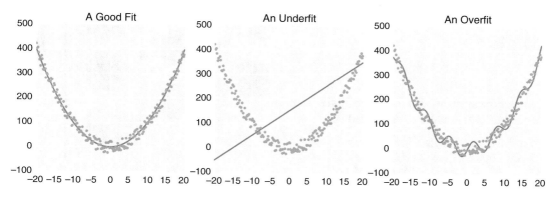

Fig. 5.5 When discussing fitting, the number of parameters should be representative of the underlying data and ignore noise. By increasing the number of fit parameters, any model can be fit with reduced error, but this reduces the predictability of future results without massive data increases

where y is an output that is dependent on the variable x as described by linear function f. The variables m and b are parameters of the function f, commonly known as "slope" and "intercept," respectively, and are generally unknown. A simple example might be the relationship between the height (y) of an individual with the width of that person's shoulders (x). Linear regression can be extended beyond a single variable—so instead of the width of shoulders being dependent on height alone, you can include other variables like considering the effects of average caloric intake.

Linear regression is process of estimating unknown parameters (m, b) given a set of observations (x_i, y_i). It is performed by minimizing the difference (or "residuals") between the measured and the model values. That is, we seek to minimize the function over

$$S(m,b) = \Sigma\left[y_i - f_{m,b}(x_i)\right]^2 = \Sigma\left[y_i - mx_i - b\right]^2$$

This minimization is found for slope m when the derivative of S with respect to m is zero, i.e., $\dfrac{\partial S(m)}{\partial m} = 0$. This formulation may not be very intuitive, but this minimization leads to the ability to predict the slope of the curve, which can be demonstrated to be [11]:

$$m = \frac{\text{Covariance}[x,y]}{\text{Variance}[x]} = \frac{\Sigma xy - \dfrac{\Sigma x \Sigma y}{n}}{\Sigma x^2 - \dfrac{(\Sigma x)^2}{n}}$$

After the slope, m, is found, the intercept, b, can then be found:

$$b = \bar{y} - m\bar{x}$$

The "goodness-of-fit" of a linear function is often referred to as "r," which is calculated as:

$$r = \frac{\Sigma(x - \bar{x})(y - \bar{y})}{\sqrt{\Sigma(x - \bar{x})^2 (y - \bar{y})^2}}$$

where $\bar{x}$ and $\bar{y}$ are sample means. When "r" approaches 1, then fitted x and y values have a good fit.

5.2.3 The Neural Network

You would undoubtedly have heard of "deep learning" and hopefully a "neural network" (Fig. 5.6). These build on the principle of a "neuron," which is a single building block in a neural network. A "*neuron*" is a linear fit of inputs (or features, usually denoted as x) that are fed into a transformation (called an activation function, which is often a nonlinear transformation) and attempts to minimize the error between its output (a predicted y) and a measured quantity (an observed y). When multiple neurons are chained together, they form a "*neural network*." When a large number of these neurons are chained together, they are considered a "deep neural network" [12].

When the outputs of a group of neurons are fed into the inputs of another group of neurons, each of these groups is considered a "*layer*." Each layer of neurons is usually referred to as a "hidden layer," with the inputs (x) and predicted outputs (y) not being hidden. A neuron individu-

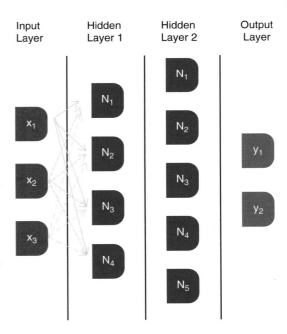

Fig. 5.6 A neural network with three inputs, two hidden layers, and two predicted outputs. Neural networks can have any number of neurons per hidden layer, as well as any number of hidden layers, provided the computational ability remains

ally has a largely linear relationship between inputs and outputs. However, by chaining neurons together with activation functions, nonlinear relationships occur that can model most complex functions. By increasing the number of layers, the model becomes more specific and less generalized, which requires more data and more specific data. A higher number of neuron layers is incredibly useful when the model has an unknown or difficult to model relationship, which occurs frequently in the arbitrary shapes that many lesions can cause.

We want to suppress the output of neurons that are not contributing to accuracy in the end prediction (Fig. 5.7). Within biology, an activation function is when a cell has minimal output until a set of inputs, such as a voltage or chemical concentration, surpass a definable limit to ensure a neuron fires only after passing the threshold of an action potential. Due to this similarity, neural networks are referred to as "artificial neural networks." In order to attenuate these computational neurons, similar to biological under-stimulation or hypersensitization, we use a similar idea encapsulated in within the "activation function." A neuron weights each of its inputs, creating a linear model, and then outputs this. This output is fed into an activation function, also known as nonlinearity, that performs a certain fixed mathematical operation on it.

Activation functions subdue or amplify the outputs of a neuron to increase or decrease its importance in a neural network. Common activation functions are in Fig. 5.8. The *sigmoid* function (or logistic curve) is a common function to "squish" a real number between 0 and 1. Very negative inputs become close to 0, very positive inputs become close to 1, and the function steadily increases or decreases around the input 0. The sigmoid function is continuously differentiable as a smooth, nonlinear step function. This function is useful for predicting probabilities. However, this is not zero-centered, which may require more data for training and can be difficult to optimize [12]. The hyperbolic tangent, *tanh*, function is sigmoid scaled to be centered around zero, and so is preferred over the sigmoid function. The most widely used activation function currently is the "rectified linear unit" or "ReLU" pictured in Fig. 5.8, used for its speed and stability. The *ReLU* has simpler mathematical operations over the *sigmoid* and *tanh* activation functions. No activation function is perfect, as the ReLU results in the a "dying ReLU problem,"

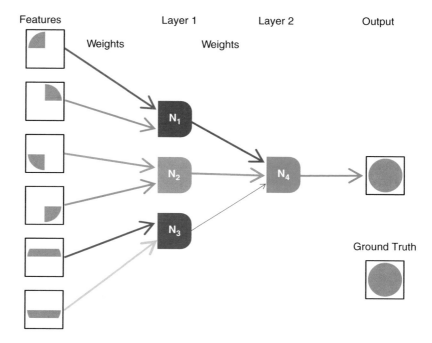

Fig. 5.7 An example of how different input "features" can combine within a network to create an output. The weights might be randomly initialized. This example shows that there may be overlaps of features, which should become less weighted with increased training

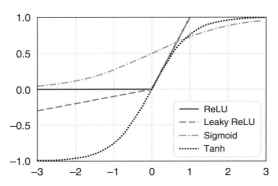

Fig. 5.8 Four activation functions are shown. A neural network weights its inputs and then based on that output, undergoes a transformation following an activation function. This amplifies neurons that contribute to the final objective

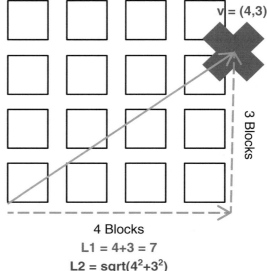

4 Blocks

L1 = 4+3 = 7

L2 = sqrt(4^2+3^2)

Fig. 5.9 A 4 × 4 tile showing the difference between an L1 norm and an L2 norm. An L1 norm is the distance it takes for a taxicab to drive to the location, which is shown as from the origin (0,0) to the point (4,3). An L2 norm is the quadratic distance, following the Pythagorean theorem for a two-dimensional plot

which is when "dead" neurons form during the learning process if their weights have progressed to zero, and no longer can be updated. The leaky ReLU is an upgraded version of ReLU, which has a small linear gradient to ensure that a neuron's weights will never reach zero and thus never become fully deactivated [13].

5.2.4   The Objective Function

The objective function is the calculated penalty between a wrong classification and prediction. In many ML problems, we wish to minimize the errors between a set of predicted outputs and the observations (often measurement data, which can include disease scores). This process of minimization is based on a so-called objective function that encodes in a single value the disagreement between predictions and observation metrics [14, 15]. The objective function can also be referred to as a "loss," "regret," or "cost" function. There are ML problems where the objective function is maximized and referred to as a "reward," "profit," "utility," or "fitness" function, although we will not consider these latter cases.

The objective or cost between a set of predicted and measured outputs could be a simple difference between these values. There is no

ideal universal "cost" between predictions and observations. Every cost function has their drawbacks and their effectiveness depends on the application. There are two frequently used cost functions, referred to as the L1 and L2 norms [16]. A norm can be thought of like an absolute value—except how does one take the absolute value of a multidimensional vector? The norm of −1 is +1. Moving to complex numbers, the norm of $1 + i$, where i is equal to the $\sqrt{-1}$ is dependent on whether one is measuring its L1 or L2 norm.

The L1 norm of a vector, v, is its distance from the origin and has the symbol $\|v\|_1$ the absolute sum of all vector values. That is, $\|v\|_1 = |v_1| + |v_2| + \cdots + |v_n|$. This is also called the "taxicab" or "Manhattan" norm because it refers to the distance it takes for a taxicab in Manhattan to reach its destination, based on a square grid (Fig. 5.9). The L1 norm of $1 + i$ is 2. The L1 norm when used in ML will be the difference between each predicted and measured output:

$$\| y \|_1 = \left| y_{1,\text{pred}} - y_{1,obs} \right| + \left| y_{2,\text{pred}} - y_{2,obs} \right| + \dots$$
$$+ \left| y_{n,\text{pred}} - y_{n,obs} \right|$$

The L2 norm of a vector is its classical distance from the origin and has the symbol $\|v\|_2$. It can also be referred to as the Euclidean norm and is the most common norm used (Fig. 5.9). It is the square root of the sum of the squared vector values. The L2 norm of $1 + i$ is $\sqrt{2}$. The L2 norm of a vector with higher dimensions is

$$\| v \|_2 = \sqrt{\left| v_1 \right|^2 + \left| v_2 \right|^2 + ? \left| v_n \right|^2}$$ or within an optimization technique:

$$\| y \|_2 = \sqrt{\left| y_{1,\text{pred}} - y_{1,obs} \right|^2 + \left| y_{2,\text{pred}} - y_{2,obs} \right|^2 + \dots \atop + \left| y_{n,\text{pred}} - y_{n,obs} \right|^2}$$

These two norms are the most commonly used cost functions. Another cost function could be the p-norm, which is the L2 norm with the power of two replaced with the power of p:

$$\| y \|_p = \sqrt[p]{\left| y_{1,\text{pred}} - y_{1,obs} \right|^p + \left| y_{2,\text{pred}} - y_{2,obs} \right|^p + \dots \atop + \left| y_{n,\text{pred}} - y_{n,obs} \right|^p}$$

State-of-the-art deep learning approaches use a variety of task-specific complex cost functions that aim to be easier to optimize [16–18], seek to capture perceptual differences between images [19–21], and even learn a cost function specific for the task [22, 23]. Irrespective of choice of cost/objective function, the training process must numerically minimize the chosen cost function to obtain the model with optimal parameters (e.g., (m, b) in the regression example above) [24, 25]. Ideally the optimization process seeks to find the "global" minima of the objective function, i.e., there does not exist any other set of parameters that can have a lower cost [26]. Finding a global minima or even verifying a candidate for global minima is a very difficult problem, especially in state-of-the-art ML approaches

that have a large number of parameters. Hence, most optimization methods use local information like derivatives and Taylor series expansion to find a "local" minima that is practically useful for the task [27–29]. "Gradient descent" is a widely used technique that uses local derivatives to find local minimum for a variety of applications [30, 31].

5.2.5   Gradient Descent

Gradient descent is a widely used iterative method to optimize an objective function. That is, it is the method for updating parameters within a neural network algorithm [30, 31].

A gradient descent algorithm can be used to optimize a continuous function. Let us say our model is quadratic, that is, $y_{\text{model}} = x^2$, and we have a set of measured values, $y_{1,\text{obs}}, y_{2,\text{obs}}, y_{3,\text{obs}}$. We want to find the x values that minimize the error between the model and the observed or measured values. While the solution to each x is trivial because we know the model (since we could easily take the square root of $y_{1,\text{obs}}, y_{2,\text{obs}},$ and $y_{3,\text{obs}}$), this is enlightening as it can help us understand models with more complicated interdependencies, such as if y_1, y_2, and y_3 were not completely independent.

The L2 norm in this model will be

$$\| y \|_2 = \sqrt{\left| y_{1,\text{pred}} - y_{1,obs} \right|^2 + \left| y_{2,\text{pred}} - y_{2,obs} \right|^2 \atop + \left| y_{3,\text{pred}} - y_{3,obs} \right|^2}$$

If we assume no knowledge of x_1, x_2, and x_3 prior to starting, we can enter in initial guesses and calculate $\|y\|_2$. However, we need a method to update these values. To do this, we can take the derivative—or gradient—of the objective function. If the gradient is large, then that parameter should change quickly. If the gradient is small, then that parameter creates a minimum or maximum value in the objective function. Gradient descent corrects for predictions or guesses that are distant from the optimum value.

Gradient descent updates each parameter with its rate of change based on the derivative of the cost function. For example, with each gradient descent step, an initial point x_1 is moved in the direction of steepest descent with a step-size α:

$$x_{1,new} = x_{1,old} - \alpha \cdot \frac{\partial \| y \|_2}{\partial x_{1,old}}$$

Alpha, α, is a "learning rate," which can be statically set or updated throughout training. Alpha is often determined empirically and can be considered a "hyperparameter." Hyperparameters are often user-definable variables that can affect training effectiveness substantially. Large-scale optimization, like that in deep learning, generally use sophisticated approaches for updating the learning rate throughout the process to quickly find the minimal point [32–35].

When applied to neural networks, the gradient descent algorithm is used to update the weights w_n and biases b_m to minimize the cost (Fig. 5.10). This process by which values are updated is called "back-propagation" because the informa-

tion gained by comparing the network's output and our observation data is propagated through the rest of the network. The minimum is found by repeatedly using the above update rule:

$$w_{n+1} = w_n - \alpha \cdot \frac{\partial \| y \|_2}{\partial w_n}$$

$$b_{m+1} = b_m - \alpha \cdot \frac{\partial \| y \|_2}{\partial b_m}$$

Neural networks will typically use "mini-batch" gradient descent, which is a combination of two other gradient descent methods: batch and stochastic gradient descent. Batch gradient descent calculates the descent for all parameters and observations but is computationally expensive especially with very large datasets. Stochastic gradient descent updates parameters using an "estimate" of the derivative computed using only a random "mini" subset of the complete observation, thus saving on computational requirements, which results in high variability in the new parameter estimates [36, 37].

5.2.6 Deep Learning with Convolutional Neural Networks

Deep learning (DL) is machine learning that occurs over many learning layers. Similar to ordinary neural networks, convolutional neural networks (CNNs) also consist of neurons that have learnable weights and biases. The main difference is that the structure of CNNs assumes matrices/images as inputs (Fig. 5.11; see also [4, 5, 12]) and are thus built accordingly to make use of convolution filters, which is fundamental to several image processing operations [38–40]. The layers of CNNs are made up of neurons arranged in three dimensions—height, width, and depth.

The core parts of any CNN are the convolutional layers (CL). As with any other layer, a CL receives an input and outputs a transformation of the input to the next layer. Inputs passing through a convolutional layer will have a set of k small $n \times n$ filters convolve (slide) across its volume

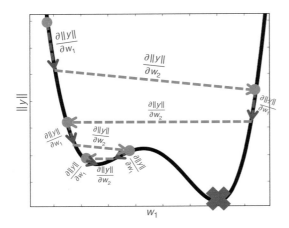

Fig. 5.10 The goal of the optimization process is to determine the weights of the system that reach the minimum value (marked with the green x). The weights can be updated with a gradient descent algorithm. New values of the system are based on the rate of change caused by each parameter. Parameters that drastically affect the system have a higher rate of change and are updated more quickly. Multiple parameters can affect a system, which is the effect shown in blue, where these might be updated each w update shown in red. A danger of optimization techniques is that local minima can be reached

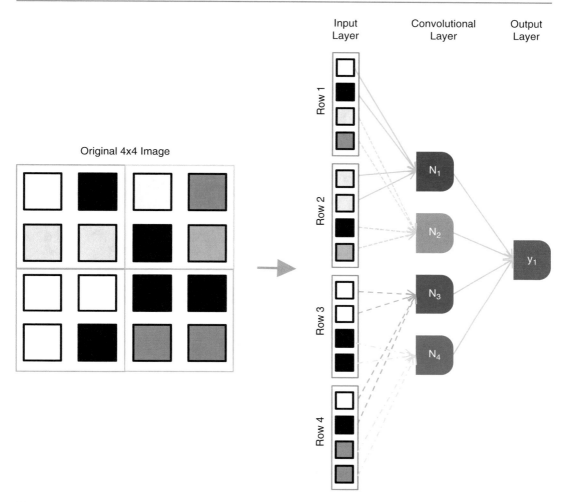

Fig. 5.11 A 4 × 4 image is unwrapped to show how it can create 16 inputs into a convolutional layer with 4 neurons. These four neurons can then weigh into a final output layer, which may be a prediction of the severity of a disease

and have the dot product between each filter and input entry calculated (Fig. 5.12). Therefore, k 2D feature maps are obtained, which are stacked across the depth dimension. The three hyper-parameters that define the output volume size are the number of filters k (depth of the CL), the stride with which the filter is convolved over the input and the size of zero-padding around the input's border. A stride of 1 means, the filter is slid pixel by pixel over the input. Zero-padding allows control over the output spatial size. By padding the borders of the input with zeros, the spatial size of the output equals the size of the input.

In addition to the convolutional layer, CNNs are made up of a series of different types of layers that either perform a transformation of the input's activations (convolutional layer, fully connected layer) or apply a fixed function (activation function layer (AF), pooling layer, batch normalization).

A fully connected layer (FCL) simply multiplies its input by a weight matrix followed by a bias offset and an activation function transformation. All the neurons from an FCL are connected to all neurons from the previous layer. FCLs are typically used at the end of CNNs designed for performing classification tasks.

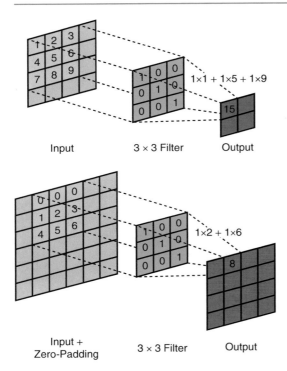

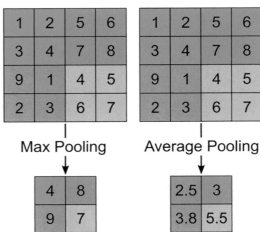

Fig. 5.13 Pooling an image or layer down-samples that image to become a smaller shape. "Max pooling" selects the maximum value within a region. "Average pooling" can also be performed, where the average of a region is selected

Fig. 5.12 (Top) A demonstration of convolution using a 3 × 3 filter (or "kernel" if in 2D) that highlights diagonal elements. (Bottom) Prior to convolution, the input image is zero padded to maintain the final image size

5.2.7 Advanced Deep Learning Architectures

The list of various deep learning architectures used in medical imaging is long and growing rapidly [44]. Here we cover a few of the most widely used models.

5.2.7.1 Autoencoders

Autoencoders learn a feature representation of unlabeled data using an unsupervised encoding–decoding approach (Fig. 5.14) [45, 46]. Typically, an input image is fed into an encoding CNN and mapped to a lower-dimensional feature representation of the input. Through this process, the input experiences a dimensionality reduction to only obtain the most important features that define the input. After encoding, the features are fed into a decoding CNN (increasing dimensionality) to reconstruct the input data. Here stems the name "autoencoding" as the network is encoding its most prominent features to be able to reconstruct itself. The network learns by comparing the reconstructed input with the original input using for instance an L2 cost function. This

Pooling layers (PL) are used intermittently between CL to reduce the spatial dimension of the feature maps [12, 41]. Common pooling operations are max pooling and average pooling of the spatial data (Fig. 5.13). Through pooling, important feature information is preserved while other less important is discarded [42]. This increases the robustness for feature extraction and controls overfitting while reducing the total number of parameters in the network and ultimately the computation time [43].

CNN architectures typically consist of a series of convolutional layer → activation function layer or convolutional layer → batch normalization layer → activation function layer stacks, while each stack is followed by a pooling layer, until the input has been spatially reduced. A final fully connected layer → activation function layer is then applied to classify each neuron.

Autoencoder

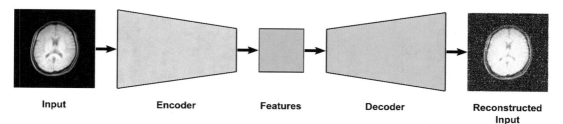

Fig. 5.14 The autoencoder consists of two neural networks, an encoder and a decoder network. The dimension of input (brain MRI) is first reduced by the encoder to a lower-dimensional feature representation followed by a dimension upsampling by the decoder to generate the output. Usually, the encoding and decoding paths are symmetric to generate an output identical to the input

learning is unsupervised as no external labeled data is used during training. After training, the decoder part of the network can be discarded while the encoder part could be used for some different task, such as to initialize a new supervised network or to provide justification [47, 48].

5.2.7.2 ResNet

The ResNet architecture was introduced in 2015 and won the ImageNet challenge in that year. It consists of so-called ResNet or residual blocks that allowed easier and faster training of very deep networks [49] by mitigating the vanishing gradient problem. When the gradient is backpropagated in very deep networks, the repetitive multiplication tends to make the gradient vanishingly small. This can lead to the accuracy of deep networks being saturated or even degraded once network convergence begins. The residual block uses skip or shortcut connections that skip one or more layers and creates a parallel branch that reuses the activations from previous layers. By skipping layers, training time and the effect of the vanishing gradient are reduced as the network uses fewer layers during initial training while preserving information as the input is fed through the layers.

5.2.7.3 U-Net

The U-Net was also introduced in 2015 and has become one of the most widely used networks for automated image segmentation (Fig. 5.15) [7]. The name is derived from its U-like appearance when its neuron layers are shown in a graph for-

mat. Within U-Net, the input is progressively down-sampled (encoder) by a typical CNN architecture described in the previous section and then up-sampled (decoder) by a series of transpose convolutional layers. By introducing additional skip-connections, features from the encoding network path are concatenated to features from the decoding network paths, enabling high-resolution segmentations.

5.2.7.4 Generative Adversarial Networks

A generative adversarial network consists of two competing neural networks that are trained simultaneously in a mini-max game to optimize a loss objective function [50]. As an example, a noise image can be fed into a network, which competes against the original input image fed into the same network for generating the best result. This relies on a generative network, G, focusing on image generation while another classification network, D, works on image discrimination. During training, D guides G to learn a translation of input images to realistic representations of the ground truth training data. D makes a binary prediction of whether the generated image is a true representation of the desired output or not, and feeds its prediction back to G to produce more accurate representations. Therefore, GANs and its conditional variant (cGANs) have been successfully applied in many image-to-image transformation tasks such as segmentation and image synthesis.

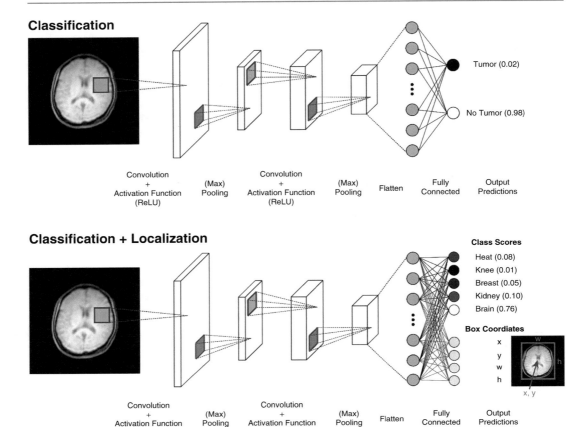

Fig. 5.15 The U-Net progressively down-samples an input (brain MRI) in an encoding path through multiple convolutional and pooling layers while increasing the number of feature representations. In a succeeding, symmetric decoding path, the features are up-sampled using up- or transpose convolutions to the original spatial size of the input. By concatenating features from the encoding to the decoding path through additional skip-connections, high-resolution segmentations are achieved

5.2.7.5 Deep Boltzmann Machines

Deep learning can also appear as "Deep Boltzmann machines" (DBMs) [51] that can perform image recognition tasks, but these differ from CNNs in several ways. A DBM is used for classification problems, whereas a CNN can be applied to more general problems. DBMs do not use gradient descent and backpropagation. Instead, DBMs use probability distributions over binary values. A Boltzmann machine can also be called a Markov random field.

5.2.8 Deep Learning in Medical Image Analysis

Over the recent years, the application of deep learning has had a significant impact on various areas of medical imaging analysis [52]. With the rapid progression and development of deep learning architectures and their subsequent application to the analysis of medical images, this section will only highlight a few applications and publications demonstrating the advances in this research field.

5.2.8.1 Classification, Localization and Detection

Image classification has become one of the most effective applications of deep learning in medical image analysis. A deep neural network classifies an image by extracting image features to predict class labels of an object in the input image. Typically, the input image is fed into a CNN that progressively down-samples the image through multiple convolutional and pooling layers and outputs a single categorical label defining the input, for example, "Tumor" or "No Tumor" to characterize tumor presence in a brain MR image (Fig. 5.16).

Deep learning has also been successfully applied to object localization in which the incidence of an object is located, and their location usually specified by a bounding box. In this network, object classification and localization are combined by adding an additional fully connected layer that outputs box coordinates, such as the width, height, and x and y coordinates of the bounding box (Fig. 5.16). In object detection, the localization task is extended to multiple objects in a single input image. All objects in an image are defined by a class label and location.

GANs have been implemented to detect abnormalities in medical images by training the network only on images of normal, "healthy" anatomy appearance. Structures that are not part of the normal distribution learned can be detected by an anomaly scoring system [53]. Furthermore, deep learning methods have been applied to medical image denoising and artifact detection. For example, an autoencoder has been shown to outperform the FSL SUSAN denoising algorithm for denoising brain MRIs with various degrees of additional Gaussian noise [54], while a CNN has been used to patch-wise detect motion artifacts in cranial and abdominal MRIs [55].

5.2.8.2 Segmentation

Region- or tissue-specific segmentation plays an important role in the analysis of medical images for disease quantification and clinical translation of new imaging techniques. Expert manual segmentation remains to be the most accurate method, however, requires a significant amount of time and is subject to inter-rater variability. Consequently, the attention has grown to develop sophisticated deep learning networks to fully automate the semantic segmentation task of medical images, i.e., labeling each pixel in an image with a class label. The most recognized CNN-based segmentation architecture applied to medical images is the previously mentioned

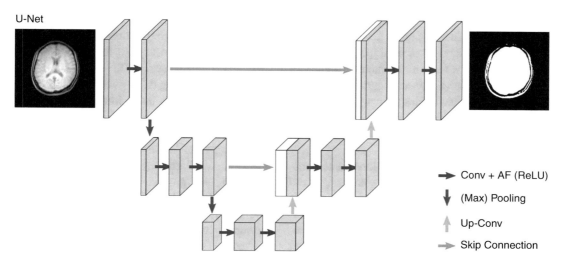

Fig. 5.16 In the classification task, the network output is a discrete label or description of the object in the input image. In the localization task, the network outputs the exact location of the object, along with the class label describing the object detected

U-Net. The majority of CNNs developed for segmentation tasks are spin-offs of the U-Net architecture such as its 3D variant, called V-Net, applying 3D convolutions [6]. GANs are also increasingly being used for automated segmentation of medical images as they are showing great promise in overcoming a spatial continuity constraint identified in U-Net-based methods. They typically employ a U-Net-based generator network for creating the segmentation image, while the GAN's discriminator network could act as a shape regulator and increase the spatial consistency in the final segmentation image. Conventionally, pixel-wise or voxel-wise objective functions are used during training. Examples are (binary) cross entropy or variants of segmentation-based evaluation metrics such as the Sørensen–Dice Similarity Coefficient [56, 57] or Jaccard Index [58].

While most segmentation strategies have been applied to single-modality images, there has been an increasing interested in multi-modality segmentation as this can provide different structural and functional information about the target simultaneously. For this purpose, the multi-modality images are usually fused as multi-channel inputs, with a single-channel segmentation map as network output. For example, Wang et al. [59] and Zhou et al. [60] fused the four MRI modalities (T1-w, T1c-w, T2-w, and FLAIR images) from the BraTS dataset [61] as the multi-channel input to a CNN for brain tumor segmentation. Zhao et al. [62] fused PET and CT images as their multi-channel input to a 3D CNN for lung cancer segmentation and achieved higher accuracies than with respective single-modality segmentation.

5.2.8.3 Registration

In medical image registration, a coordinate transformation is determined from one image and applied to another to spatially align both. CNNs employed for registration tasks often use traditionally used registration metric such as a similarity measure between two images from different imaging modalities as the cost function during network training. Conditional GANs can also be used for medical image registration. In this case, the cGAN generator could determine the transformation parameters or the transformed image while the discriminator classifies between aligned and unaligned image sets. Deep learning methods have been applied for various multi-modality image registration tasks, such as unsupervised affine and deformable image registration of CTs and MRIs [63–65]. These methods have shown to be significantly faster than conventional image registration methods.

5.2.8.4 Image Synthesis

Deep learning networks have also shown their benefit in cross-modality image synthesis where the desired image modality is either expensive or infeasible to acquire. For this, CNNs are used to convert an image acquired with one modality into an image of another. The pooling layer is usually absent in CNNs used for image synthesis, with down-sampling occurring through convolutions. GANs in particular have shown great promise in the field of synthetic image generation producing realistic images in supervised and unsupervised cross-modality settings. GANs have been used to generate cross-modality medical images between MR, CT, and PET. While the majority of studies have been focused on generating synthetic images of the brain (MR → CT [66]; CT → MR [67]; MR → PET [68], PET → MR [69]), image synthesis using GANs has also been applied to musculoskeletal (MR → CT [70]), heart (MR → CT [71]), liver (CT → [72]), and lung (CT → MR [73]) images.

In image synthesis tasks, image quality is traditionally assessed by calculating the mean absolute error (MAE), mean squared error (MSE), (peak) signal to noise ratio ((P)SNR), or the structural similarity (SSIM) index between generated and ground truth reference image. While MAE, MSE, and (P)SNR assess pixel-wise intensity differences, SSIM additionally measures contrast and structural differences between the synthetic and reference image [20].

5.2.9 Federated Learning

An emerging method for ML training is called "federated learning." Federated learning ties computers across multiple sites, even internationally, and enables distributed learning [74, 75]. This allows individual centers learn a "local" model weights using their data, which is then sent to central locations that can then create a "global" model based on local inputs. The advantage of this is that data can remain within a center, which is a consideration to ensure patient privacy by reducing the amount of identifiable data. This also leverages the ability of varied patient groups, datasets, and computational capabilities to provide a more general model than can be achieved within a single center. Researchers are actively exploring use of federated learning with homomorphic encryption [76], which can enable distributed learning while maintaining complete privacy [74, 77–79].

As ML becomes increasingly prevalent in medicine and in other aspects of our lives, it may be that we will eventually possess models and weights based on global datasets and trained from federated learning projects on our phones—if our phones are not participating in these projects!

References

1. Haralick RM, Dinstein I, Shanmugam K. Textural features for image classification. IEEE Trans Syst Man Cybern. 1973;SMC-3:610–21. https://doi.org/10.1109/TSMC.1973.4309314.
2. Jain AK, Farrokhnia F. Unsupervised texture segmentation using Gabor filters. In: 1990 IEEE international conference on systems, man and cybernetics conference and proceedings. IEEE, 1990. https://doi.org/10.1016/0031-3203(91)90143-S.
3. Khotanzad A, Chen J-Y. Unsupervised segmentation of textured images by edge detection in multidimensional feature. IEEE Trans Pattern Anal Mach Intell. 1989;11:414–21. https://doi.org/10.1109/34.19038.
4. Lawrence S, Giles CL, Tsoi AC, Back AD. Face recognition: a convolutional neural-network approach. IEEE Trans Neural Netw. 1997;8:98–113. https://doi.org/10.1109/72.554195.
5. LeCun Y, Boser BE, Denker JS, Henderson D, Howard RE, Hubbard WE, Jackel LD. Handwritten digit recognition with a back-propagation network. Adv Neural Inf Proces Syst. 1990;2:396–404.
6. Milletari F, Navab N, Ahmadi SA. V-net: fully convolutional neural networks for volumetric medical image segmentation. In: Proceedings of the 4th international conference on 3D vision, 3DV 2016, 2016, p. 565–71. https://doi.org/10.1109/3DV.2016.79.
7. Ronneberger O, Fischer P, Brox T. U-net: convolutional networks for biomedical image segmentation. arXiv Prepr. arXiv1505.04597v1, 2015, p. 1–8.
8. Girshick R, Donahue J, Darrell T, Malik J. Rich feature hierarchies for accurate object detection and semantic segmentation. In: Proceedings of the IEEE computer society conference on computer vision and pattern recognition, 2014, p. 580–7. https://doi.org/10.1109/CVPR.2014.81.
9. Horvitz E, Apacible J. Learning and reasoning about interruption. In: Proceedings of the 5th international conference on multimodal interfaces, 2003, p. 20–7. https://doi.org/10.1145/958432.958440.
10. Arlot S, Celisse A. A survey of cross-validation procedures for model selection. Stat Surv. 2010;4:40–79. https://doi.org/10.1214/09-SS054.
11. Montgomery DC, Peck EA, Vining GG. Introduction to linear regression analysis. 5th ed. Boca Raton: Wiley; 2012.
12. Goodfellow I, Bengio Y, Courville A. Deep learning. Cambridge: MIT Press; 2016.
13. Maas AL, Hannun AY, Ng AY. Rectifier nonlinearities improve neural network acoustic models. In: ICML workshop on deep learning for audio, speech and language processing, 2013.
14. Botchkarev A. Performance metrics (error measures) in machine learning regression, forecasting and prognostics: properties and typology. arXiv Prepr. arXiv 1809.03006, 2018. p. 1–37.
15. Hossin M, Sulaiman MN. A review on evaluation metrics for data classification evaluations. Int J Data Min Knowl Manag Process. 2015;5:1–11. https://doi.org/10.5121/ijdkp.2015.5201.
16. Janocha K, Czarnecki WM. On loss functions for deep neural networks in classification. arXiv Prepr. arXiv 1702.05659, 2017. https://doi.org/10.4467/20838476SI.16.004.6185.
17. Bishop CM. Neural networks for pattern recognition. Oxford: Oxford University Press; 1995.
18. Reed R, MarksII RJ. Neural smithing: supervised learning in feedforward artificial neural networks. Cambridge: MIT Press; 1999.
19. Heusel M, Ramsauer H, Unterthiner T, Nessler B, Hochreiter S. GANs trained by a two time-scale update rule converge to a local Nash equilibrium. In: Advances in neural information processing systems, 2017, p. 6627–38.
20. Horé A, Ziou D. Image quality metrics: PSNR vs. SSIM. In: Proceedings of the 20th international conference on pattern recognition, 2010, p. 2366–9. https://doi.org/10.1109/ICPR.2010.579.
21. Johnson J, Alahi A, Fei-Fei L. Perceptual losses for style transfer and super-resolution. In: European con-

ference on computer vision, 2016, p. 694–711. https://doi.org/10.1007/978-3-319-46475-6_43.

22. Isola P, Zhu JY, Zhou T, Efros AA. Image-to-image translation with conditional adversarial networks. In: Proceedings of the 30th IEEE conference on computer vision and pattern recognition, CVPR 2017, 2017, p. 5967–76. https://doi.org/10.1109/CVPR.2017.632.

23. Maximo A, Bhushan C. Conditional adversarial network for segmentation with simple loss function. In: Proceedings of the 27th annual meet. ISMRM, Montreal, Canada, vol. 4737, 2019.

24. Shrestha A, Mahmood A. Review of deep learning algorithms and architectures. IEEE Access. 2019;7:53040–65. https://doi.org/10.1109/ACCESS.2019.2912200.

25. Sun S, Cao Z, Zhu H, Zhao J. A survey of optimization methods from a machine learning perspective. IEEE Trans Cybern. 2020;50:3668–81. https://doi.org/10.1109/tcyb.2019.2950779.

26. Törn A, Zilinskas A. Global optimization. Berlin: Springer-Verlag; 1989. https://doi.org/10.1007/3-540-50871-6.

27. Heath MT. Scientific computing: an introductory survey, revised. 2nd ed. Philadelphia: Society for Industrial and Applied Mathematics; 2018.

28. Horst R, Pardalos PM. Handbook of global optimization. Boston: Springer; 1995. https://doi.org/10.1007/978-1-4615-2025-2.

29. Nocedal J, Wright SJ. Numerical optimization, springer series in operations research and financial engineering. New York: Springer; 2006. https://doi.org/10.1007/978-0-387-40065-5.

30. Cauchy A-L. Méthode générale pour la résolution des systèmes d'équations simultanées. C R Hebd Seances Acad Sci. 1847;25:536–8.

31. Le QV, Ngiam J, Coates A, Lahiri A, Prochnow B, Ng AY. On optimization methods for deep learning. In: Proceedings of the 28th international conference on machine learning, 2011, p. 129–32.

32. Behera L, Kumar S, Patnaik A. On adaptive learning rate that guarantees convergence in feedforward networks. IEEE Trans Neural Netw. 2006;17:1116–25. https://doi.org/10.1109/TNN.2006.878121.

33. Yu C-C, Liu B-D. A backpropagation algorithm with adaptive learning rate and momentum coefficient. In: Proceedings of the 2002 international joint conference on neural networks, IJCNN'02 (Cat. No.02CH37290). IEEE, 2002, p. 1218–23. https://doi.org/10.1109/IJCNN.2002.1007668.

34. Kingma DP, Ba JL. Adam: a method for stochastic optimization. In: 3rd international conference on learning representations (ICLR), San Diego, USA, 2015, p. 1–15.

35. Luo Z-Q. On the convergence of the LMS algorithm with adaptive learning rate for linear feedforward networks. Neural Comput. 1991;3:226–45. https://doi.org/10.1162/neco.1991.3.2.226.

36. Bottou L. Online learning and stochastic approximations. On-line Learn Neural Netw. 1998;17.

37. Sra S, Nowozin S, Wright SJ, editors. Optimization for machine learning. Cambridge: MIT Press; 2011.

38. Duda RO, Hart PE. Pattern classification and scene analysis. 1st ed. Boca Raton: Wiley; 1973.

39. Gonzalez RC, Woods RE, Eddins SL. Digital image processing using MATLAB. 3rd ed. Upper Saddle River: Pearson Prentice Hall; 2020.

40. Shapiro L. Computer vision and image processing. 1st ed. Boston: Academic Press; 1992.

41. Nagi J, Ducatelle F, Di Caro GA, Cireşan D, Meier U, Giusti A, Nagi F, Schmidhuber J, Gambardella LM. Max-pooling convolutional neural networks for vision-based hand gesture recognition. In: 2011 IEEE international conference on signal and image processing applications, ICSIPA, 2011, p. 342–7. https://doi.org/10.1109/ICSIPA.2011.6144164.

42. Boureau Y-L, Ponce J, LeCun Y. A theoretical analysis of feature pooling in visual recognition. In: Proceedings of the 27th international conference on machine learning, Haifa, Israel, 2010.

43. Guo T, Dong J, Li H, Gao Y. Simple convolutional neural network on image classification. In: IEEE 2nd international conference on big data analysis, 2017, p. 721–724. https://doi.org/10.1109/ICBDA.2017.8078730.

44. Emmert-Streib F, Yang Z, Feng H, Tripathi S, Dehmer M. An introductory review of deep learning for prediction models with big data. Front Artif Intell. 2020;3:1–23. https://doi.org/10.3389/frai.2020.00004.

45. Vincent P, Larochelle H, Bengio Y, Manzagol P-A. Extracting and composing robust features with denoising autoencoders. In: Proceedings of the 25th international conference on machine learning, ACM, 2008, p. 1096–103.

46. Vincent P, Larochelle H, Lajoie I, Bengio Y, Manzagol PA. Stacked denoising autoencoders: learning useful representations in a deep network with a local denoising criterion. J Mach Learn Res. 2010;11:3371–408.

47. An J, Cho S. Variational autoencoder based anomaly detection using reconstruction probability. Spec Lect IE. 2015;2(1):1–18.

48. Bhushan C, Yang Z, Virani N, Iyer N. Variational encoder-based reliable classification. In: IEEE international conference on image process; 2020.

49. He K, Zhang X, Ren S, Sun J. Deep residual learning for image recognition. arXiv Prepr. arXiv1512.03385v1, 2015, p. 1–17. https://doi.org/10.1007/s11042-017-4440-4.

50. Goodfellow IJ, Pouget-Abadie J, Mirza M, Xu B, Warde-Farley D, Ozair S, Courville A, Bengio Y. Generative adversarial networks. arXiv Prepr. arXiv1406.2661v1, 2014, p. 1–9. https://doi.org/10.1001/jamainternmed.2016.8245.

51. Salakhutdinov R, Hinton G. Deep Boltzmann machines. J Mach Learn Res. 2009;5:448–55.

52. Lee J-G, Jun S, Cho Y-W, Lee H, Kim GB, Seo JB, Kim N. Deep learning in medical imaging: general overview. Korean J Radiol. 2017;18:570–84. https://doi.org/10.3348/kjr.2017.18.4.570.

53. Schlegl T, Seeböck P, Waldstein SM, Langs G, Schmidt-Erfurth U. F-AnoGAN: fast unsupervised anomaly detection with generative adversarial networks. Med Image Anal. 2019;54:30–44. https://doi.org/10.1016/j.media.2019.01.010.

54. Bermudez C, Plassard AJ, Davis LT, Newton AT, Resnick SM, Landman BA. Learning implicit brain MRI manifolds with deep learning. In: Proceedings of SPIE 10574, medical imaging 2018 image processing, vol. 56, 2018. https://doi.org/10.1117/12.2293515.

55. Küstner T, Liebgott A, Mauch L, Martirosian P, Bamberg F, Nikolaou K, Yang B, Schick F, Gatidis S. Automated reference-free detection of motion artifacts in magnetic resonance images. Magn Reson Mater Phys Biol Med. 2018;31:243–56. https://doi.org/10.1007/s10334-017-0650-z.

56. Dice LR. Measures of the amount of ecologic association between species. Ecology. 1945;26:297–302. https://doi.org/10.2307/1932409.

57. Sørensen TJ. A method of establishing groups of equal amplitude in plant sociology based on similarity of species and its application to analyses of the vegetation on Danish commons. Biol Skr. 1948;5:1–34.

58. Jaccard P. Distribution de la Flore Alpine dans le Bassin des Dranses et dans quelques régions voisines. Bull la Société vaudoise des Sci Nat. 1901;37:241–72. https://doi.org/10.5169/seals-266440.

59. Wang G, Li W, Ourselin S, Vercauteren T. Automatic brain tumor segmentation using cascaded anisotropic convolutional neural networks. In: Lecture notes in computer science (including subseries lecture notes in artificial intelligence. Lecture notes in bioinformatics) 10670 LNCS, 2018, p. 178–90. https://doi.org/10.1007/978-3-319-75238-9_16.

60. Zhou C, Ding C, Wang X, Lu Z, Tao D. One-pass multi-task networks with cross-task guided attention for brain tumor segmentation. IEEE Trans Image Process. 2020;29:4516–29. https://doi.org/10.1109/TIP.2020.2973510.

61. Menze BH, Jakab A, Bauer S, Kalpathy-Cramer J, Farahani K, Kirby J, Burren Y, Porz N, Slotboom J, Wiest R, Lanczi L, Gerstner E, Weber MA, Arbel T, Avants BB, Ayache N, Buendia P, Collins DL, Cordier N, Corso JJ, Criminisi A, Das T, Delingette H, Demiralp Ç, Durst CR, Dojat M, Doyle S, Festa J, Forbes F, Geremia E, Glocker B, Golland P, Guo X, Hamamci A, Iftekharuddin KM, Jena R, John NM, Konukoglu E, Lashkari D, Mariz JA, Meier R, Pereira S, Precup D, Price SJ, Raviv TR, Reza SMS, Ryan M, Sarikaya D, Schwartz L, Shin HC, Shotton J, Silva CA, Sousa N, Subbanna NK, Szekely G, Taylor TJ, Thomas OM, Tustison NJ, Unal G, Vasseur F, Wintermark M, Ye DH, Zhao L, Zhao B, Zikic D, Prastawa M, Reyes M, Van Leemput K. The multimodal brain tumor image segmentation benchmark (BRATS). IEEE Trans Med Imaging. 2015;34:1993–2024. https://doi.org/10.1109/TMI.2014.2377694.

62. Zhao X, Li L, Lu W, Tan S. Tumor co-segmentation in PET/CT using multi-tumor co-segmentation in PET/CT using multi-modality fully convolutional neural network. Phys Med Biol. 2019;64:015011, 15pp. https://doi.org/10.1088/1361-6560/aaf44b.

63. Balakrishnan G, Zhao A, Sabuncu MR, Dalca AV, Guttag J. An unsupervised learning model for deformable medical image registration. In: 2018 IEEE/CVF conference on computer vision on pattern recognition, 2018, p. 9252–60. https://doi.org/10.1109/CVPR.2018.00964.

64. de Vos BD, Berendsen FF, Viergever MA, Sokooti H, Staring M, Išgum I. A deep learning framework for unsupervised affine and deformable image registration. Med Image Anal. 2019;52:128–43. https://doi.org/10.1016/j.media.2018.11.010.

65. Shan S, Yan W, Guo X, Chang EI-C, Fan Y, Xu Y. Unsupervised end-to-end learning for deformable medical image registration. arXiv Prepr. arXiv 1711.08608v2, 2018, p. 1–12.

66. Emami H, Dong M, Nejad-Davarani SP, Glide-Hurst CK. Generating synthetic CTs from magnetic resonance images using generative adversarial networks. Med Phys. 2018;45:3627–36. https://doi.org/10.1002/mp.13047.

67. Jin CB, Kim H, Liu M, Jung W, Joo S, Park E, Ahn YS, Han IH, Lee JI, Cui X. Deep CT to MR synthesis using paired and unpaired data. Sensors (Switzerland). 2019;19:1–19. https://doi.org/10.3390/s19102361.

68. Pan Y, Liu M, Lian C, Zhou T, Xia Y, Shen D. Synthesizing missing PET from MRI with cycle-consistent generative adversarial networks for Alzheimer's disease diagnosis. In: Frangi A, Schnabel J, Davatzikos C, Alberola-López C, Fichtinger G, editors. Medical image computing and computer assisted intervention – MICCAI 2018. Lecture notes in computer science, vol. 11072, 2018, p. 595–602. https://doi.org/10.1007/978-3-030-00931-1_52.

69. Choi H, Lee DS. Generation of structural MR images from amyloid PET: application to MR-less quantification. J Nucl Med. 2018;59:1111–7. https://doi.org/10.2967/jnumed.117.199414.

70. Hiasa Y, Otake Y, Takao M, Matsuoka T, Takashima K, Carass A, Prince JL, Sugano N, Sato Y. Cross-modality image synthesis from unpaired data using CycleGAN. In: Simulation and synthesis in medical imaging, SASHIMI 2018. Lecture notes in computer science, vol. 11037 LNCS, 2018, p. 31–41. https://doi.org/10.1007/978-3-030-00536-8_4.

71. Chartsias A, Joyce T, Dharmakumar R, Tsaftaris SA. Adversarial image synthesis for unpaired multi-modal CardiacData. In: Simulation and synthesis in medical imaging, SASHIMI 2017. Lecture notes in computer science, vol. 10557 LNCS, 2017. https://doi.org/10.1007/978-3-319-68127-6_1.

72. Ben-Cohen A, Klang E, Raskin SP, Soffer S, Ben-Haim S, Konen E, Amitai MM, Greenspan H. Cross-modality synthesis from CT to PET using FCN and GAN networks for improved automated lesion detection. Eng Appl Artif Intell. 2019;78:186–94. https://doi.org/10.1016/j.engappai.2018.11.013.

73. Jiang J, Hu Y-C, Tyagi N, Zhang P, Rimner A, Mageras GS, Deasy JO, Veeraraghavan H. Tumor-

aware, adversarial domain adaptation from CT to MRI for lung cancer segmentation. In: Frangi A, Schnabel J, Davatzikos C, Alberola-López C, Fichtinger G, editors. Medical image computing and computer assisted intervention – MICCAI 2018. Lecture notes in computer science, vol. 11071 LNCS, 2018. https://doi.org/10.1007/978-3-030-00934-2_86.

74. Li T, Sahu AK, Talwalkar A, Smith V. Federated learning: challenges, methods, and future directions. IEEE Signal Process Mag. 2020;37:50–60. https://doi.org/10.1109/MSP.2020.2975749.

75. Yang Q, Liu Y, Chen T, Tong Y. Federated machine learning: concept and applications. ACM Trans Intell Syst Technol. 2019;10:1–19. https://doi.org/10.1145/3298981.

76. Gentry C, Boneh D. A fully homomorphic encryption scheme. Ph.D. Diss., Stanford University, 2009. https://doi.org/10.5555/18349540.

77. Cheng K, Fan T, Jin Y, Liu Y, Chen T, Yang Q. SecureBoost: a lossless federated learning framework. arXiv Prepr. arXiv 1901.08755v1; 2019.

78. Kairouz P, McMahan HB, Avent B, Bellet A, Bennis M, Bhagoji AN, Bonawitz K, Charles Z, Cormode G, Cummings R, D'Oliveira RGL, El Rouayheb S, Evans D, Gardner J, Garrett Z, Gascón A, Ghazi B, Gibbons PB, Gruteser M, Harchaoui Z, He C, He L, Huo Z, Hutchinson B, Hsu J, Jaggi M, Javidi T, Joshi G, Khodak M, Konečný J, Korolova A, Koushanfar F, Koyejo S, Lepoint T, Liu Y, Mittal P, Mohri M, Nock R, Özgür A, Pagh R, Raykova M, Qi H, Ramage D, Raskar R, Song D, Song W, Stich SU, Sun Z, Suresh AT, Tramèr F, Vepakomma P, Wang J, Xiong L, Xu Z, Yang Q, Yu FX, Yu H, Zhao S. Advances and open problems in federated learning. arXiv Prepr. arXiv 1912.04977v1, 2019, p. 1–105.

79. Xu G, Li H, Liu S, Yang K, Lin X. VerifyNet: secure and verifiable federated learning. IEEE Trans Inf Forensics Secur. 2020;15:911–26. https://doi.org/10.1109/TIFS.2019.2929409.

Part II

Clinical Applications

Imaging Biomarkers and Their Meaning for Molecular Imaging

6

Angel Alberich-Bayarri, Ana Jiménez-Pastor, and Irene Mayorga-Ruiz

Contents

6.1   Introduction

The famous quote from Lord Kelvin "When you can measure what you are speaking about, and express it in numbers, you know something about it, when you cannot express it in numbers, your knowledge is of a meager and unsatisfactory kind; it may be the beginning of knowledge, but you have scarely, in your thoughts advanced to the stage of science" is a really inspiring statement for the explanation of the imaging biomarker concept. Imaging biomarkers can be defined as characteristics extracted from the images of an individual that can be objectively measured and act as indicators of a normal biological process, a disease, or a response to a therapeutic intervention. Biomarkers have been shown to be useful as a complement to the traditional radiological diagnosis to detect a specific disorder or lesion, quantify its biological situation, evaluate its progression, stratify phenotypic abnormalities, and assess the treatment response [1–6].

Despite the evolution of image processing platforms and image quantification solutions to cover unmet clinical needs, their application in daily practice is still work in progress in many aspects. In the field of radiology, a wide variety of algorithms for neuroimaging to be applied to magnetic resonance imaging (MRI) have been developed as well as other solutions for computerized tomography (CT), some of them based on artificial intelligence pipelines, such as lung nodule detection and characterization. Although not being an absolute but a relative quantification, in molecular imaging, the concept of imaging biomarker has been present since the use of standardized uptake value (SUV). Furthermore, workstations and other solutions have been mainly addressed to provide quantitative analysis tools in a patient-specific basis, but not to store

A. Alberich-Bayarri (✉) · A. Jiménez-Pastor
I. Mayorga-Ruiz
Quantitative Imaging Biomarkers in Medicine,
Quibim SL, Valencia, Spain
e-mail: angel@quibim.com

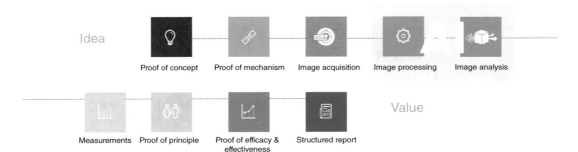

Fig. 6.1 Stepwise development of imaging biomarkers to convert a clinical idea into value for clinical practice. The AI section refers to the components that can be improved with the use of convolutional neural networks (CNN), image processing, and image analysis steps

quantitative data in databases for the posterior data mining and scientific research in imaging biomarkers. As an example, although the technology is already there [1], today pipelines, like automatically detect the lesions in lymphoma, extract their SUV values as well as their metabolic tumor volume (MTV) and store in a structured report in the PACS are still not available.

In this chapter, we introduce the concept of imaging biomarker and explain the main characteristics of the development process and validation to finally detail how the process can be applied in hybrid modalities where it is highly relevant to combine the spatial information with the functional one.

6.2 Imaging Biomarkers, Paradigm Shift in Medical Imaging

Imaging biomarkers allow to measure subtle tissue changes, either at a structural or at a function level [7]. They are the main enabler of quantitative imaging and the key for the paradigm shift in medical imaging. They can be classified in different types depending on their main application across different clinical scenarios. Imaging biomarkers can be used to extract patient phenotypes, either independently or together with other clinical or genomic variables. The main applications of imaging biomarkers are:

- Detection imaging biomarkers: use as a tool to find high levels of a specific measure in a tissue or organ that can indicate the presence of a disease.
- Diagnostic imaging biomarkers: use as a tool for the identification of the specific disease suffered by the patient.
- Staging imaging biomarkers: use as a tool for grading of the disease severity or extent.
- Predictive/prognostic imaging biomarkers: use as a tool to forecast the progression of the disease and its potential relapse.
- Follow-up imaging biomarkers: use as a tool for monitoring treatment response and disease progression in the patient.

The most supported process for the development of imaging biomarkers, converting a clinical idea or need into clinical value is described in [2] and also proposed in [4], which is divided into different steps (Fig. 6.1).

The first step is the proof of concept, which is usually a small test to solve an unmet clinical need of a specific pathology that can be evaluated with current image acquisition modalities and image processing techniques. The proof of mechanism establishes a link (in magnitude and direction) between the parameter under study and the existence, staging, and evolution of the disease. Thereafter, a design on the most appropriate image acquisition protocol to ensure appropriate image quality is performed; the images needed to extract the biomarker must be technically adequate (signal-to-noise ratio, spatial resolution, contrast-to-noise ratio, uniformity, among others). The following preprocessing step aims to improve the image quality before the analysis (with techniques such as filtering, interpolation, registration, movement correction, and segmentation). Segmentation is one of the processes that has been significantly improved with the use of artificial intelligence approaches such as the application of convolutional neural networks (CNN). The development of network architectures such as U-Net has permitted the segmentation of organs and structures clearly outperforming traditional computer vision algorithms [8]. The analysis and modeling of the signal is the process by which the quantitative or objective information is extracted from the images. This information can represent structural or functional properties of the tissue. Those imaging biomarkers that can be calculated voxel-wise allow for the representation of the spatial distribution in parametric maps, defined as derived images (secondary) in which the value of a specific parameter is placed as the pixel value. In general, imaging biomarkers have specific measurement units; however, due to the nature of the calculation process, some parameters may be measured in arbitrary units (a.u.). This is the case of radiomics features or parameters such as the fractal dimension. An additional layer of multivariate post-processing applied to the imaging biomarkers allows for the combination of the most relevant features into indicators representing disease status that can be plotted in new parametric images called nosological maps. Measurements of imaging biomarkers in specific lesions or tissues must be optimized to the physiological phenomena under study. A clear example is the conventional approach in the measurements of SUV, consisting of the extraction of the maximum value (SUV_{max}) of the region (instead of average, median, or other histogram descriptors). Automation and AI can allow for the seamless extraction of a wide variety of measurements for a specific imaging biomarker beyond the conventional ones. An exploratory example in molecular imaging that is

demonstrating an important evidence with the outcome in lymphoma patients consists of the extraction of metabolic heterogeneity from lesions, beyond the maximum values of SUV, that is, the current standard of care [9]. Finally, after the technical process for the extraction and measurement of the imaging biomarker is clear, a pilot test in the way of a Proof of Principle must be performed in a controlled cohort of subjects to evaluate potential biases related to sex, age, or others. This also serves as a preliminary validation of the method. Comprehensive proofs of efficacy and effectiveness on external, larger, and well-characterized series of subjects will show the ability of a biomarker to really measure (even if it is in a surrogate manner) the clinical endpoint.

6.3 Imaging Biomarkers in Hybrid Molecular Imaging

The imaging biomarkers that can be extracted in molecular imaging are related to the imaging modalities used in the examination. Generally speaking, the imaging biomarkers that can be extracted from the molecular imaging components of the modality (see Table 6.1, considering only those ones based on PET) are the standardized uptake value (SUV), related to the metabolic activity, the metabolic tumor volume (MTV), which is related to the size of the metabolic region within the lesion, the total lesion glycolysis (TLG), derived from the multiplication of the MTV by the average metabolic activity, the delta-, which calculates the difference in a given imaging biomarker between two specific timepoints in the longitudinal course of the disease. Finally, lesion heterogeneity can be characterized both in the anatomical-structural component of the modality, that is, the CT or the MR images, and in the PET component. For the structural or metabolic heterogeneity estimation of lesion, different textural (radiomics) features can be extracted by the use of standard first-order histogram analysis or more advanced second-order techniques: gray level co-occurrence matrix (GLCLM),   gray   level   run-length   matrix

Table 6.1 Most relevant imaging biomarkers in molecular imaging, objective of their quantification and specific units

Objective	Modality	Imaging biomarker	Units
Metabolic activity	PET/CT & PET/MR	Standardized uptake value (SUV)	a.u.
Tumoral burden	PET/CT & PET/MR	Metabolic tumor volume (MTV)	mL
Tumoral burden + metabolic activity	PET/CT & PET/MR	Total lesion glycolysis (TLG)	g
Change in metabolic activity	PET/CT & PET/MR	Delta-SUV (ΔSUV), averaged or voxel-wise	a.u.
Lesion heterogeneity	CT, MR, PET/CT, & PET/MR	Textures—radiomics	a.u.

(GLRLM), gray level size zone matrix (GLSZM), gray level dependence matrix (GLDM), neighboring gray tone difference matrix (NGTDM), among others. In total, thousands of descriptors can be obtained, expressing the heterogeneity of a single lesion. Furthermore, these features can be obtained from either a 2D or 3D analysis.

References

1. Martí Bonmatí L, Alberich-Bayarri A, García-Martí G, Sanz Requena R, Pérez Castillo C, Carot Sierra JM, Manjón Herrera JV. Biomarcadores de imagen, imagen cuantitativa y bioingeniería [Imaging biomarkers, quantitative imaging, and bioengineering]. Radiologia. 2012;54(3):269–78. https://doi.org/10.1016/j.rx.2010.12.013. Spanish. Epub 2011 Jul 5. PMID: 21733539.
2. Alberich-Bayarri Á, Hernández-Navarro R, Ruiz-Martínez E, García-Castro F, García-Juan D, Martí-Bonmatí L. Development of imaging biomarkers and generation of big data. Radiol Med. 2017;122(6):444–8. https://doi.org/10.1007/s11547-017-0742-x. Epub 2017 Feb 21. PMID: 28224398.
3. Biomarkers Definitions Working Group. Biomarkers and surrogate endpoints: preferred definitions and conceptual framework. Clin Pharmacol Ther. 2001;69:89–95.
4. European Society of Radiology (ESR). ESR statement on the stepwise development of imaging biomarkers. Insights Imaging. 2013;4:147–52.
5. European Society of Radiology. White paper on imaging biomarkers. Insights Imaging. 2010;1:42–5.
6. Martí-Bonmatí L. Introduction to the stepwise development of imaging biomarkers. In: Marti-Bonmatí L, Alberich-Bayarri A, editors. Imaging biomarkers, development and clinical integration. Cham: Springer; 2017. p. 9–27. ISBN 978-3-319-43504-6.
7. Alberich-Bayarri A, Neri E, Marti-Bonmatí L. Imaging biomarkers and imaging biobanks. In: Ranschaert E, Morozov S, Algra PR, editors. Artificial intelligence in medical imaging: opportunities, applications and risks. Cham: Springer; 2019. p. 119–26. ISBN 978-3-319-94877-5.
8. Ronneberger O, Fischer P, Brox T. U-Net: convolutional networks for biomedical image segmentation, MICCAI, LNCS, vol. 9351. Cham: Springer; 2015. p. 234–41. Available at arXiv:1505.04597.
9. Ceriani L, Milan L, Martelli M, Ferreri AJM, Cascione L, Zinzani PL, Di Rocco A, Conconi A, Stathis A, Cavalli F, Bellei M, Cozens K, Porro E, Giovanella L, Johnson PW, Zucca E. Metabolic heterogeneity on baseline 18FDG-PET/CT scan is a predictor of outcome in primary mediastinal B-cell lymphoma. Blood. 2018;132(2):179–86. https://doi.org/10.1182/blood-2018-01-826958. Epub 2018 May 2. PMID: 29720487.

Integration of Artificial Intelligence, Machine Learning, and Deep Learning into Clinically Routine Molecular Imaging

7

Geoffrey Currie and Eric Rohren

Contents

7.1 Introduction

Assimilation of AI into clinical practice heralds an exciting era with the reimagining of precision nuclear medicine and molecular imaging capabilities. AI has a long history in nuclear medicine and molecular imaging, although perhaps not using that language. Consider the use of automated region of interest production for generation of circumferential profiles and risk scores associated with 201-Thallium chloride planar myocardial perfusion scans or the auto contouring and production of functional parameters and phase/paradox images for gated blood pool scans. This rudimentary form of AI using expert systems or knowledge graphs might also be obvious in bone mineral density contouring, regions and fracture risk scoring. The emergence of quantitative software and polar maps for single photon emission computed tomography (SPECT) myocardial perfusions studies is a more advanced example of AI via expert systems. There are early examples of ML in nuclear medicine also. ML involves learning from large amounts of data that

G. Currie (✉) · E. Rohren
School of Dentistry and Medical Sciences, Charles Sturt University, Wagga Wagga, NSW, Australia

Baylor College of Medicine, Houston, TX, USA
e-mail: gcurrie@csu.edu.au

perform a task without explicit instruction; the artificial neural network (ANN) being the main platform to do so. An early example was the application of a 15 node ANN in 1993 evaluating 28 input features in ventilation perfusion lung scans against experienced physicians [1]. In molecular imaging, feature extraction, and radiomic feature extraction can be integrated into ML and DL algorithms based on big data to enhance precision nuclear medicine but this requires clinically validated models (Fig. 7.1). In visual or image-based DL, the convolutional neural network (CNN) is designed for and tasked with four basic operations: classification/object recognition, classification/localization, object detection, and instance segmentation (Fig. 7.2).

The role of AI in the general community, medicine broadly, and specifically in molecular imaging sparks considerable debate. Anecdotally, molecular imaging folk sit in one of several AI camps. There are those that believe AI will displace human resources producing professional anarchy (dystopians) in contrast to those that think AI will improve our ability to perform our jobs, improve outcomes and free up time from menial tasks to provide better patient care (utopians). There are also optimists who think AI is exciting and may emerge to improve our systems (poised to be fast followers), pessimists who think AI is hype or a hoax designed to raise revenue (skeptics), and realists thinking AI is a crucial part of the landscape but also understand not everyone will be expert. In lower numbers there are also a few conspiracy theorists claiming AI is just another tool being used by the government to spy on or control us, those who worry about the emergence of AI and doubt their ability to assimilate into an AI augmented world (metathesiophobics), and those that fear relinquishing control if AI diverts some perceived power, control, or attention from those performing amazing things without AI to those breaking new ground with AI (narcissists).

Much of the disconnection comes from a lack of understanding. AI is part of molecular imaging now and will be a growing part tomorrow. Individuals need to upskill, not so they can

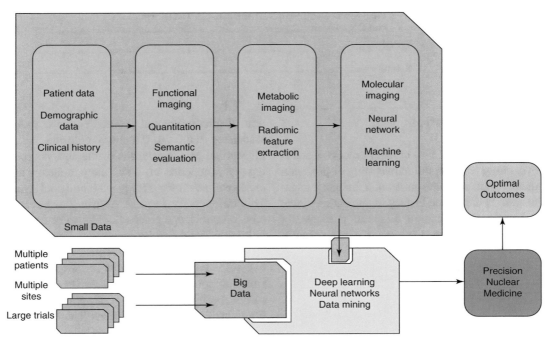

Fig. 7.1 Schematic representation of the semantic evaluation of imaging data, addition of radiomic feature extraction and ANN analysis to produce small data and the potential to integrate with big data to enhance outcomes and drive precision nuclear medicine. (Reprinted with permission [2])

Classification and Object Recognition	Classification and Localization	Object Detection	Instance Segmentation

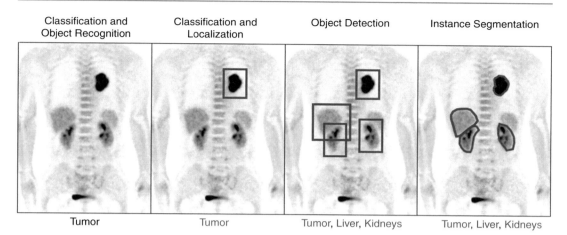

Tumor	Tumor	Tumor, Liver, Kidneys	Tumor, Liver, Kidneys

Fig. 7.2 Schematic representation of the difference between image recognition tasks in DL

conduct ML or DL research projects, but so they can implement developments and devise strategy for clinical AI in an informed position. Careful consideration needs to be given to how AI will assimilate into mainstream clinical practice. Advanced planning needs invested stakeholders who have ownership in the plan and technology. AI may see emergence of new roles, recrafting of some responsibilities and, potentially, role redundancy. Organizational change management is critical to manage these possibilities. This implementation needs to be done within an ethical and legal framework [3]. At the same time, improving the language used in this space may decrease misunderstanding and associated antagonism. Recognizing AI is not new to nuclear medicine, being precise about using ML or DL instead of AI when appropriate, diverging from generalized use of term like AI in preference for greater precise and more meaningful terms when appropriate like "engineered learning" or "intelligent imaging", and recognizing that AI is neither artificial nor intelligent.

7.2   Classification

Classification is an interesting problem to solve in molecular imaging. Suppose we have a simple situation where there are two features of interest. These are depicted in Fig. 7.3. For simplicity, the data is represented in a two-dimensional plot but obviously in molecular imaging the data is significantly more dense and may be in four dimensions (three-dimensional space and time). Clear boundaries between data distribution is not always obvious. Support vector machines use vectors (purple arrows) to determine the line that best separates the known classifications. Consider this data the training set (blue and green circles) with grounded truth labels. If we introduced a new unclassified data point (yellow dot), then we classify it as a blue dot because it lies below the line. This approach may not work as well if the boundaries between classifications are not as obvious or linear; including linear regression approaches. Another approach is the K-nearest-neighbors where the K represents the number of nearest neighbors considered in the classification. As shown in Fig. 7.4, the purple circles are centered on the new unclassified data point. Using $K = 1$, the single nearest neighbor would see the new data point classified as blue. Using a $K = 9$, more data points are considered, random chance is averaged, and now the yellow dot would be classified as green (6 green and 3 blue in the purple nearest neighbor circle). Clustering methods adopt an iterative approach that begins with random assignment of class to data points and determining the geometric center of each cluster. The second iteration applies a new classification based on position relative to the geometric center of the first iteration clusters, and uses the new points to

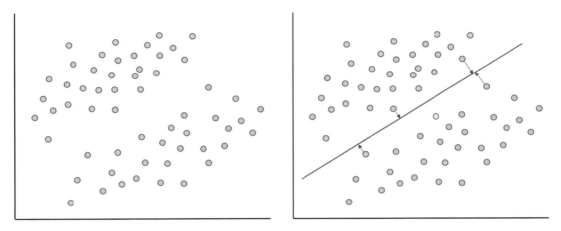

Fig. 7.3 Schematic representation of linear approaches to classification with the purple arrows representing the vector for separation and the new data point (yellow) being classified based on which side of the fit line it is located

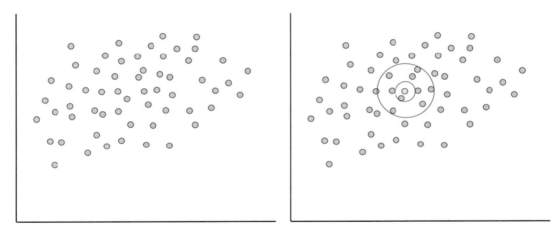

Fig. 7.4 Schematic representation of nearest neighbor approaches to classification with the purple circles representing the number of neighbors included in the calculation for the new data point (yellow)

adjust the geometric centers of clusters. This iterative process continues until the geometric centers of the clusters no longer change. New data points are then classified based on proximity to the final geometric centers of clusters. The artificial neural network approach is a nonlinear solution based on changes to weights on individual perceptrons to optimize the correct answers (Fig. 7.5). The training data defines the nonlinear demarcation between classifications which also highlights the value of larger training sets in providing more accurate classification differentiators (Fig. 7.6). The inferential phase would see new data points assigned classifications based on this.

7.3 Segmentation

Image segmentation is not a new application in molecular imaging. Segmentation is a method for partitioning one or more parts of an image from the other parts. We do this to simplify the image or to enhance the representation of parts of the image of most interest. During reconstruction of myocardial perfusion SPECT or brain SPECT images, for example, the boundaries of the area of interest are set and information outside that window are truncated out of the image. On a bone scan a region may be drawn (manually or automatically) around the bladder

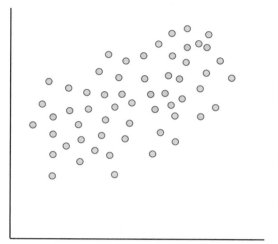

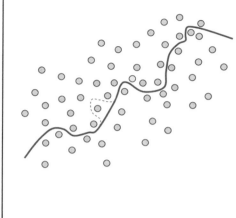

Fig. 7.5 Schematic representation of nonlinear approaches to classification using neural analysis for separation and the new data point (yellow) being classified based on which side of the fit line it is located. The red dashed line represents the position of the fit line with over fitting

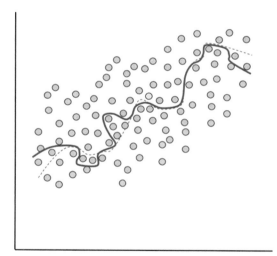

Fig. 7.6 Schematic representation of nonlinear approaches to classification using neural analysis for separation and the new data point (yellow) being classified based on which side of the fit line it is located. The red dashed line represents line determined in Fig. 7.4 while the solid red line is the position of the fit line with the addition of more data points

to suppress the contribution of bladder counts to the image. Adjusting the windowing on a computed tomography (CT) image from soft tissue to bone provides a means for segmenting parts of the image of interest. From a computing perspective, true segmentation is identifying every pixel in the image in a manner that all pixels segmented together have the same label identifying that pixel. In nuclear medicine, CT and magnetic resonance imaging (MRI), segmentation can be used to enhance an object of interest in a complex scene. A very simple example of segmentation is the use of specific color scales for nuclear medicine images. The step 10 color palette for viewing SPECT reconstructions partitions every pixel in the image into one of ten labels, each corresponding to a specific color, and each sequentially representing 10% of the minimum to maximum count range. More complex examples of segmentation include the co-registration of positron emission tomography (PET) and CT images with a lesion of interest segmented from surrounding tissues both anatomically (CT) and physiologically (PET). In CNN and DL, segmentation is critical for identification and characterization of target tissues, and radiomic feature extraction. On CT for example, the volume, size, shape, and texture of a lung tumor will change as the constraints that define the segmentation vary. Similarly, the standardized uptake value (SUV) will change as the constraints of the lesion segmentation are altered. An important role of AI tools is to provide accurate and reproducible segmentation in an automated fashion.

There are many approaches to segmentation. Here several of the more common approaches encountered in molecular imaging segmentation are discussed. As already mentioned, thresholding is a very simple way to segment an image. This might be windowing or truncating the count scale (color scale) on nuclear medicine images or switching between windows (bone/soft tissue) on CT. This is referred to as region-based segmentation or threshold segmentation and uses the individual pixel values (numerical value that represents a color, count density, attenuation, or other value). Setting a specific threshold (or more than one threshold) allows segmentation of pixels based on their position relative to the threshold (above or below). Images that contain high contrast have differences between these values that can be exploited (Fig. 7.7). A global threshold is used to segment the image into two partitions; the object or structure of interest and background. Multiple local thresholds can be used to segment multiple objects of interest from background.

Edge detection segmentation is a convolutional process. The image is segmented based on the edge between different parts of the image. These partitions or edges may represent a change in contrast, count density, or color. Discontinuity within an image identifies an edge (e.g., edge of myocardium and ventricular lumen or a tumor compared to surrounding tissue). Using a filter or kernel that enhances the edges of data on hori-zontal planes (Fig. 7.8) combined with a similar kernel for the vertical plane allow contouring between objects.

Clustering methods are the same approach as outlined for classification. Clustering is an iterative approach that begins with random assignment of class to data points and determining the geometric center of each cluster. The second iteration applies a new classification based on position relative to the geometric center of the first iterations clusters, and uses the new points to adjust the geometric centers of clusters. This iterative process continues until the geometric centers of the clusters no longer changes. Data points are then classified based on proximity to the final geometric centers of clusters. Each cluster might be represented as a different gray scale or color, or some clusters may be eliminated from the image (Fig. 7.9).

The last approach discussed here is the DL approach referred to as Mask R-CNN or instance segmentation. It is not the only DL approach and is used commonly in social media (origins in Facebook). The R represents region signifying object detection. The mask aspect differentiates this approach from other R-CNNs by adding in parallel a convolution branch that employs a region of interest. In essence, a small convolutional network applied to each region of interest (Fig. 7.10). While threshold segmentation is fast and simple, there may be no significant boundary or, indeed, overlap between partitions. Edge

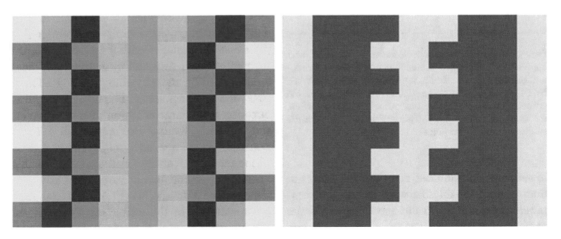

Fig. 7.7 Schematic representation of a threshold segmentation partitioning an image into regions above or below a predefined threshold

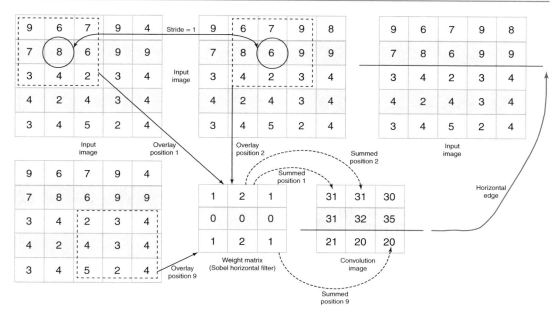

Fig. 7.8 Schematic representation of an edge detection segmentation partitioning an image into regions based on identifying the edges between objects within the image. The kernel is applied in a weighted fashion to each pixel to create the convolution image, in this case for the horizontal edge. (Reprinted with permission [4])

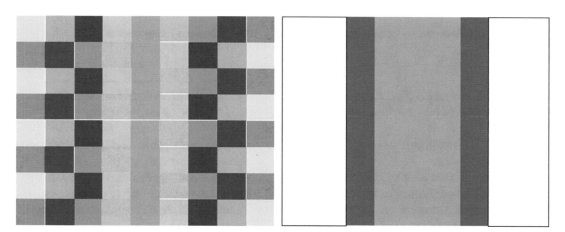

Fig. 7.9 Schematic representation of a cluster-based segmentation partitioning an image into regions based on *K*-means with clusters identified by color or eliminated from the image

detection segmentation is useful when there is good image contrast but is confounded by complex images containing numerous edges/partitions. Cluster-based segmentation is useful for small datasets but can be computationally demanding for larger data sets. Instance segmentation is simple and flexible but requires substantial and time-consuming neural network training.

7.4 Detection and Localization

An important area of computer vision algorithms and certainly in applications in nuclear medicine is object detection. CNNs and DL play an integral role in this capability. Clearly, segmentation is the underlying principle of detection and local-

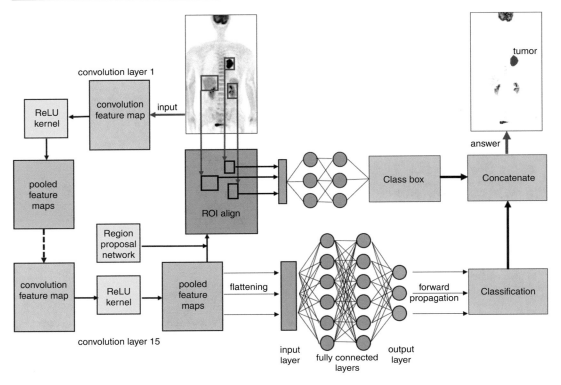

Fig. 7.10 Schematic representation of instance segmentation (red bounding boxes) using mask R-CNN

ization, and classification (Fig. 7.2). It is useful to simplify the process into the three major tasks:

- Image classification predicts the class of an object in an image.
- Object localization uses a bounding box and defined spatial parameters to locate an object.
- Object detection determines the presence of objects in an image and applies a class label.

Computer aided detection (CADe) is a system for detection of objects on medical images and consists of four main steps: segmentation of the region of interest, detection of the object of interest, analysis of object features, and classification against potential false positives (Fig. 7.11 excluding the green box). Computer aided diagnosis (CADx) is a system that extracts the image features and uses a classifier to predict what the object of interest is (Fig. 7.11).

7.5 Applications of ML and DL in Molecular Imaging

The research applications of AI, ML, and DL in molecular imaging are growing quickly. The opportunities and applications can be divided into several broad categories; potential clinical applications and physics applications. Physics and instrumentation applications include attenuation correction from pseudo-CT [5–9], scatter correction [10], motion correction, image reconstruction [11–13], co-registration, low dose imaging [14–17], noise reduction [18], and radiation dosimetry [19, 20]. Much of the recent clinical literature relates to CNNs and DL offering potential solutions in automated disease detection [21], classification [22, 23], triage, segmentation [24], guide therapy [25], and assisted diagnosis [26]. It is important to recognize that AI and ML also have significant benefits to clini-

Fig. 7.11 Flow diagram of the process for detection and localization on medical images. The entire process represents CADx while truncation before the final step are the limits of CADe

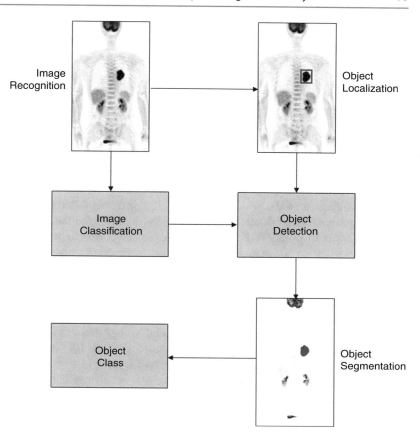

cal practice without the use of CNN and DL. At a rudimentary level, an ANN can be used in parallel to conventional statistical approaches to glean deeper insights into features or combinations of features that provide the greatest predictive power [27, 28]. Despite the breadth of AI, ML, and DL applications published in the literature, there are few that have transitioned to general implementation in clinical practice. This, in part, relates to the regulatory framework for software as a medical device (SaMD). Among the US FDA approved SaMDs are the following molecular imaging-related AI applications or AI platforms:

- Aidoc BriefCase-PE is a CNN algorithm for analysis of CTPA to triage based on the probability of pulmonary embolism with reported sensitivity of 91% and specificity of 90%.
- AI-Rad Companion-Cardiovascular is a CNN algorithm for segmentation and coronary calcium scoring of the heart.

- cNeuro cMRI is a CNN algorithm for annotation, segmentation, and quantitation of neurological MRI.
- Arterys Cardio DL is an AI platform for post-processing analysis and quantitation of cardiac MRI.
- HealthCCS is an AI algorithm for calculating cardiac risk based on coronary artery plaque calcification on CT.
- IB Neuro is an AI algorithm for post-processing image registration of serial brain MRI with generation of parametric perfusion maps.
- Icobrain is an AI pipeline for annotation, segmentation, and quantitation of serial brain MRI.
- NeuroQuant is an AI platform for annotation, segmentation, and quantitation of brain MRI.
- Quantib Brain provides an AI driven platform for MRI segmentation, quantitation, and classification.

- SubtlePET is image processing software for data management and noise reduction for PET scans.

Among the emerging AI applications in molecular imaging, those associated with auto-contouring and segmentation, radiomic feature extraction, triage and second reporters, attenuation correction, reconstruction, dose reduction and radiation dosimetry are perhaps the most important and most likely to transition to more widespread clinical utility.

An important area of development for molecular imaging is in pseudo-CT attenuation maps (Fig. 7.12) that could reduce radiation dose. There are a number of limitations in estimating an attenuation map from MRI for SPECT/MRI or PET/MRI hybrid systems. CNNs may overcome the limitations of maximum likelihood reconstruction of activity and attenuation (MLAA) and provide accurate attenuation maps without transmission studies. Hwang et al. [5] evaluated deep CNNs to produce an attenuation map that closely modeled the CT-based grounded truth and this

was supported in PET/MRI using a deep neural network work [6]. Torrado-Carvajal et al. [7] integrated the Dixon method with a CNN to generate pseudo-CT for pelvic PET/MRI scans with less than 2% variation from the CT map. A deep CNN combined with zero-echo-time Dixon pseudo-CT was also used to produce more accurate attenuation maps than traditional MRI pseudo-CT methods [8]. DL approaches can produce pseudo-CT attenuation maps from the sinogram of 18F FDG brain PET with less than 1% error reported over CT [9].

Despite the advances associated with iterative reconstruction algorithms, CNN/DL-based reconstruction approaches have been a number of positive reports in the literature. Zhu et al. [11] employed a deep neural network to produce reconstructed data direct from the sinogram of brain MRI and PET data with less noise and artefact. Haggstrom et al. [12] used a DL encoder-decoder CNN on PET data (Fig. 7.13) to reconstruct higher quality images compared to iterative and backprojection methods. The root mean square error was 11% lower than for ordered subset expectation

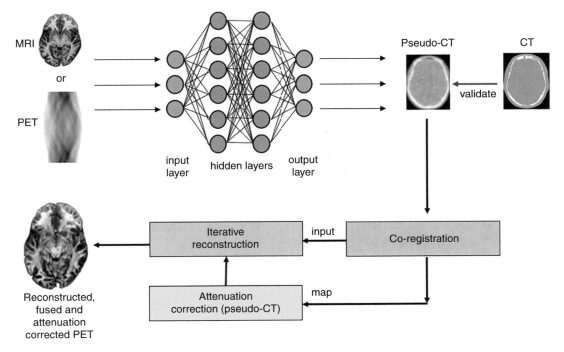

Fig. 7.12 Model for potentially using CNN for improved pseudo-CT attenuation correction in PET/MRI. (Adapted and reprinted with permission [4])

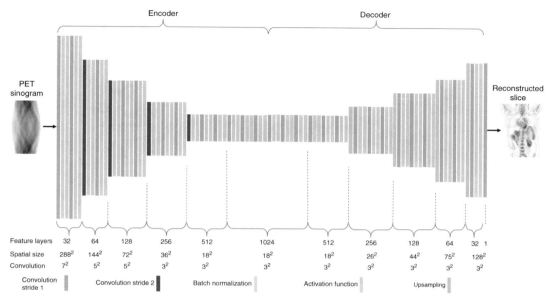

Encoder						Decoder				

PET sinogram → Reconstructed slice

Feature layers	32	64	128	256	512	1024	512	256	128	64	32 1
Spatial size	288^2	144^2	72^2	36^2	18^2	18^2	18^2	26^2	44^2	75^2	128^2
Convolution	7^2	5^2	5^2	3^2	3^2	3^2	3^2	3^2	3^2	3^2	3^2

Convolution stride 1 | Convolution stride 2 | Batch normalization | Activation function | Upsampling

Fig. 7.13 Schematic representation of the DeepPET convolutional encoder-decoder network

maximization (OSEM) and 53% lower than filtered backprojection (FBP). The DL approach also produced better structural similarity index and signal-to-noise ratio. Jiao et al. [13] adopted a CNN approach using the back-projection image of the sinogram data as the input tensor to reconstruct 18F choline and 18F florbetapir brain PET images with faster processing times. There remains much work to be done in this space.

An important consideration in medical imaging and for nuclear medicine specifically is dose reduction. A number of dose reduction strategies have been employed to maintain image quality and diagnostic integrity but with low doses administered to patients. This addresses not only the issues of radiation dose and safety but also the sustainable use of scarce and expensive resources. With the emergence of hybrid imaging technology, dose reduction where feasible is critical. A number of advances have facilitated dose reduction including more sensitive detector systems and improved reconstruction algorithms. CNNs and DL may also play a role in dose reduction and this is an important domain for DL focus. Indeed, there are two concepts to consider; dose reduction to minimize the dose without compromising the quality of imaging, and dose optimi-

zation focused on calculating the ideal dose for diagnostic or therapeutic outcomes. Xu et al. [14] adopted a similar coder-decoder architecture described in Fig. 7.14 except the inputs are multiple low count PET slices. They reported superior image quality for reconstructing ultra-low dose PET through the encoder-decoder CNN than standard dose using conventional reconstruction techniques. Similar approaches have been reported by several authors using T1 weighted MRI. Kaplan and Zhu [15] used a CNN to reduce the noise associated with low dose PET scans and reported a final result of comparable performance metrics to the grounded truth (full dose scan). Ouyang et al. [16] used an encoder-decoder generative adversarial network (GAN) in amyloid brain PET to train low dose (1%) scans down-sampled from list mode data against the 100% reconstruction as grounded truth. Outside the brain, Lei et al. [17] employed a cycle-consistent GAN to estimate whole-body PET images from low count data following inverse transformation. The method improved the mean error and normalized means square error from 5.6% and 3.5% to −0.1% and 0.5% respectively.

Excluding low dose PET and SPECT scans, molecular images are generally noisy. CNN and

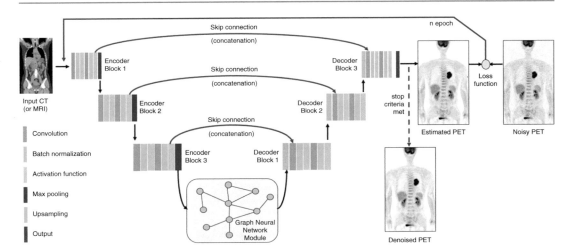

Fig. 7.14 Schematic representation of the encoder-decoder GNN in the U-net architecture used with CT or MRI to denoise PET images

DL can be used to reduce the noise in nuclear medicine images. One approach is to use an encoder-decoder architecture with a built-in graph neural network (GNN) module (Fig. 7.14). A CT or MRI can be used as an input and an iterative process undertaken comparing the loss function after each epoch until stop criteria are satisfied. Cui et al. [18] employed a process similar to this using CT or MRI to reduce noise on PET scans. The contrast-to-noise ratio (CNR) was superior to other methods (iterative reconstruction, Gaussian filtering) of noise reduction.

CNN and DL are used in radiation therapy for auto-contouring, auto-planning and decision support to optimize treatment outcomes and better manage radiation dosimetry. It makes sense that radionuclide therapy and theranostics adopt CNN/DL approaches to optimize patient dose and dosimetry to target tissues versus non-target tissues. An area of particular interest in radiation dosimetry is associated with 177Lu-lutate and 177Lu-PSMA therapy. Post therapy, 177Lu allows gamma imaging for whole-body distribution and dosimetry calculations. This data can be subsequently used to measure tumor burden during therapy, dose burden to non-target tissues and also optimization of subsequent rounds of radionuclide therapy. A trained CNN could not only automate dosimetry calculations but could reduce the error for individual tissues calculations com-

pared to the population-based estimations. Indeed, there is potential to train a CNN against the original 68Ga PET scan, the serial 177Lu gamma distributions to provide dosimetry estimates first by the 68Ga PET (allowing immediate optimization of the therapy dose), and then corrected based on the first 177Lu gamma image. This field is not advancing very fast because the first step is to develop rigorous CNN approaches for multiple lesion detection and segmentation. Zhao et al. [19] developed a U-net based deep CNN for automatic characterization of lesions on 68Ga PSMA PET/CT and calculate tumor burden with the intention of further developing the algorithm for optimizing radionuclide therapy. Precision was reported to be 99% in bone lesions and 94% in lymph nodes but segmentation accuracy was lower than detection. Jackson et al. [20] trained a CNN to automatically contour for kidney regions for radiation dose estimation in radionuclide therapy with 177Lu PSMA. While no differences were seen in the dosimetry estimations associated with manual versus CNN regions, automation improves the time cost. Nonetheless, the study also revealed some confounding for the CNN based on anatomical or pathological anomalies of the renal system (e.g., polycystic kidneys). With developments focused on foundations, Fig. 7.15 provides a schematic of processes that may be on the horizon.

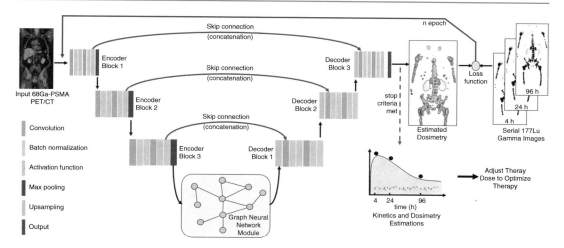

Fig. 7.15 Schematic representation of an encoder-decoder GNN in the U-net architecture that could be used to develop dosimetry-based optimization of therapy doses of 177Lu based on the 68Ga PET/CT. (PSMA images courtesy of [29])

With respect to clinical applications, an ANN was trained against six expert nuclear cardiologists to provide superior 17 segment defect scoring in myocardial perfusion scans [21]. In a multicenter trial [22] using a deep CNN produced a statistically significant improvement over total perfusion defect scores. The report provided an insight into how AI outcomes could be integrated into conventional image display using a polar map display (Fig. 7.16). ML has also been used to predict major cardiac events (MACE) on myocardial perfusion SPECT with superiority over expert readers and automated quantitative software [23].

Unsupervised DL was used on 18F-FDG PET to differentiate Alzheimer's disease and was able to identify abnormal patterns in 60% of studies classified as normal by expert visualization [26]. DL has also been successfully used to identify nasopharyngeal carcinoma patients most likely to benefit from induction chemotherapy on PET/CT [25]. DL on quantitative SPECT/CT has provided automated volume of interest segmentation on CT that can then be applied to the SPECT data for calculation of glomeruli filtration rate [24]. There is a diverse array of emerging DL and CNN based literature in clinical molecular imaging including radiomic feature extraction and segmentation on PET or PET/CT in a variety of tumors (e.g., lung, head/neck), brain studies (e.g.,

Parkinson's, beta amyloid, and 18F-FDG Alzheimer's), myocardial perfusion studies (SPECT and PET), and the thyroid. There is a very diverse array of clinical applications of DL producing a rapidly growing body of literature.

7.6 Internal Department Applications

There are also opportunities for data rich departments to train an ANN or CNN for a specific internal purpose [30, 31]. This could produce internally valid algorithms that can reliably perform the prescribed task to enhance internal processes. Clearly, commercialization of these algorithms would require navigation of regulatory frameworks associated with data sharing, privacy and security yet the major barrier would be local bias in the data [3]. There may also be specific parameter or equipment biases in the algorithm unique to the developing department that do not hold when parameters or equipment change. Changing the acquisition or reconstruction parameters is also likely to produce variations in performance of the trained algorithm. Over and above these technical specifics, there is likely to be a local population bias that threatens external validity of a trained algorithm.

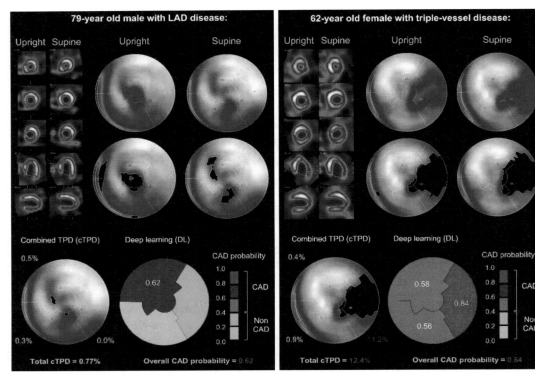

Fig. 7.16 Prediction of CAD with integration of DL outputs into polar maps provides an insight into how AI outcomes will be integrated into radiomic outputs. (Reprinted with permission [23])

In addition to the site-specific characteristics that may act as barriers to the expansion of an internally developed AI process to more general usage, there are operational and logistical challenges that must be considered, as well. First, the electronic ecosystems in which medical data resides is widely varied across institutions. In part this is reflective of the variety of information technology (IT) solutions available in the marketplace, but even in cases in which the same vendor solution is deployed, there are often site-specific customizations and modifications that may make direct translation of algorithms and processes a challenge. These same issues present challenges to the commercialization of AI technology, since the ideal commercial product should be vendor agnostic both with regards to scanner technology (input) as well as IT infrastructure (processing and output). This provides an insight into the discrepancy between the enormous potential applications of ML and DL in molecular imaging, and the actual number of commercially available algorithms approved by the US FDA. Thus, there is an opportunity for departments to develop internal AI tools that enhance outcomes and performance.

To illustrate the thinking and process, consider simple theoretical applications and projects with particular consideration to how the ML or DL could be integrated into existing graphical outputs as highlighted by Figure 7.16. The addition of CNN risk stratification to pre-existing commercial software for quantitation, radiomic feature extraction and display offers an intuitive and seamless approach. Consider a CNN risk score for pulmonary embolism summarized and displayed in a simple format (Fig. 7.17). This could offer perfusion SPECT segmentation against the accompanying low-dose CT to predict pulmonary embolism (Fig. 7.18). A similar

Fig. 7.17 Mock summary output for a CNN-based risk algorithm for pulmonary embolism using ventilation and perfusion mismatch. (Reprinted with permission [32])

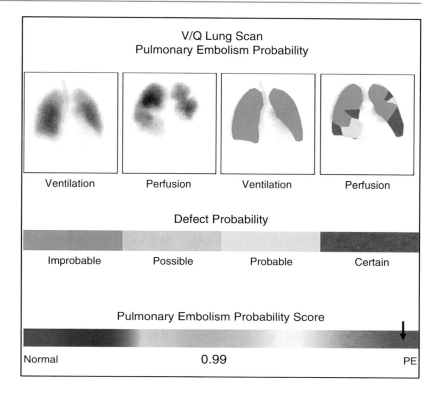

approach to segmentation, risk scoring of individual lesions and mapping total disease burden might be helpful for patients presenting for evaluation of metastatic spread to bone (Fig. 7.19). While these mock-examples provoke ideas of what is potentially possible, the value is immediately transparent. The emergence, for example, of parametric images in PET offers a perfect opportunity to incorporate AI driven outputs into image display.

7.7   A Glance at Tomorrow

AI, ML, and DL today provide opportunity to improve efficiency and improve efficacy [2, 31, 33, 34]. Fully realized, tomorrow this capability has the potential to optimize patient management and drive precision nuclear medicine. This may see AI initiatives move from segmentation and classification to fully integrated tools in theranostics, image guided therapy, and radiation dosimetry. Harnessed properly, DL affords the tools for improving outcomes, reducing radiation dose

burden and enhancing precision medicine. Integration of images and radiomic features of current AI applications (e.g., myocardial perfusion SPECT software) to include DL predictions integrated into the reporting display will become the norm across all procedures undertaken in nuclear medicine (Fig. 7.16).

Increasingly, AI will play an important role in patient management and business administration. Consider the possibilities for improved outcomes of, for example, a patient presenting to nuclear medicine for 68Ga PSMA and 177Lu PSMA where facial recognition software not only identifies the patient and registers them in the clinic, but also retrieves the patients' medical records and previous imaging as they walk through the waiting room door. DL algorithms automatically evaluate all previous scans, segmenting critical organs and target tissues, individualizing the diagnostic radiopharmaceutical dose to optimize the image quality as a trade-off against radiation dosimetry. DL/GAN based iterative reconstruction with segmentation and radiomic feature extraction would include auto-mapping all

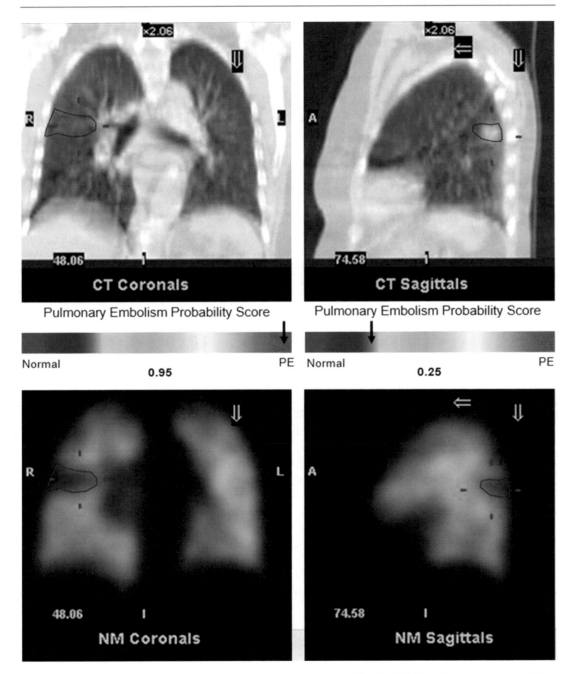

Fig. 7.18 Mock summary output for a CNN-based risk algorithm for pulmonary embolism using low-dose CT and perfusion SPECT mismatch. The coronal and digital slices represent two different patients; one with mismatch consistent with a high likelihood of pulmonary embolism (left) and the other matching defect associated with lower likelihood of pulmonary embolism (right). (Reprinted with permission [32])

Bone Scan
Metastatic Disease Probability

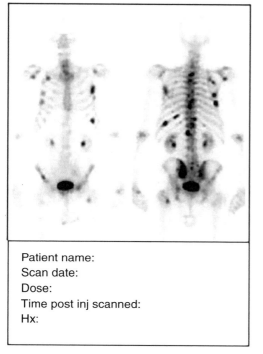

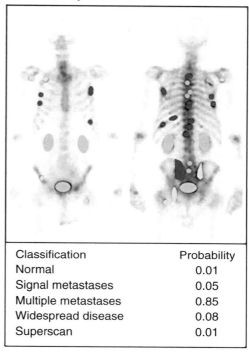

Patient name:		
Scan date:		
Dose:		
Time post inj scanned:		
Hx:		

Classification	Probability
Normal	0.01
Signal metastases	0.05
Multiple metastases	0.85
Widespread disease	0.08
Superscan	0.01

Defect Probability

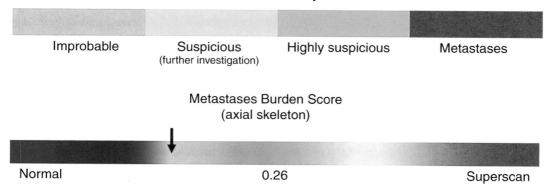

| Improbable | Suspicious (further investigation) | Highly suspicious | Metastases |

Metastases Burden Score
(axial skeleton)

| Normal | 0.26 | Superscan |

Fig. 7.19 Mock summary output for a CNN-based risk algorithm for skeletal metastases with probability classification for various outcomes and risk assessment for individual lesions. (Reprinted with permission [32])

lesions in the patients' series. An ML algorithm might evaluate radiomic inputs and other patient records and personalize the therapeutic approach. ML and DL algorithms built to model the specific insight and expertise of specialists (from anywhere in the world), could provide expert second reader systems for image reporting. DL/GAN algorithm co-registers whole body PET with gamma camera scans used to image therapy distribution to segment and extract radiomic features and determine dosimetry.

Back-office operations could also be substantially streamlined. From the point of conception that a particular imaging study or therapy may be clinically useful for a particular patient, an integrated AI system could assess the application of the proposed procedure with the patient's medical record, including clinical histories, laboratory values, and prior imaging, and compare with available literature and appropriate use criteria (AUC) recommendations. Furthermore, such a system could recommend alternate imaging or therapy as justified by the clinical scenario. In addition to the potential enhancement to clinical care, such an upstream integration of AI technology would facilitate the interface between health systems and payers, both governmental and third-party, where AUC and medical need statements are being increasingly employed. AI technology focused on aiding medical justification and rationale would greatly improve the experience for the referring clinicians, decreasing the time spent on administrative activities. The possibilities are limitless but there are significant barriers to overcome.

7.8 Workforce; Redundancy, Displacement, Transformation, and Opportunity

Perhaps the greatest speculation, hysteria, and resistance around AI in radiology has been the impact on the workforce. At one extreme are the doomsday predictors foreshadowing the extinction of radiologists as a species while on the opposite end of the spectrum lies those who deny the emerging capability of AI and see no role for it in radiology. The reality lies across a broad central band depending on a variety of factors relating to work function.

The speculation around the impact of AI on the role of radiologists is perplexing and warrants discussion and consideration in relation to nuclear medicine. At best, CNN and DL programs provide fantastic triage and second reader systems that support the physician,

improve efficiency, and decrease error rates. But the judgment of the physician remains essential. In some ways, automating some of the more menial tasks makes better use of a physician's time for the skill set they have trained extensively to have. Automation of menial tasks in nuclear medicine has been rolled out over many decades (e.g., auto-contours for region of interest identification) without a sense of doom associated with employment displacement or redundancy.

Concurrently, there has been very little discussion about the impact of AI on the technologist or physicist. It is entirely conceivable that an AI system could be designed that simply requires a "concierge" to direct the patient to the X-ray room; threatening the role of the radiographer. The nature of higher order imaging procedures in nuclear medicine represents a deep moat and high wall protecting the responsibilities of the nuclear medicine technologist from AI automation. Nonetheless, image analysis and reconstruction will have an increasing AI presence and many of the radiopharmacy responsibilities may be automated where there is potential for robotic AI. Perhaps more importantly, the triage capability of AI is a direct threat to the role of technical staff providing interim reports.

In nuclear medicine, the emergence of capabilities of ML and DL will challenge the patient care paradigm and drive a shift toward improved patient care (and outcomes) and greater satisfaction amongst physicians. The paradigm shift is unlikely to have any significant impact on the role and responsibilities of the nuclear medicine physician. Efficiencies created by ML and DL are more likely to have a direct impact on nuclear medicine technologists and scientists/physicists who take responsibility for data curation and stewardship. Here, there is potential for role expansion beyond current roles in PACs administration/management to new roles in

Table 7.1 Hypothetical nuclear medicine department workforce and the associated probable changes to workforce structure associated with a deep assimilation of AI

Role/position	Number in traditional department	Workforce transformation in fully immersive AI department
Physician	4	4
Physicist	2	1
Data Scientist	0	2
Radiopharmacist	1	1
Technologist	9.5	8.5
PACS/Data Manager	0.5	1.5
Nurse	2	2
Research Fellow	2	4
PhD Candidates	2	6

data management and data science. Indeed, the workforce of a department may expand rather than contract with an increased research and development footprint (Table 7.1).

A critical consideration as one imagines a future nuclear medicine department with fully integrated AI technology is the importance of the human element. Although medicine is in a large part a science, there also exists elements of art and culture. Dispassionate and data-driven decisions may be laudable in the intellectual sense, but these terms are seldom used to describe the ideal way to interact with patients. Rather, terms such as caring, empathetic, and understanding paint the picture of the trusted physician or healthcare team member. Illustrative of this is the increasing focus on patient experience factors in the assessment of healthcare systems, which in some cases are beginning to lead to financial rewards or penalties. In fact, patients themselves may be significant drivers in the appropriate adoption of AI enhancements into practice. Consider the scenario in which an AI algorithm is brought online to aid in the evaluation of cardiac perfusion scans. Patient A may come to the conclu-

sion that their hospital is using new technology to help the doctors make the best decisions to enhance their outcomes consistent with precision medicine. Patient B may come to the conclusion that the hospital is merely using computer programs to save themselves time and effort undermining the nature of personalized medicine. From a system perspective, the viewpoint of Patient A is obviously much more preferable, to be seen as a patient-centered system layering the latest technologies over the core of personalized care.

As a result of all these factors, AI may reshape the nuclear medicine workforce but workforce changes themselves could be minor and redundancy rare. Uncertainty may be fueled by the emergence of digital technology that saw redundancy of the dark room technician. For AI, however, displacement of work functions in nuclear medicine is less likely. Yet AI is a disruptive technology and the impact on clinical and research practice may see those with AI capability or literacy displace those without.

7.9 Summary

ML and DL are rich tools for evaluating the large volume of radiomic features extracted from molecular imaging data sets. Moreover, ML and DL can be valuable in identifying those radiomic features that should be used alone or in combination in decision making. ML and DL has the capability to uncover relationships amongst features and outcomes that may not be apparent in the standard combination of semantic reporting (Fig. 7.20). While ML and DL are unlikely to cause job redundancy, there is an opportunity to enhance patient outcomes, reporting accuracy, and efficiency. In particular, AI and DL are part of the inventory required to capitalise on high data density image sets, enhance image quality, extract abstract features and allow advances in radiation dosimetry.

Fig. 7.20 A number of models for integration of AI into radiology have been proposed, but in nuclear medicine, perhaps the most appropriate model captures the best of each domain. (Reprinted with permission [2])

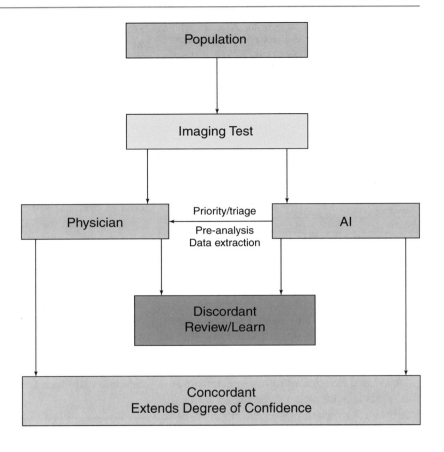

The emergence of AI in molecular imaging heralds an era of disruptive technology with the potential to reinvigorate the ecosystem of and reengineer the landscape in which, clinical molecular imaging is practiced. While AI is not new in molecular imaging, more recent developments and applications of ML and DL create refreshed interest in the architecture, operation, and implementation of AI. As a profession, nuclear medicine and molecular imaging has provided leadership across several genera- tions in the development and implementation of AI; without perhaps using the language associated with AI. This leaves nuclear medicine and molecular imaging well placed to assimilated ML and DL into clinical practice to enhance precision medicine (Fig. 7.21). The disruptive revolution of AI in molecular imaging is upon us so for those colleagues eager to grow with our profession, it is timely to craft a position in the AI space today and for tomorrow.

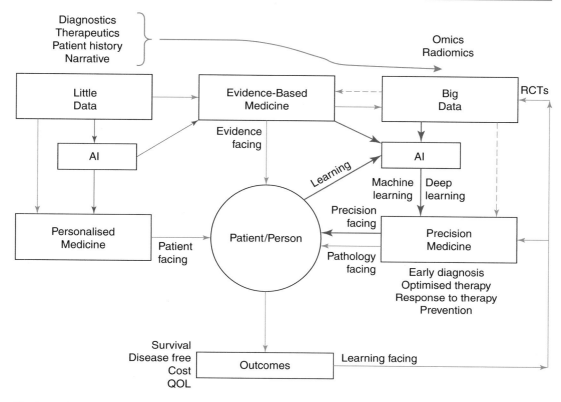

Fig. 7.21 Schematic representation of the role of big data, radiomics, and AI (ML and DL) in enhancing precision medicine

References

1. Scott J, Palmer E. Neural network analysis of ventilation-perfusion lung scans. Radiology. 1993;186(3):661–4.
2. Currie G. Intelligent imaging: artificial intelligence augmented nuclear medicine. J Nucl Med Technol. 2019;47(3):217–22.
3. Currie G, Hawk KE, Rohren E. Ethical principles for the application of artificial intelligence (AI) in nuclear medicine and molecular imaging. Eur J Nucl Med Mol Imaging. 2020;47(4):748–52. https://doi.org/10.1007/s00259-020-04678-1.
4. Currie G. Artificial intelligence in nuclear medicine: a primer for scientists and technologists. Reston: SNMMI Publishing; 2022.
5. Hwang, et al. Improving the accuracy of simultaneously reconstructed activity and attenuation maps using deep learning. J Nucl Med. 2018;59:1624–9.
6. Hwang D, Kang SK, Kim KY, Seo S, Paeng JC, Lee DS, Lee JS. Generation of PET attenuation map for whole-body time-of-flight ^{18}F-FDG PET/MRI using a deep neural network trained with simultaneously reconstructed activity and attenuation maps. J Nucl Med. 2019;60(8):1183–9. https://doi.org/10.2967/jnumed.118.219493. pii: jnumed.118.219493.
7. Torrado-Carvajal A, Vera-Olmos J, Izquierdo-Garcia D, Catalano OA, Morales MA, Margolin J, Soricelli A, Salvatore M, Malpica N, Catana C. Dixon-VIBE deep learning (DIVIDE) pseudo-CT synthesis for pelvis PET/MR attenuation correction. J Nucl Med. 2019;60(3):429–35. https://doi.org/10.2967/jnumed.118.209288. Epub 2018 Aug 30.
8. Leynes A, et al. Zero-echo-time and dixon deep pseudo-CT (ZeDD CT): direct generation of pseudo-CT images for pelvic PET/MRI attenuation correction using deep convolutional neural networks with multi-parametric MRI. J Nucl Med. 2018;59:852–8.
9. Liu F, Jang H, Kijowski R, Zhao G, Bradshaw T, McMillan AB. A deep learning approach for ^{18}F-FDG PET attenuation correction. EJNMMI Phys. 2018;5(1):24. https://doi.org/10.1186/s40658-018-0225-8.
10. Qian H, Rui X, Ahn S, IEEE. Deep learning models for PhT scatter estimations. In: IEEE nuclear science symposium and medical imaging conference. New York: IEEE; 2017. p. 2017.

11. Zhu B, Liu JZ, Cauley SF, Rosen BR, Rosen MS. Image reconstruction by domain-transform manifold learning. Nature. 2018;555(7697):487–92.

12. Haggstrom I, Schmidtlein CR, Campanella G, Fuchs TJ. DeepPET: a deep encoder-decoder network for directly solving the PET image reconstruction inverse problem. Med Image Anal. 2019;54:253–62.

13. Jiao J, Ourselin S. Fast PET reconstruction using multi-scale fully convolutional neural networks; 2017.

14. Xu J, Gong E, Pauly J, Zaharchuk G. 200x low-dose PET reconstruction using deep learning; 2017.

15. Kaplan S, Zhu Y-M. Full-dose PET image estimation from low-dose PET image using deep learning: a pilot study. J Digit Imaging. 2019;32(5):773–8.

16. Ouyang J, Chen KT, Gong E, Pauly J, Zaharchuk G. Ultra-low-dose PET reconstruction using generative adversarial network with feature matching and task-specific perceptual loss. Med Phys. 2019;46(8):3555–64.

17. Lei Y, Dong X, Wang T, et al. Whole-body PET estimation from low count statistics using cycle consistent generative adversarial networks. Phys Med Biol. 2019;64(21):215017.

18. Cui JN, Gong K, Guo N, et al. PET image denoising using unsupervised deep learning. Eur J Nucl Med Mol Imaging. 2019;46(13):2780–9.

19. Zhao Y, Gafita A, Vollnberg B, et al. Deep neural network for automatic characterization of lesions on ^{68}Ga-PSMA-11 PET/CT. Eur J Nucl Med Mol Imaging. 2020;47:603–13. https://doi.org/10.1007/s00259-019-04606-y.

20. Jackson P, Hardcastle N, Dawe N, Kron T, Hofman MS, Hicks RJ. Deep learning renal segmentation for fully automated radiation dose estimation in unsealed source therapy. Front Oncol. 2018;8:215. https://doi.org/10.3389/fonc.2018.00215. eCollection 2018.

21. Nakajima K, Kudo T, Nakata T, Kiso K, Kasai T, Taniguchi Y, Matsuo S, Momose M, Nakagawa M, Sarai M, Hida S, Tanaka H, Yokoyama K, Okuda K, Edenbrandt L. Diagnostic accuracy of an artificial neural network compared with statistical quantitation of myocardial perfusion images: a Japanese multicenter study. Eur J Nucl Med Mol Imaging. 2017;44(13):2280–9.

22. Betancur J, Hu LH, Commandeur F, Sharir T, Einstein AJ, Fish MB, Ruddy TD, Kaufmann PA, Sinusas AJ, Miller EJ, Bateman TM, Dorbala S, Di Carli M, Germano G, Otaki Y, Liang JX, Tamarappoo BK, Dey D, Berman DS, Slomka PJ. Deep learning analysis of upright-supine high-efficiency SPECT myocardial perfusion imaging for prediction of obstructive coronary artery disease: a multicenter trial. J Nucl Med. 2019;60(5):664–70.

23. Betancur J, Otaki Y, Motwani M, Fish MB, Lemley M, Dey D, Gransar H, Tamarappoo B, Germano G, Sharir T, Berman DS, Slomka PJ. Prognostic value of combined clinical and myocardial perfusion imaging data using machine learning. JACC Cardiovasc Imaging. 2018;11(7):1000–9. https://doi.org/10.1016/j.jcmg.2017.07.024. Epub 2017 Oct 18.

24. Park J, Bae S, Seo S, Park S, Bang JI, Han JH, Lee WW, Lee JS. Measurement of glomerular filtration rate using quantitative SPECT/CT and deep-learning-based kidney segmentation. Sci Rep. 2019;9(1):4223. https://doi.org/10.1038/s41598-019-40710-7.

25. Peng H, Dong D, Fang MJ, Li L, Tang LL, Chen L, Li WF, Mao YP, Fan W, Liu LZ, Tian L, Lin AH, Sun Y, Tian J, Ma J. Prognostic value of deep learning PET/CT-based radiomics: potential role for future individual induction chemotherapy in advanced nasopharyngeal carcinoma. Clin Cancer Res. 2019;25(14):4271–9. https://doi.org/10.1158/1078-0432.CCR-18-3065.

26. Choi H, Ha S, Kang H, Lee H, Lee DS. Deep learning only by normal brain PET identify unheralded brain anomalies. EBioMedicine. 2019;43:447–53. https://doi.org/10.1016/j.ebiom.2019.04.022. Epub 2019 Apr 16.

27. Currie G, Iqbal B, Kiat H. Intelligent imaging: radiomics and artificial neural networks in heart failure. J Med Imaging Radiat Sci. 2019;50(4):571–4.

28. Currie G, Sanchez S. Topical sensor metrics for 18F-FDG positron emission tomography dose extravasation. Radiography. 2020;27:178–86.

29. Violet J, Jackson P, Ferdinandus J, Sandhu S, Akhurst T, Iravani A, Kong G, Kumar A, Thang S, Eu P, Scalzo M, Murphy D, Williams S, Hicks R, Hofman M. Dosimetry of ^{177}Lu-PSMA-617 in metastatic castration-resistant prostate cancer: correlations between pretherapeutic imaging and whole-body tumor dosimetry with treatment outcomes. J Nucl Med. 2019;60:517–23.

30. Currie G. Intelligent imaging: anatomy of machine learning and deep learning. J Nucl Med Technol. 2019;47(4):273–81.

31. Currie G, Hawk KE, Rohren E, Vial A, Klein R. Machine learning and deep learning in medical imaging: intelligent imaging. J Med Imaging Radiat Sci. 2019;50(4):477–87.

32. Currie G. Intelligent imaging: developing a machine learning project. J Nucl Med Technol. 2021;49(1):44–8.

33. Uribe C, et al. Machine learning in nuclear medicine: part 1—introduction. J Jucl Med. 2019;60:451–6.

34. Nensa F, Demircioglu A, Rischpler C. Artificial intelligence in nuclear medicine. J Nucl Med. 2020;60:29S–37S.

Imaging Biobanks for Molecular Imaging: How to Integrate ML/AI into Our Databases

8

Angel Alberich-Bayarri, Ana Jiménez-Pastor,
Blanca Ferrer, María José Terol,
and Irene Mayorga-Ruiz

Contents

8.1 Introduction

Biobanks are collections, repositories of all types of human biological samples, such as blood, tissues, cells or DNA and/or related data such as the associated clinical and research data, as well as biomolecular resources, including model- and micro-organisms that might contribute to the understanding of the physiology and diseases of humans [1]. At a European level, the main infrastructure of biobanks is BBMRI-ERIC (Biobanking and BioMolecular resources Research Infrastructure) (http://bbmri-eric.eu).

A. Alberich-Bayarri (✉) · A. Jiménez-Pastor
I. Mayorga-Ruiz
Quantitative Imaging Biomarkers in Medicine,
Quibim SL, Valencia, Spain
e-mail: angel@quibim.com

B. Ferrer · M. J. Terol
Hematology Department, Clinic University Hospital
of Valencia, Valencia, Spain

Although medical images can be considered as digital and immortal samples of the organs and tissues of the human body, their inclusion in biobanks has not been straightforward by design. Indeed, many discussions have been held around the biobank concept and its suitability for the management of imaging data. The European Society of Radiology (ESR) initiated an Imaging Biobanks Working Group in 2014, with the focus to provide guidelines for the creation of imaging biobanks and the integration of image repositories into existing biobanks initiatives. The definition of imaging biobanks according to the working group guidelines was "organized databases of medical images, and associated imaging biomarkers (radiology and beyond), shared among multiple researchers, linked to other biorepositories" [2].

Thereafter, a memorandum of understanding was signed in November 11, 2015, between the ESR and BBMRI-ERIC [3]. The reason for these efforts on integration is that medical images generated in radiology and nuclear medicine are not only pictures, but quantitative data, provided in the form of imaging biomarkers that can be derived from the digital images acquired in an individual using modalities such as Computed Tomography (CT), Magnetic Resonance Imaging (MRI), X-rays, ultrasounds, and related to the topic of this chapter, also positron emission tomography (PET), single-photon emission computed tomography (SPECT) as well as hybrid modalities (PET/CT and PET/MRI) [4, 5].

There are several technological solutions for the creation of biobanks for medical imaging in general and that can be perfectly adapted to the molecular imaging space [6]. Image processing algorithms for molecular imaging have emerged to cover unmet clinical needs but their application to clinical routine in an optimized manner is still not straightforward, since it requires frequent manual interactions. Furthermore, standalone software and other solutions have been mainly addressed to provide quantitative analysis tools in a patient-specific basis, but not to populate databases for the posterior scientific research and data mining in imaging biomarkers. As an example, although the technology is available, today pipelines like quantifying the metabolic tumor volume (MTV) or total lesion glycolysis (TLG) of lymphoma lesions, storing the obtained results in the PACS, and obtaining its metabolic heterogeneity in a seamless way in clinical routine are still not available.

Artificial Intelligence, Machine Learning, and more specifically, the use of convolutional neural networks (CNN), also called Deep Learning, have allowed for the development of AI models that might help to streamline organ segmentation, lesion detection and quantification processes [7–9]. Despite the high number of research initiatives on deep learning, the integration of AI models in clinical routine requires the accomplishment of regulatory and technical challenges.

From the regulatory perspective, the model needs to be cleared as a Medical Device product by relevant organisms such as the Food and Drug Administration (FDA) and notified bodies clearing CE mark for Medical Devices on behalf of the European Commission. This regulatory requires comprehensive validation studies, including multi-center data and large cohorts of patients in which the algorithm obtains excellent performance.

With regard to the seamless integration in current information technology (IT) infrastructures existing in hospitals, AI modules should be inferenced in a software platform that can be interoperable with the current healthcare information systems (i.e., understanding standards such as DICOM communication with PACS, HL7 messaging, XML) and that incorporates automated analysis pipelines execution.

This chapter addresses the main specifications for the creation of imaging biobanks for molecular imaging as well as the strategies for the integration of AI/ML models to streamline the data extraction from the images.

8.2 Imaging Biobanks in Molecular Imaging

Imaging biobanks are not formed exclusively by images but also by associated data in the form of imaging biomarkers that can be extracted from them after the application of the appropriate image processing techniques. Imaging biomarkers are defined as characteristics extracted from the images of an individual that can be objectively measured and act as indicators of a normal biological process, a disease, or a response to a therapeutic intervention. Imaging biomarkers are complementary to conventional radiological readings either to detect a specific disease or lesion; quantify its biological situation; evaluate its progression; stratify phenotypic abnormalities; and assess the treatment response [6, 10–12]. An illustrative example of derived imaging biomarkers from molecular imaging is the calculation of the standardized uptake value (SUV), which depends on the images, the injected radiotracer dose, and the patient weight. Therefore, in the design of imaging biobanks for molecular imaging field, it is of utmost importance to collect information about the patient preparation and doses of the radiotracer that might be needed for

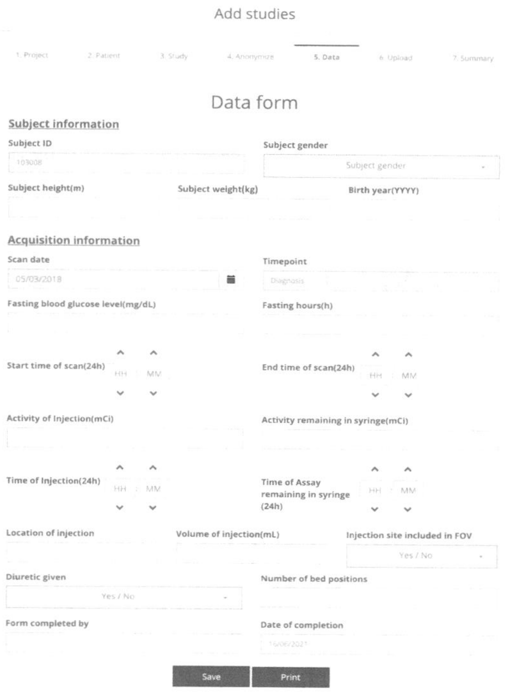

Add studies

1. Project   2. Patient   3. Study   4. Anonymize   5. Data   6. Upload   7. Summary

Data form

Subject information

Subject ID
103008

Subject gender
Subject gender

Subject height(m)   Subject weight(kg)   Birth year(YYYY)

Acquisition information

Scan date
05/03/2018

Timepoint
Diagnosis

Fasting blood glucose level(mg/dL)   Fasting hours(h)

Start time of scan(24h)   HH   MM

End time of scan(24h)   HH   MM

Activity of Injection(mCi)   Activity remaining in syringe(mCi)

Time of Injection(24h)   HH   MM

Time of Assay remaining in syringe (24h)   HH   MM

Location of injection   Volume of injection(mL)   Injection site included in FOV
Yes / No

Diuretic given
Yes / No

Number of bed positions

Form completed by   Date of completion
14/06/2021

Save   Print

Fig. 8.1 Example of data transmittal form associated to a PET asking for additional information that is not present in the DICOM headers and is needed to preserve the imaging information with high-quality standards

the calculation of imaging biomarkers (Fig. 8.1). Although the DICOM standard is designed to incorporate in the metadata specific characteristics of the patient and the examination characteristics, much of the information needed for molecular imaging analysis is not included.

Quantitative imaging biomarkers should be linked to other information from the patient, such as next generation sequencing (NGS) data, proteomics, blood test data, as well as clinical information [2].

With regard to the subjects and associated pathologies being registered in the imaging biobank, two different strategies exist: the creation of population-based imaging biobanks, that are the ones created to collect data from general population with the purpose of identifying risk factors in the development of specific diseases and help in the early detection and the disease-oriented imaging biobanks, which consist of the ones developed to collect multi-omics data from

a specific disease with the purpose of creating appropriate models of the tissues, organs, and the patient [13]. As an example, such models will be used to predict the risk of disease progression in diseases like lymphoma, and to tailor treatment based on individual response to novel therapeutic approaches [14]. Focusing on the current imaging biomarkers available, solid tumors (breast, lung, colorectal, and prostate cancer) and hematological malignancies (lymphoma, multiple myeloma) are the ideal scenarios to develop disease-oriented imaging biobanks. Nevertheless, scalability of the infrastructure would allow their inclusion of other clinical scenarios (rare tumors, neuroblastoma, glioblastoma, among others).

From the technological viewpoint, an imaging biobank should have an optimized software architecture for the massive extraction of quantitative imaging data and its association to other variables. The main users of the platform are not only medical doctors but any collaborator from transversal disciplines such as biology, biotechnology, and biomedical engineering. Considering the scenario of use of the imaging biobank, the main functional requirements can be summarized in the following:

- **Integration**: The imaging biobank software platform should be adapted to current healthcare information systems (i.e., understanding standards like DICOM communication with PACS, XML, HL7 messaging) and to be structured in conventional cells & tissues biobanks data formats (Minimum Information About Biobank Data Sharing, MIABIS).
- **Modularity**: structured in different components (medical images visualization, inference of image analysis algorithms and AI models, database searching engines and data mining capabilities, reports generator, back-end, front-end) and layers able to work as whole infrastructure.
- **Scalability**: infrastructure ready to grow with peaks of demand either on the storage or in the computing fronts through elastic architectures, allowing for the wake up process of new storage units or servers when an increase demand exists.

- **Accessibility**: The imaging biobank should be built in a client-server approach to be reachable from any place by simply using a web browser.
- **Vendor-agnostic**: The imaging biobank should be able to manage images and data from any manufacturer.
- **Inference of AI models and algorithms:** The imaging biobank architecture would allow to integrate scripts or software components developed by researchers in languages such as Python, R and embedded in Docker containers, in order to apply analysis pipelines to the data.
- **Data mining**: The infrastructure should allow for Big Data management and scientific exploitation.

8.3   Bioethical Issues

Biobanks must preserve the human and legal rights of each person that offers biomaterial for research [15]. Data privacy and security is a key factor to consider in the creation of imaging biobanks. Recent initiatives in medical imaging research such as the big consortiums on AI and medical imaging include an open data policy in their data management plans. As an example, the European Commission aims to accelerate Europe's innovation capacity through data sharing and by following the principle of open access to research results. The availability of open, high-quality and large-scale imaging biobanks and processing facilities in terms of data, services, and resources will radically simplify access to knowledge, improve interoperability and standardization and will help consolidate the medical imaging research community and foster multi-disciplinary collaboration at European level [16]. One of the keys to success in the European medical research and innovation field is to find the compromise between ensuring that medical and scientific network collaboration is not hindered while keeping a strict and high level of information security.

Biomedical imaging will become one of the major data producers, and researchers working in this domain will have to face the burden of data management and analysis within shared imaging biobanks [16].

The General Data Protection Regulation (EU) 2016/679 (GDPR) is a regulation in EU law on data protection and privacy in the European Union (EU) and the European Economic Area (EEA) and represents one of the most comprehensive and strict legal guidelines existing worldwide. GDPR sets the definition and establishes the difference between pseudonymization and anonymization of personal data, which is summarized in Fig. 8.2.

All the data incorporated into biobanks in general requires the approval of the research project by an ethics committee and the corresponding informed consent in which the patient confirms whether accepts to participate in a research program. In the case of observational non-interventional projects, mainly retrospective studies based on data collection for their storage in a biobank, the informed consent can be waived by the ethics committee.

Molecular images from modalities such as PET or SPECT, as in other medical imaging modalities are stored in DICOM format, combining the pixel data component (the image) and the associated information (the metadata). A standard process in research projects and the creation of imaging biobanks is the appropriate pseudonymization or anonymization of the images. An example of pseudonymization consists of assigning a code to the patient information that could be linked afterwards with the real patient identity by any individual (even if the code assignment information is stored in the source hospital and can only be linked by the healthcare professionals managing the patient). An example of anonymization consists of completely deleting all patient information in the images metadata and on the file folders so that the images cannot be linked back with the patient identity by any person. There exists controversy on whether the images themselves are considered personal data or not, since it could be considered that these are unique and different for every patient. Nevertheless, taking into account that the effort required to identify an individual from an image is disproportionate (taking the anonymized image

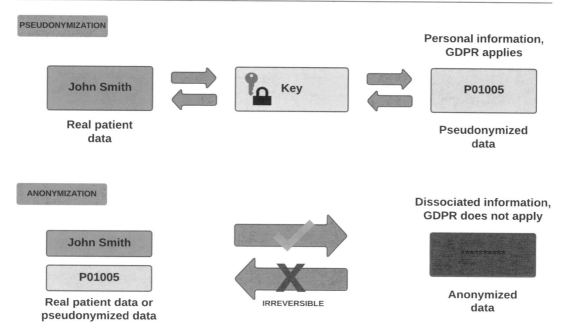

Fig. 8.2 Difference between pseudonymization and anonymization as per General Data Protection Regulation (GDPR)

and applying a brute-force correlation algorithm with the identified images of a hospital to find the match) due to the combination of steps that need to be undertaken, most current legal advisors exclude anonymized medical images from being considered personal data. Care has to be taken when managing high resolution medical images of the head, with modalities such as CT or MRI, since 3D reconstructions allow to visualize the face of the patients and eventually identify them [17]. The best approach in this case is to apply facial blurring or removal techniques before their storage in an imaging biobank.

8.4   Proposed Architecture

Imaging biobanks are not simple collections of medical images associated with patient data. In fact, architectures for the creation of medical imaging and also molecular imaging biobanks must incorporate advanced high performance computing capabilities where medical images, metadata, and other information associated to the images can be used for imaging biomarkers

extraction [18]. They must also allow to analyze these features extracted from medical images at a population level (radiomics), aiming to find prospective disease biomarkers and to combine them with other molecular biology and genomics data (radiogenomics) [19].

One of the aspects that must be clearly defined before the low-level architecture definition is the data ingestion and flow, checking whether manual and automated uploads will be allowed and the strategy for making the biobank accessible to worldwide researchers. Imaging biobanks are originated in research projects in which a group of partners participate, and images are mainly managed in a pseudonymized domain. Once the biobank has been created and populated with data, it is usually released to public domain after complete anonymization (Fig. 8.3).

The architecture of a molecular imaging biobank is organized in three different layers, the front-end, the back-end services and the data persistence layer. The following components can be found in software platforms used for imaging biobanks such as Quibim Precision® (Quibim SL, Valencia, Spain) (Fig. 8.4):

Imaging Biobanks - Data entry and flow

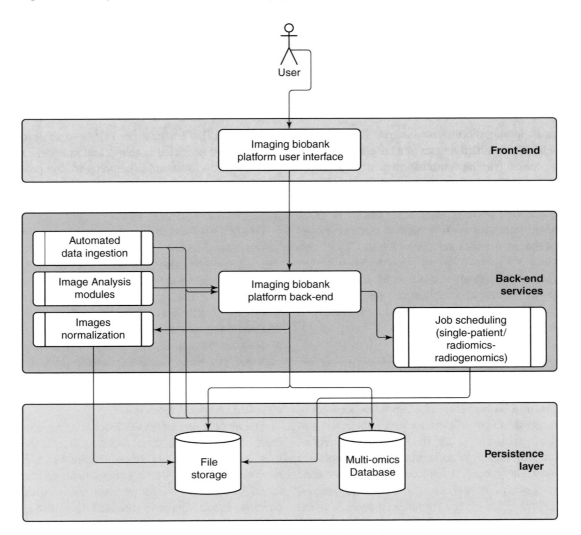

Fig. 8.3 Data entry and flow in the creation of an imaging biobank

Fig. 8.4 Architecture of the Quibim Precision® (Quibim SL, Valencia, Spain) software platform, used for the creation of imaging biobanks

- *Front-end layer*: This layer is directly exposed to the final user to interact with the software using the web user interface. Users can access to this user interface typically through a URL that opens the web application.
- *Back-end layer*: This layer is built by different services that processes requests from the user interface, external applications, and the interaction between the services. At this stage, three main components are present:
  - Imaging biobank platform back-end: This component handles all the requests related to the front-end and serves the code of the application. Besides, it provides common data to other services such as molecular imaging analysis algorithms and external applications.
  - Automated data ingestion: This component handles the connection between the imaging biobank platform and the local repositories (PACS) using the DICOM protocol.
  - Job scheduler: This service is used to schedule the execution of image analysis modules. The platform needs to incorporate a simple and flexible orchestrator (Nomad, Kubernetes) to deploy and manage image analysis algorithms in containers (Docker).
- Persistence layer: This layer is used to persist the non-volatile information of the software, that is, the data. This layer is composed of:
  - Multi-omics database: a relational SQL or non-relational NoSQL database where the application persists the structured information.
  - File storage: the application persists all the files (imaging studies, results, configuration files, ...) in a local or cloud repository.

The images analysis modules that can be implemented and integrated within an Imaging Biobank platform architecture must include all the image processing and quantification steps desired to meet the clinical and research needs. The programming language of these algorithms will vary depending on the expertise of the developers although the three most frequently used languages in the field of molecular imaging are: Python, Matlab, and R, among others.

As an illustrative example, given a molecular imaging biobank in which a specific project is dedicated to manage diffuse large B-cell lymphoma cases, including the PET/CT examinations together with the associated clinical data, an image analysis pipeline can be focused in applying a systematic analysis methodology to a batch of examinations (Fig. 8.5). The image analysis pipeline is embedded in a Docker container and integrated within the imaging biobank platform.

PET/CT analysis pipeline
(metabolic tumor volume & texture analysis – metabolic heterogeneity)

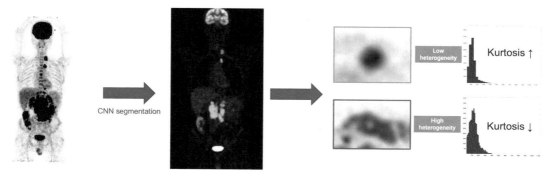

Fig. 8.5 Molecular imaging analysis pipeline dedicated to the estimation of metabolic tumor volume of individual lesions detected as well as quantification of histogram and textural properties to measure metabolic heterogeneity

References

1. BBMRI-ERIC Statutes, Article 1(1). https://www.bbmri-eric.eu/wp-content/uploads/2016/12/BBMRI-ERIC_Statutes_Rev2_for_website.pdf. Visited 15 May 2021.
2. European Society of Radiology (ESR). ESR position paper on imaging biobanks. Insights Imaging. 2015;6:403–10.
3. https://www.myesr.org/article/145. Visited 15 May 2021.
4. O'Connor JP, Aboagye EO, Adams JE, et al. Consensus statement. Imaging biomarkers roadmap for cancer studies. Nat Rev Clin Oncol. 2017;14(3):169–86. https://doi.org/10.1038/nrclinonc.2016.162. Epub 2016 Oct 11.
5. Gillies RJ, Kinahan PE, Hricak H. Radiomics: images are more than pictures, they are data. Radiology. 2016;278(2):563–77. https://doi.org/10.1148/radiol.2015151169. Epub 2015 Nov 18. PMID: 26579733; PMCID: PMC4734157.
6. Alberich-Bayarri Á, Hernández-Navarro R, Ruiz-Martínez E, García-Castro F, García-Juan D, Martí-Bonmatí L. Development of imaging biomarkers and generation of big data. Radiol Med. 2017;122(6):444–8. https://doi.org/10.1007/s11547-017-0742-x. Epub 2017 Feb 21. PMID: 28224398.
7. Blanc-Durand P, Jégou S, Kanoun S, Berriolo-Riedinger A, Bodet-Milin C, Kraeber-Bodéré F, Carlier T, Le Gouill S, Casasnovas RO, Meignan M, Itti E. Fully automatic segmentation of diffuse large B cell lymphoma lesions on 3D FDG-PET/CT for total metabolic tumour volume prediction using a convolutional neural network. Eur J Nucl Med Mol Imaging. 2021;48(5):1362–70. https://doi.org/10.1007/s00259-020-05080-7. Epub 2020 Oct 24. PMID: 33097974.
8. Naser MA, van Dijk LV, He R, Wahid KA, Fuller CD. Tumor segmentation in patients with head and neck cancers using deep learning based-on multimodality PET/CT images. Head Neck Tumor Segm (2020). 2021;12603:85–98. https://doi.org/10.1007/978-3-030-67194-5_10. Epub 2021 Jan 13. PMID: 33724743; PMCID: PMC7929493.
9. Arabi H, AkhavanAllaf A, Sanaat A, Shiri I, Zaidi H. The promise of artificial intelligence and deep learning in PET and SPECT imaging. Phys Med. 2021;83:122–37. https://doi.org/10.1016/j.ejmp.2021.03.008. Epub 2021 Mar 22. PMID: 33765602.
10. Marti-Bonmati L, Alberich-Bayarri A, Garcia-Marti G, Sanz-Requena R, Perez Castillo C, Carot Sierra JM, Manjon Herrera JV. Imaging biomarkers, quantitative imaging and bioengineering. Radiologia. 2012;54:269–78.
11. Biomarkers Definitions Working Group. Biomarkers and surrogate endpoints: preferred definitions and conceptual framework. Clin Pharmacol Ther. 2001;69:89–95.
12. European Society of Radiology (ESR). ESR statement on the stepwise development of imaging biomarkers. Insights Imaging. 2013;4:147–52.
13. Alberich-Bayarri A, Neri E, Marti-Bonmati L. Imaging biomarkers and imaging biobanks. In: Ranschaert E, et al., editors. Artificial intelligence in medical imaging. London: Springer Nature; 2019. p. 119–26. https://doi.org/10.1007/978-3-319-94878-2.
14. Ferrer Lores B, Mayorga-Ruiz I, Alberich Bayarri A, Morello-González D, Pastor-Galán I, Navarro-Cubells B, Serrano A, Teruel AI, Dosdá-Muñoz R, Solano C, Marti-Bonmati L, Terol MJ. Prognostic value of radiomics signature by diagnostic 18F-FDG PET/CT analysis in aggressive non-Hodgkin's lymphoma. Blood. 2018;132(Suppl 1):1703. https://doi.org/10.1182/blood-2018-99-119851.
15. Coppola L, Cianflone A, Grimaldi AM, Incoronato M, Bevilacqua P, Messina F, Baselice S, Soricelli A, Mirabelli P, Salvatore M. Biobanking in health care: evolution and future directions. J Transl Med. 2019;17(1):172. https://doi.org/10.1186/s12967-019-1922-3. PMID: 31118074; PMCID: PMC6532145.
16. ESR statement on data protection regulation. https://www.myesr.org/sites/default/files/ESR%20Statement%20on%20EC%27s%20proposal%20on%20Data%20Protection%20Regulation_1.pdf. Visited 15 May 2021.
17. Schwarz CG, Kremers WK, Therneau TM, Sharp RR, Gunter JL, Vemuri P, Arani A, Spychalla AJ, Kantarci K, Knopman DS, Petersen RC, Jack CR Jr. Identification of anonymous MRI research participants with face-recognition software. N Engl J Med. 2019;381(17):1684–6. https://doi.org/10.1056/NEJMc1908881. PMID: 31644852; PMCID: PMC7091256.
18. Martí-Bonmatí L, Alberich-Bayarri Á, Ladenstein R, Blanquer I, Segrelles JD, Cerdá-Alberich L, Gkontra P, Hero B, García-Aznar JM, Keim D, Jentner W, Seymour K, Jiménez-Pastor A, González-Valverde I, de Las M, Heras B, Essiaf S, Walker D, Rochette M, Bubak M, Mestres J, Viceconti M, Martí-Besa G, Cañete A, Richmond P, Wertheim KY, Gubala T, Kasztelnik M, Meizner J, Nowakowski P, Gilpérez S, Suárez A, Aznar M, Restante G, Neri E. PRIMAGE project: predictive in silico multiscale analytics to support childhood cancer personalised evaluation empowered by imaging biomarkers. Eur Radiol Exp. 2020;4(1):22. https://doi.org/10.1186/s41747-020-00150-9. PMID: 32246291; PMCID: PMC7125275.
19. Neri E, Regge D. Imaging biobanks in oncology: European perspective. Future Oncol. 2017;13(5):433–41. https://doi.org/10.2217/fon-2016-0239. Epub 2016 Oct 28. PMID: 27788586.

Artificial Intelligence/Machine Learning in Nuclear Medicine

9

Sangwon Lee, Kyeong Taek Oh, Yong Choi,
Sun K. Yoo, and Mijin Yun

Contents

9.1   Introduction

Though the diagnosis of neurodegenerative diseases is mainly based on clinical criteria, neuroimaging in nuclear medicine plays important supportive roles in diagnosis and differential diagnosis of neurodegenerative diseases and prediction of disease progression [1, 2]. Different from magnetic resonance imaging (MRI) dependent on morphological changes of cortical and subcortical structures, positron emission tomography/computed tomography (PET/CT) provides quantitative evaluation of functional or molecular changes related to metabolism, proteinopathy, enzyme expression, transporter, or receptor. In addition to visual analysis, quantitative image analysis is essential to investigate clinical significance of neuroimaging. Of them, voxel-based analysis and region-of-interest (ROI) or volume-of-interest (VOI) analysis are widely used for comparison between control (or normal) and patient groups. Statistical parametric mapping (SPM) is the most popular voxel-based approach, which demonstrates areas of the brain with a significant difference between normal controls and patients [3, 4]. ROI or VOI-based image analysis

S. Lee · M. Yun (✉)
Department of Nuclear Medicine, Yonsei University
College of Medicine, Seoul, South Korea
e-mail: LSW0423@yuhs.ac; YUNMIJIN@yuhs.ac

K. T. Oh · S. K. Yoo
Department of Medical Engineering, Yonsei
University College of Medicine, Seoul, South Korea
e-mail: OKT2704@yuhs.ac; SUNKYOO@yuhs.ac

Y. Choi
Department of Electronics Engineering, Sogang
University, Seoul, South Korea
e-mail: Ychoi@sogang.ac.kr

© The Author(s), under exclusive license to Springer Nature Switzerland AG 2022
P. Veit-Haibach, K. Herrmann (eds.), *Artificial Intelligence/Machine Learning in Nuclear Medicine and Hybrid Imaging*, https://doi.org/10.1007/978-3-031-00119-2_9

performs the calculation in the pixels of each ROI or VOI. Manual, semi-automatic, and automatic method can be used to draw a region or volume. Although accurate, manual drawing is time-consuming, operator dependent, and less reproducible. On the contrary, accurate region segmentation by automatic drawing should be guaranteed in each patient for robustness and reliability of data analysis.

Different from traditional image analysis, machine learning as a subset of the artificial intelligence finds patterns through big data. Based on the training data, it builds a mathematical model to make prediction. A learning method can be unsupervised, semi-supervised, or supervised. Supervised learning requires labeled data to find the pattern, whereas unsupervised learning uses unlabeled data and semi-supervised learning needs a small labeled data and a large unlabeled data. Machine learning is trained using a large number of input data with high reproducibility to extract the feature of clinical significance. After extraction, feature selection removes unnecessary features to reduce the training time and the possibility of overfitting, and avoid the dimensionality issues. Then, a classifier algorithm such as support vector machine, random forest, or artificial neural network is performed to map the feature for the classification of disease.

As a part of the machine learning, deep learning is consisted of the artificial neural networks with multiple convolutional layers and nodes. Unlike traditional machine learning, deep learning performs the feature extraction and learning by itself. For the feature extraction and transformation, the techniques of deep learning are based on a cascade of multiple layers of nonlinear processing units. High-quality data and labels are most important to train and test the deep learning models. Dataset is typically composed of training, validation, and test set. The training data are used to train a network that loss function calculates the loss values in the forward propagation and learnable parameters are updated via back-propagation. The validation data are to fine-tune hyper-parameters and the test data to evaluate the performance of the model. This chapter will focus on artificial intelligence used for neuroim-aging in nuclear medicine including classification of diseases, segmentation of ROI or VOI, denoising, image reconstruction, and low-dose imaging.

9.2 Classification

9.2.1 Alzheimer's Disease

Alzheimer's disease (AD) is a neurodegenerative disease characterized by a decline in cognitive function. It mostly affects older people so that the prevalence of AD is increasing with the growth of the elderly population. Early diagnosis of AD before the symptoms become severe is of utmost clinical importance since it may provide opportunities for effective treatment. ^{18}F-FDG PET/CT is one of the most useful modalities to support the clinical diagnosis of dementia including AD. It shows changes in glucose metabolism of the brain over various disease entities related to dementia with high sensitivity and specificity. In patients with AD, the reduction of glucose metabolism is expected stating from the mesial temporal to posterior cingulate cortex (PCC), lateral temporal, inferior parietal, and prefrontal regions to help diagnose [5].

Deep learning methods have been studied for the evaluation of patients with AD. Several auto-encoders with multi-layered neural network to combine multimodal features were applied for AD classification [6]. In a study with a stacked auto-encoder to extract high-level features of multimodal ROI and an SVM classifier, the proposed method was 95.9%, 85.0%, and 75.8% accurate for AD, MCI, and MCI-converter diagnosis, respectively, using the ADNI dataset [7]. Recently, CNN methods with 2D or 3D volume data of PET/CT or MRI scans were applied for AD classification [8–11]. In 2D CNN models, the features from the specific slices of axial, coronal, and sagittal scans were concatenated and used for AD classification. Using MRI volume data, skull stripping and gray matter segmentation were performed and the slices with gray matter information were used as CNN model input. Compared to 2D CNN models, studies have used 3D volume data with promising results. Using the Alzheimer's Disease Neuroimaging Initiative (ADNI) MRI dataset without skull-stripping pre-processing, Hosseini-Asl et al. built a deep 3D Convolutional Neural Network (3D-CNN) upon a convolutional auto-encoder, which was pre-trained to capture anatomical shape variations in structural brain MRI scans for source domain [8]. Then, fully connected upper layers of the 3D-CNN were fine-tuned for each task-specific AD classification in target domain. The proposed 3D deeply supervised adaptable CNN outperformed several proposed approaches, including 3D-CNN model, other CNN-based methods, and conventional classifiers by accuracy and robustness. Liu et al. used cascaded convolutional neural networks (CNNs) to learn the multi-level and multimodal features of MRI and PET brain images for AD classification [10]. In the method, multiple deep 3D-CNNs were applied on different local image patches to transform the local brain image into more compact high-level features. Then, an upper high-level 2D-CNN followed by softmax layer was cascaded to ensemble the high-level features and generate the latent multimodal correlation features for classification task. Finally, a fully connected layer followed by softmax layer combined these learned features for AD classification. Without image segmentation and rigid registration, the method could automatically learn the generic multi-level and multimodal features from multiple imaging modalities for classification. With ADNI MRI and PET dataset from 397 subjects including 93 AD patients, 204 mild cognitive impairment (MCI, 76 MCI converters +128 MCI non-converters) and 100 normal controls (NC), the proposed method demonstrated promising performance of an accuracy of 93.26% for classification of AD vs. NC and 82.95% for classification MCI converters vs. NC.

Although studies have shown that various deep learning methods were effective for AD classification, the model performance of external validation compared to the training dataset is an issue to be resolved. In fact, the qualities and properties of medical images could be affected by the image-acquisition environment including the imaging acquisition system, acquisition protocol, reconstruction method, etc. Therefore, there is a need for a model with enhanced generalization performance to improve clinical utility of a proposed method. In a recent study using FDG PET/CT, instead of 3D volume data, slice-selective learning using a BEGAN-based model was constructed to solve the above (Fig. 9.1) [9]. The model was trained with an ADNI dataset, then performed external validation with their own dataset. A range was set to cover the most important AD-related regions and searched for the most appropriate slices for classification. The model learned the generalized features of AD and NC for external validation when appropriate slices were selected. The slice range that covered the PCC using double slices showed the best performance. The accuracy, sensitivity, and specificity was 94.33%, 91.78%, and 97.06% using their own dataset and 94.82%, 92.11%, and 97.45% using the ADNI dataset. The performance on the two independent datasets showed no statistical difference. The study showed the feasibility of the model with consistent performance when tested using datasets acquired from a variety of image-acquisition environments.

Despite remarkable diagnostic accuracy of deep learning, the correlation between the features extracted by deep learning model and diseases is hard to explain. Several studies proposed the methods for solving this problem by providing the feature map and input data responsible for the result of prediction. Class activation map (CAM) has been widely used to understand where the deep learning model evaluate for classes and to explain how deep learning models predict the outputs [12–14]. Choi et al. demonstrated that brain regions where the CNN model evaluated for AD with decreased cognitive function using CAM method, which can generate the heat map with the probability of AD [15]. However, CAM-based interpretation should be cautious because deep learning models may classify diseases by the regions that cannot be explained by the known knowledge.

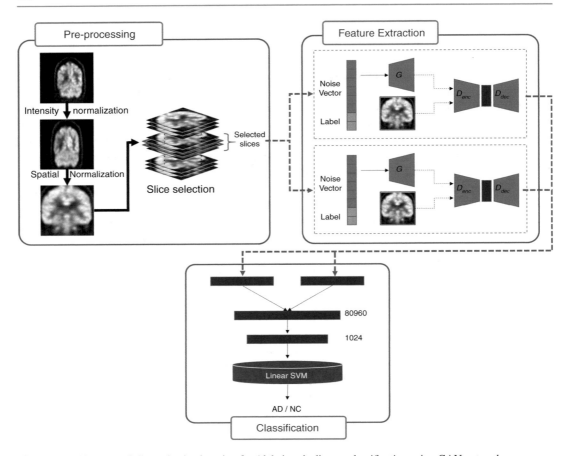

Fig. 9.1 Architecture of slice-selective learning for Alzheimer's disease classification using GAN network

9.2.2 Parkinson's Disease

Parkinson's disease (PD) is the second most common of neurodegenerative diseases which is mainly a movement disorder, such as resting tremor, bradykinesia, and rigidity [16, 17]. Alpha-synuclein aggregates, the primary PD pathology, are known to promote the dopaminergic loss [18]. Although non-invasive direct PET imaging of alpha-synuclein aggregates in the brain is limited, the quantification of presynaptic transporters of the nigrostriatal dopaminergic neurons can be performed with PET and SPECT using either ^{18}F or ^{123}I N-(3-Fluoropropyl)-2β-carbon ethoxy-3β-(4-iodophenyl) Nortropane (FP-CIT) [19, 20]. Dopamine transporter (DAT) in PET/CT has been widely used for the early diagnosis of PD and the discrimination between PD and other diseases showing parkinsonism.

Machine learning has been applied to diagnose PD using DAT-SPECT or PET scan [21–27]. The extracted feature from deep learning methods has outstanding diagnostic results. However, the clinical correlation between disease and deep learning methods needs further explanation and verification since low-level features extracted from deep learning methods may not reflect the neuropathological heterogeneity of PD. Shiiba et al. used semi-quantitative indicators and shape feature acquired on DAT-SPECT to train the model of machine learning for classification between PD and normal controls (NC) [28]. Striatum binding ratio (SBR) as semi-quantitative indicators and circularity index of shape were combined as a feature for machine learning. The performance of classification was significantly improved by using both SBR and circularity than by the one of SBR or circularity index (AUC for

SBR and circularity: 0.995, AUC for circularity only: 0.990, and AUC for SBR: 0.973).

FDG PET/CT is also actively used for the evaluation of patients with parkinsonism, especially for the differentiation between idiopathic PD and atypical parkinsonism [29]. Wu et al. used support vector machine to classify PD patients and NC using radiomics features on ^{18}F-FDG PET [21]. The proposed method showed that the accuracy of classification between PD and NC was $90.97 \pm 4.66\%$ and $88.08 \pm 5.27\%$ in Huashan and Wuxi test sets, respectively. In addition, several studies showed that the deep learning methods were also effective for classification between PD patients and NC [30, 31]. Zhao et al. developed a 3D deep residual CNN for automated differential diagnosis of idiopathic PD (IPD) and atypical parkinsonism (APD) [30]. With dataset from 920 patients including 502 IPD patients, 239 multiple system atrophy (MSA) patients, and 179 progressive supranuclear palsy (PSP) patients, the proposed method demonstrated the performance of 97.7% sensitivity, 94.1% specificity, 95.5% PPV, and 97.0% NPV for the classification of IPD, versus 96.8%, 99.5%, 98.7%, and 98.7% for the classification of MSA, and 83.3%, 98.3%, 90.0%, and 97.8% for the classification of PSP, respectively.

9.3 Segmentation

Despite the sensitivity of PET/CT is usually much higher than conventional structural images such as CT of MRI, it is considered difficult to extract anatomical information from PET/CT images because they are not well-distinguishable from low-resolution images of PET/CT [32]. So far, there are limited studies to segment anatomical structures on PET images using deep learning methods, especially in the diseases related to the brain. A 3D U-net shaped CNN has been used to segment cerebral gliomas on F-18 fluoroethyltyrosine (^{18}F-FET) PET [33]. Of the deep learning methods, generative adversarial network (GAN) model received great attention due to the ability to generate data without explicitly modeling probability density functions. It has been applied

to many tasks with excellent performance such as image-to-image translation, semantic segmentation, and resolution translation from low to high [34]. In particular, GAN models have been promising in the field of segmentation. Of the PET/CT studies, there is only one study applied pix2pix framework of GAN to segment normal white matter (WM) on ^{18}F-FDG PET/CT [35]. The DSC of segmenting WM from ^{18}F-FDG PET/CT was 0.82 on average. Despite the low resolution of ^{18}F-FDG PET/CT, the results showed similar results compared to MRI [36, 37]. The study showed a feasibility of using ^{18}F-FDG PET/CT in segmenting WM volumes.

In the WM, there are foci or areas called as white matter hyper-intensities (WMH) since they show increased signal intensity on T2-weighted fluid attenuated inversion recovery (FLAIR) on MRI. Despite seen in healthy elderly subjects, WMH are associated with greater hippocampal atrophy in non-demented elderly and cognitive decline in patients with CI [38–40]. Therefore, MRI has been invaluable in the assessment of WMH [41]. As mentioned, ^{18}F-FDG PET/CT is useful in assessing the glucose metabolism in the cortex or subcortical neurons. However, the low spatial resolution and low glucose metabolism have limited the evaluation of the WM and WMH on ^{18}F-FDG PET/CT. In our group, we applied a GAN framework to segment WMH on ^{18}F-FDG PET/CT (In Fig. 9.2, unpublished data). A dataset of mild, moderate, and severe groups of WMH according to the Fazekas scoring system was used to train and test a deep learning model. Using WMH on FLAIR MRI as gold standard, a GAN method was used to segment WMH on MRI. The dice similarity coefficient (DSC) values were closely dependent on WMH volumes on MRI. With more than 60 mL of volume, the DSC values were above 0.7 with a mean value of 0.751 ± 0.048. With a volume of 60 mL or less, the mean value of DSC was only 0.362 ± 0.263. For WMH volume estimation, GAN showed excellent correlation with WMH volume on MRI ($r = 0.998$ in severe group, 0.983 in moderate group, and 0.908 in mild group). Although it is limited to evaluate WMH on ^{18}F-FDG PET/CT by visual analysis, they are important vascular

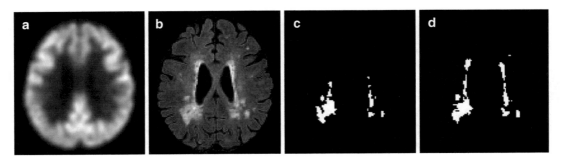

Fig. 9.2 Deep learning-based, GAN, FLAIR image synthesized using PET/CT. ^{18}F-FDG PET/CT (**a**), T2-weighted FLAIR image (**b**), predicted WMH volume (**c**), and manually segmented WMH volume (**d**)

component contributing to dementia. Our GAN method showed a feasibility to automatically segment and estimate volumes of WMH on ^{18}F-FDG PET/CT which will increase values of ^{18}F-FDG PET/CT in evaluating patients with CI.

9.4   Image Generation and Processing

Artificial intelligence in nuclear medicine is also widely used in image processing technology, such as image reconstruction and attenuation correction. For PET/MRI, attenuation correction by making pseudo CT images from MRI has compared to CT-based methods [42–46]. In a method using Dixon sequence, PET activity in bone structure is underestimated in attenuation map [43, 44]. Despite many approaches, MR-based attenuation correction methods are considered lower performance than CT-based method for PET/CT. Recently, deep learning methods have been applied to the attenuation correction for PET/MRI. Hwang et al. [47] proposed a deep learning-based whole-body PET/MRI attenuation correction, which is more accurate than Dixon-based 4-segment method. The proposed deep learning method used activity and attenuation maps estimated using the maximum-likelihood reconstruction of activity and attenuation (MLAA) algorithm as inputs to a CNN to learn a CT-derived attenuation map. The attenuation map generated from CNN showed better bone identification than MLAA and aver-

age DSC for bone region was 0.77, which was significantly higher than MLAA-derived attenuation map (0.36). Liu et al. also demonstrated that deep learning approach to generate pseudo CT from MR image reduced PET reconstruction error compared to CT-based method [48]. With the retrospective T1-weighted MR images from 40 subjects, deep convolutional auto-encoder (CAE) network was trained with 30 datasets and then evaluated in 10 dataset by comparing the generated pseudo CT to a ground-truth of CT scan. The results of this study showed that the DSC for air region of 0.97, soft tissue of 0.94, and bone of 0.80.

A generation of MRI from CT or CT from MRI has been performed by a lot of researchers, but very few studies have been carried out for the generation of MR images from PET/CT. Choi et al. [49] built GAN model, based on image-to-image translation, to generate MR images from florbetapir PET images. The generated MR images are used for quantification of florbetapir PET and measured value was highly correlated with real MR-based quantification method. Although there was a high structural similarity of 0.91 ± 0.04 between real MR image and generated MR image, the differentiation between gray and white matter was difficult and there was blurring of the detailed structures in the generated MR. In our group, cycle GAN based deep learning method was applied for generating FLAIR images from ^{18}F-FDG PET/CT. As shown in Fig. 9.3 (unpublished data), the generated FLAIR images from our method had excellent visual quality.

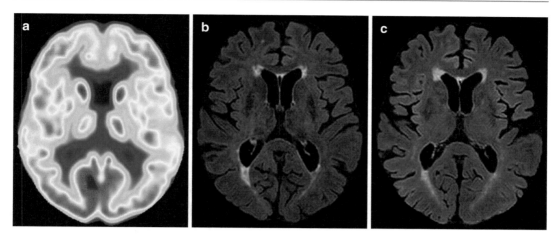

Fig. 9.3 Representative images of ^{18}F-FDG PET/CT as an input to deep learning model (**a**), real FLAIR (**b**), and the generated FLAIR image by deep learning model (**c**) (unpublished data)

9.5 Low-Dose Imaging

High-quality PET images need a large number of gamma events either from high-dose injection or long scan time. Long scan time can result in patient motion artifacts and inconvenience, while high-dose administration increases radiation exposure to patients. To overcome these issues, the development of technology has concentrated on increasing the PET scanner sensitivity to detect a large number of coincidence events. A newer PET system with an axial field-of-view covering the whole body in a single bed position has shown a 40-fold improvement in effective sensitivity [50, 51]. In addition, numerous image reconstruction and noise reduction algorithm have improved spatial resolution and signal-to-noise ratio (SNR) of PET image [52, 53]. Ordered subset expectation maximization (OSEM) with modeling of the point spread function has been used to reconstruct gamma event for high-resolution PET imaging.

With deep learning method, convolutional neural network (CNN) models have been used to learn the relationship between full-dose and low-dose PET images [54–56]. Xu et al. [56] proposed a deep learning method, an encoder-decoder structure with concatenate skip connection with residual learning framework, to reduce dose of radioactive tracer in ^{18}F-FDG PET imaging. They

achieved significantly better performance compared with reconstructed by denoising algorithms (nonlocal means, block-matching 3D, and auto-context network) from 0.005 of the standard dose.

Chen et al. [57] proposed a method to reconstruct full-dose amyloid PET/MR using ^{18}F-florbetaben (^{18}F-FBB) image from low-dose image. Compared with low-dose image, the synthesized images using CNN model showed marked improvement on all quality metrics, such as peak signal-to-noise ratio (PSNR), structural similarity, and room mean square error (RMSE). In a visual reading of amyloid burden of synthesized FBB image using CNN model, accuracy for amyloid status was 89%. In addition, the CNN model showed the smallest mean and variance for standardized uptake value ratio (SUVR) difference to full-dose images. Ouyang et al. [58] also reported a generative adversarial network (GAN) model to reconstruct the full-dose PET image from low-dose image, which significantly outperformed Chen et al.'s method with the same input by 1.87 dB in PSNR, 2.04% in SSIM, and 24.75% in RMSE.

In our group, a CNN model with a residual learning framework was applied for predicting full-time ^{18}F-FBB PET/CT images from short-time scan of 1 to 5 min with excellent image quality (Fig. 9.4, unpublished data). In amyloid

Fig. 9.4 ^{18}F-FBB PET/
CT images reconstructed
with different scan time
(left column) and the
predicted ^{18}F-FBB PET/
CT images by deep
learning method from
short scan time (right
column). Amyloid status
of negative (**a**) and
positive case (**b**) were
shown

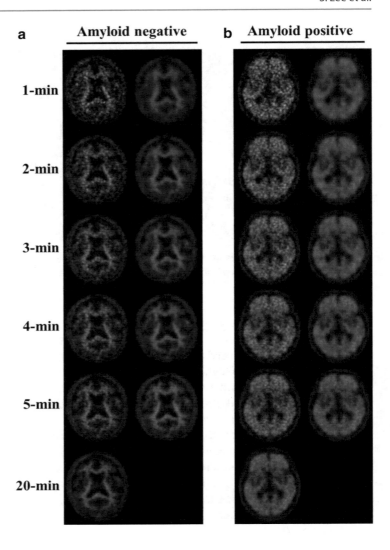

imaging, amyloid positivity can be measured by quantitative analysis of SUVR, which were normalized to the mean value in the cerebellar cortex. The results of our ROC analyses showed that the cut-off values for amyloid positivity deduced from the images predicted from the CNN models using low-dose images from 1 to 5 min remained unchanged as compared with those obtained from the ground-truth images.

Scan time reduction using low-dose imaging has been tried for ^{18}F-FDG PET/CT imaging. Kim et al. [59] proposed that deep learning method to synthesize the PET images with high SNR acquired for typical scan durations from

short scan time PET images with low SNR using deep learning with a concatenated connection and residual learning framework (Fig. 9.5). The list-mode PET data were formatted into 10, 30, 60, and 120 s to investigate the effect of scan time on the quality of synthesized PET images. The PSNRs and NRMSEs of the synthesized ^{18}F-FDG PET images were significantly superior to those of the short scan images for all scan times. As the scan time increased from 10 to 120 s, the PSNRs and NRMSEs of the synthesized ^{18}F-FDG PET images were improved by an average of 21.6 ± 3.8% and 47.0 ± 5.5%, respectively.

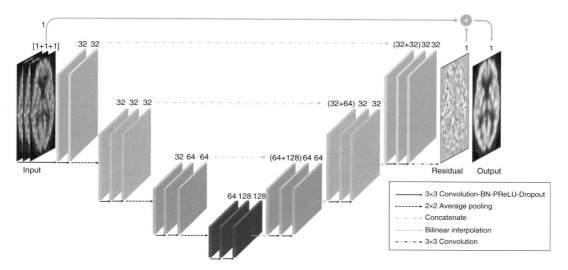

Fig. 9.5 A schematic of the encoder-decoder convolutional neural network for predicting the full-time scan from short-time scan of ¹⁸F-FDG PET/CT

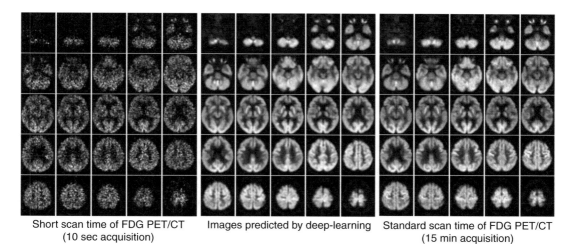

Short scan time of FDG PET/CT   Images predicted by deep-learning   Standard scan time of FDG PET/CT
(10 sec acquisition)   (15 min acquisition)

Fig. 9.6 Representative ¹⁸F-FDG PET/CT images in 62-year-old female with normal control, with short-time scan (10 sec, left), predicted images by CNN with residual learning framework (middle), and full-time scan (15 min, right)

As shown in Fig. 9.6, high quality of PET image generated using deep learning model with low count data and/or short scan time can have practical impact on reducing radiation exposure. It will provide new opportunities for PET/CT for those patients such as children, pregnant women, and patients prone to motion artifacts.

References

1. Staffaroni AM, Elahi FM, McDermott D, Marton K, Karageorgiou E, Sacco S, et al. Neuroimaging in dementia. Semin Neurol. 2017;37(5):510–37. https://doi.org/10.1055/s-0037-1608808.
2. Nasrallah I, Dubroff J. An overview of PET neuroimaging. Semin Nucl Med. 2013;43(6):449–61. https://doi.org/10.1053/j.semnuclmed.2013.06.003.
3. Friston KJ, Frith CD, Liddle PF, Frackowiak RS. Comparing functional (PET) images: the assessment of significant change. J Cereb Blood Flow Metab. 1991;11(4):690–9. https://doi.org/10.1038/jcbfm.1991.122.
4. Friston KJ, Frith CD, Liddle PF, Dolan RJ, Lammertsma AA, Frackowiak RS. The relationship between global and local changes in PET scans. J Cereb Blood Flow Metab. 1990;10(4):458–66. https://doi.org/10.1038/jcbfm.1990.88.
5. Nestor PJ, Altomare D, Festari C, Drzezga A, Rivolta J, Walker Z, et al. Clinical utility of FDG-PET for the differential diagnosis among the main forms of dementia. Eur J Nucl Med Mol Imaging. 2018;45(9):1509–25. https://doi.org/10.1007/s00259-018-4035-y.
6. Liu S, Liu S, Cai W, Che H, Pujol S, Kikinis R, et al. Multimodal neuroimaging feature learning for multiclass diagnosis of Alzheimer's disease. IEEE Trans Biomed Eng. 2015;62(4):1132–40. https://doi.org/10.1109/tbme.2014.2372011.
7. Suk HI, Shen D. Deep learning-based feature representation for AD/MCI classification. Med Image Comput Comput Assist Interv. 2013;16(Pt 2):583–90. https://doi.org/10.1007/978-3-642-40763-5_72.
8. Hosseini-Asl E, Ghazal M, Mahmoud A, Aslantas A, Shalaby AM, Casanova MF, et al. Alzheimer's disease diagnostics by a 3D deeply supervised adaptable convolutional network. Front Biosci (Landmark Ed). 2018;23:584–96. https://doi.org/10.2741/4606.
9. Kim HW, Lee HE, Lee S, Oh KT, Yun M, Yoo SK. Slice-selective learning for Alzheimer's disease classification using a generative adversarial network: a feasibility study of external validation. Eur J Nucl Med Mol Imaging. 2020;47(9):2197–206. https://doi.org/10.1007/s00259-019-04676-y.
10. Liu M, Cheng D, Wang K, Wang Y. Multi-modality cascaded convolutional neural networks for Alzheimer's disease diagnosis. Neuroinformatics. 2018;16(3–4):295–308. https://doi.org/10.1007/s12021-018-9370-4.
11. Mehmood A, Maqsood M, Bashir M, Shuyuan Y. A deep siamese convolution neural network for multiclass classification of Alzheimer disease. Brain Sci. 2020;10(2) https://doi.org/10.3390/brainsci10020084.
12. Rajpurkar P, Irvin J, Zhu K, Yang B, Mehta H, Duan T, et al. Chexnet: radiologist-level pneumonia detection on chest x-rays with deep learning. arXiv preprint arXiv:171105225. 2017.
13. Zhou B, Khosla A, Lapedriza A, Oliva A, Torralba A. Learning deep features for discriminative localization. In: Proceedings of the IEEE conference on computer vision and pattern recognition; 2016. p. 2921–9.
14. Zintgraf LM, Cohen TS, Adel T, Welling M. Visualizing deep neural network decisions: prediction difference analysis. arXiv preprint arXiv:170204595. 2017.
15. Choi H, Kim YK, Yoon EJ, Lee JY, Lee DS. Cognitive signature of brain FDG PET based on deep learning: domain transfer from Alzheimer's disease to Parkinson's disease. Eur J Nucl Med Mol Imaging. 2020;47(2):403–12. https://doi.org/10.1007/s00259-019-04538-7.
16. Dorsey ER, Constantinescu R, Thompson JP, Biglan KM, Holloway RG, Kieburtz K, et al. Projected number of people with Parkinson disease in the most populous nations, 2005 through 2030. Neurology. 2007;68(5):384–6. https://doi.org/10.1212/01.wnl.0000247740.47667.03.
17. Jankovic J. Parkinson's disease: clinical features and diagnosis. J Neurol Neurosurg Psychiatry. 2008;79(4):368–76. https://doi.org/10.1136/jnnp.2007.131045.
18. Gratwicke J, Jahanshahi M, Foltynie T. Parkinson's disease dementia: a neural networks perspective. Brain J Neurol. 2015;138(Pt 6):1454–76. https://doi.org/10.1093/brain/awv104.
19. Brooks DJ. Molecular imaging of dopamine transporters. Ageing Res Rev. 2016;30:114–21. https://doi.org/10.1016/j.arr.2015.12.009.
20. Brücke T, Djamshidian S, Bencsits G, Pirker W, Asenbaum S, Podreka I. SPECT and PET imaging of the dopaminergic system in Parkinson's disease. J Neurol. 2000;247(Suppl 4):Iv/2-7. https://doi.org/10.1007/pl00007769.
21. Wu Y, Jiang JH, Chen L, Lu JY, Ge JJ, Liu FT, et al. Use of radiomic features and support vector machine to distinguish Parkinson's disease cases from normal controls. Ann Translat Med. 2019;7(23):773. https://doi.org/10.21037/atm.2019.11.26.
22. Katako A, Shelton P, Goertzen AL, Levin D, Bybel B, Aljuaid M, et al. Machine learning identified an Alzheimer's disease-related FDG-PET pattern which is also expressed in Lewy body dementia and Parkinson's disease dementia. Sci Rep. 2018;8(1):13236. https://doi.org/10.1038/s41598-018-31653-6.
23. Zhang YC, Kagen AC. Machine learning interface for medical image analysis. J Digit Imaging. 2017;30(5):615–21. https://doi.org/10.1007/s10278-016-9910-0.
24. Augimeri A, Cherubini A, Cascini GL, Galea D, Caligiuri ME, Barbagallo G, et al. CADA-computer-aided DaTSCAN analysis. EJNMMI Phys. 2016;3(1):4. https://doi.org/10.1186/s40658-016-0140-9.
25. Oliveira FP, Castelo-Branco M. Computer-aided diagnosis of Parkinson's disease based on [(123)I]FP-CIT SPECT binding potential images, using the voxels-as-features approach and support vector machines. J Neural Eng. 2015;12(2):026008. https://doi.org/10.1088/1741-2560/12/2/026008.
26. Huertas-Fernández I, García-Gómez FJ, García-Solís D, Benítez-Rivero S, Marín-Oyaga VA, Jesús S, et al. Machine learning models for the differential diagnosis of vascular parkinsonism and Parkinson's disease using [(123)I]FP-CIT SPECT. Eur J Nucl Med Mol

Imaging. 2015;42(1):112–9. https://doi.org/10.1007/s00259-014-2882-8.

27. Illan IA, Gorrz JM, Ramirez J, Segovia F, Jimenez-Hoyuela JM, Ortega Lozano SJ. Automatic assistance to Parkinson's disease diagnosis in DaTSCAN SPECT imaging. Med Phys. 2012;39(10):5971–80. https://doi.org/10.1118/1.4742055.

28. Shiiba T, Arimura Y, Nagano M, Takahashi T, Takaki A. Improvement of classification performance of Parkinson's disease using shape features for machine learning on dopamine transporter single photon emission computed tomography. PLoS One. 2020;15(1):e0228289. https://doi.org/10.1371/journal.pone.0228289.

29. Walker Z, Gandolfo F, Orini S, Garibotto V, Agosta F, Arbizu J, et al. Clinical utility of FDG PET in Parkinson's disease and atypical parkinsonism associated with dementia. Eur J Nucl Med Mol Imaging. 2018;45(9):1534–45. https://doi.org/10.1007/s00259-018-4031-2.

30. Zhao Y, Cumming P, Rominger A, Zuo C, Shi K, Wu P, et al. A 3D deep residual convolutional neural network for differential diagnosis of parkinsonian syndromes on (18)F-FDG PET images. In: Conference proceedings: annual international conference of the IEEE engineering in medicine and biology society IEEE engineering in medicine and biology society annual conference. 2019; p. 3531–4. https://doi.org/10.1109/embc.2019.8856747.

31. Shen T, Jiang J, Lin W, Ge J, Wu P, Zhou Y, et al. Use of overlapping group LASSO sparse deep belief network to discriminate Parkinson's disease and normal control. Front Neurosci. 2019;13:396. https://doi.org/10.3389/fnins.2019.00396.

32. Bouter C, Henniges P, Franke TN, Irwin C, Sahlmann CO, Sichler ME, et al. (18)F-FDG-PET detects drastic changes in brain metabolism in the Tg4-42 model of Alzheimer's disease. Front Aging Neurosci. 2018;10:425. https://doi.org/10.3389/fnagi.2018.00425.

33. Blanc-Durand P, Van Der Gucht A, Schaefer N, Itti E, Prior JO. Automatic lesion detection and segmentation of 18F-FET PET in gliomas: a full 3D U-net convolutional neural network study. PLoS One. 2018;13(4):e0195798. https://doi.org/10.1371/journal.pone.0195798.

34. Yi X, Walia E, Babyn P. Generative adversarial network in medical imaging: a review. Med Image Anal. 2019;58:101552. https://doi.org/10.1016/j.media.2019.101552.

35. Oh KT, Lee S, Lee H, Yun M, Yoo SK. Semantic segmentation of white matter in FDG-PET using generative adversarial network. J Digit Imaging. 2020;33(4):816–25. https://doi.org/10.1007/s10278-020-00321-5.

36. Nie D, Wang L, Gao Y, Shen D. Fully convolutional networks for multi-modality isointense infant brain image segmentation. Proc IEEE Int Symp Biomed Imag. 2016;2016:1342–5. https://doi.org/10.1109/isbi.2016.7493515.

37. Zhang W, Li R, Deng H, Wang L, Lin W, Ji S, et al. Deep convolutional neural networks for multi-modality isointense infant brain image segmenta-tion. NeuroImage. 2015;108:214–24. https://doi.org/10.1016/j.neuroimage.2014.12.061.

38. Erten-Lyons D, Woltjer R, Kaye J, Mattek N, Dodge HH, Green S, et al. Neuropathologic basis of white matter hyperintensity accumulation with advanced age. Neurology. 2013;81(11):977–83. https://doi.org/10.1212/WNL.0b013e3182a43e45.

39. Fiford CM, Manning EN, Bartlett JW, Cash DM, Malone IB, Ridgway GR, et al. White matter hyperintensities are associated with disproportionate progressive hippocampal atrophy. Hippocampus. 2017;27(3):249–62. https://doi.org/10.1002/hipo.22690.

40. Liu CK, Miller BL, Cummings JL, Mehringer CM, Goldberg MA, Howng SL, et al. A quantitative MRI study of vascular dementia. Neurology. 1992;42(1):138–43. https://doi.org/10.1212/wnl.42.1.138.

41. Scheltens P, Barkhof F, Leys D, Pruvo JP, Nauta JJ, Vermersch P, et al. A semiquantitative rating scale for the assessment of signal hyperintensities on magnetic resonance imaging. J Neurol Sci. 1993;114(1):7–12. https://doi.org/10.1016/0022-510x(93)90041-v.

42. An HJ, Seo S, Kang H, Choi H, Cheon GJ, Kim HJ, et al. MRI-based attenuation correction for PET/MRI using multiphase level-set method. J Nucl Med. 2016;57(4):587–93. https://doi.org/10.2967/jnumed.115.163550.

43. Keereman V, Fierens Y, Broux T, De Deene Y, Lonneux M, Vandenberghe S. MRI-based attenuation correction for PET/MRI using ultrashort echo time sequences. J Nucl Med. 2010;51(5):812–8. https://doi.org/10.2967/jnumed.109.065425.

44. Rausch I, Rust P, DiFranco MD, Lassen M, Stadlbauer A, Mayerhoefer ME, et al. Reproducibility of MRI Dixon-based attenuation correction in combined PET/MR with applications for lean body mass estimation. J Nucl Med. 2016;57(7):1096–101. https://doi.org/10.2967/jnumed.115.168294.

45. Sekine T, Ter Voert EE, Warnock G, Buck A, Huellner M, Veit-Haibach P, et al. Clinical evaluation of zero-echo-time attenuation correction for brain 18F-FDG PET/MRI: comparison with atlas attenuation correction. J Nucl Med. 2016;57(12):1927–32. https://doi.org/10.2967/jnumed.116.175398.

46. Vandenberghe S, Marsden PK. PET-MRI: a review of challenges and solutions in the development of integrated multimodality imaging. Phys Med Biol. 2015;60(4):R115–54. https://doi.org/10.1088/0031-9155/60/4/r115.

47. Hwang D, Kang SK, Kim KY, Seo S, Paeng JC, Lee DS, et al. Generation of PET attenuation map for whole-body time-of-flight (18)F-FDG PET/MRI using a deep neural network trained with simultaneously reconstructed activity and attenuation maps. J Nucl Med. 2019;60(8):1183–9. https://doi.org/10.2967/jnumed.118.219493.

48. Liu F, Jang H, Kijowski R, Bradshaw T, McMillan AB. Deep learning MR imaging-based attenuation correction for PET/MR imaging. Radiology. 2018;286(2):676–84. https://doi.org/10.1148/radiol.2017170700.

49. Choi H, Lee DS. Generation of structural MR images from amyloid PET: application to MR-less quantification. J Nucl Med. 2018;59(7):1111–7. https://doi.org/10.2967/jnumed.117.199414.

50. Badawi RD, Shi H, Hu P, Chen S, Xu T, Price PM, et al. First human imaging studies with the EXPLORER total-body PET scanner. J Nucl Med. 2019;60(3):299–303. https://doi.org/10.2967/jnumed.119.226498.

51. Cherry SR, Jones T, Karp JS, Qi J, Moses WW, Badawi RD. Total-body PET: maximizing sensitivity to create new opportunities for clinical research and patient care. J Nucl Med. 2018;59(1):3–12. https://doi.org/10.2967/jnumed.116.184028.

52. Caribe P, Koole M, D'Asseler Y, Van Den Broeck B, Vandenberghe S. Noise reduction using a Bayesian penalized-likelihood reconstruction algorithm on a time-of-flight PET-CT scanner. EJNMMI Phys. 2019;6(1):22. https://doi.org/10.1186/s40658-019-0264-9.

53. Ashrafinia S, Mohy-Ud-Din H, Karakatsanis NA, Jha AK, Casey ME, Kadrmas DJ, et al. Generalized PSF modeling for optimized quantitation in PET imaging. Phys Med Biol. 2017;62(12):5149–79. https://doi.org/10.1088/1361-6560/aa6911.

54. Liu CC, Qi J. Higher SNR PET image prediction using a deep learning model and MRI image.

Phys Med Biol. 2019;64(11):115004. https://doi.org/10.1088/1361-6560/ab0dc0.

55. Kaplan S, Zhu YM. Full-dose PET image estimation from low-dose PET image using deep learning: a pilot study. J Digit Imaging. 2019;32(5):773–8. https://doi.org/10.1007/s10278-018-0150-3.

56. Xu J, Gong E, Pauly J, Zaharchuk G. 200x low-dose PET reconstruction using deep learning. arXiv preprint arXiv:171204119. 2017.

57. Chen KT, Gong E, de Carvalho Macruz FB, Xu J, Boumis A, Khalighi M, et al. Ultra-low-dose (18) F-florbetaben amyloid PET imaging using deep learning with multi-contrast MRI inputs. Radiology. 2019;290(3):649–56. https://doi.org/10.1148/radiol.2018180940.

58. Ouyang J, Chen KT, Gong E, Pauly J, Zaharchuk G. Ultra-low-dose PET reconstruction using generative adversarial network with feature matching and task-specific perceptual loss. Med Phys. 2019;46(8):3555–64. https://doi.org/10.1002/mp.13626.

59. Kim J, Kang S, Lee K, Jung JH, Kim G, Lim HK, et al. Effect of scan time on neuro 18 F-fluorodeoxyglucose positron emission tomography image generated using deep learning. J Med Imag Health In. 2020;10:1–7. https://doi.org/10.1166/jmihi.2020.3316.

AI/ML Imaging Applications in Body Oncology

10

Robert Seifert and Peter Herhaus

Contents

R. Seifert (✉)
Department of Nuclear Medicine,
University Hospital Essen, Essen, Germany
e-mail: robert.seifert@uk-essen.de

P. Herhaus
Internal Medicine III, Hematology and Medical
Oncology, Technische Universität München,
Munich, Germany

10.1 General Principles

In the following, the structure of the chapter is outlined and general principles as well as issues of artificial intelligence (AI) in nuclear medicine are discussed. There is no clear definition of AI in medical imaging nor a clear demarcation to conventional analysis techniques. Thus, other advanced image analysis methods like radiomics are summarized in this chapter as well.

© The Author(s), under exclusive license to Springer Nature Switzerland AG 2022
P. Veit-Haibach, K. Herrmann (eds.), *Artificial Intelligence/Machine Learning in Nuclear Medicine and Hybrid Imaging*, https://doi.org/10.1007/978-3-031-00119-2_10

The utilization of AI for detecting diseases in medical image data is rapidly emerging [1]. Consequently, AI in nuclear medicine has been widely employed for image data, and also for electronic health record data [2]. When applied to image data, AI may be used to determine the stage according to an existing staging system (like the bone scan index), to improve an existing staging system (e.g. by simplification of TIRADS), to generate new staging systems that are to complex or too time-consuming to be performed by medical experts (e.g. whole-body tumor volume quantification in PET-CTs) or to directly predict a clinically relevant endpoint (e.g. estimate grading of tumor, predict overall survival time). When applied to electronic health record data, AI may be used to predict endpoints as well. Additional approaches seem promising, like the utilization of artificial intelligence to form real-world control groups for image centric trial, as has been demonstrated for therapeutic trials [3].

An organ-wise structure is chosen to organize this chapter, as it focuses on the application of AI to oncological imaging. However, as AI is emerging in the field of nuclear medicine, two underlying trends can be observed: whole-body tumor volume quantification and individual lesion delineation. Quantification of the molecular whole-body tumor volume (e.g. ^{18}F-FDG or PSMA avid tumor parts in contrast to morphological tumor volume) is feasible using semi-automated approaches that facilitate the quantification by AI methods. Yet, medial expert interaction is still needed to obtain valid results. Such quantification approaches are clinically needed, as the whole-body tumor volume might be a more precise parameter to assess the extent of an oncological disease [4]. Moreover, quantifying of the whole-body tumor volume might enable more precise therapy response monitoring. The second trend is to automatically delineate and grade malignancy suspicious lesions in nuclear medicine imaging by employing AI. This is a more complex and error prone task, compared to just providing assistance to medical experts. However, several studies that are presented here could demonstrate extremely promising results (e.g. fully automatic delineation of all malignancy suspicious lesions). Therefore, both the tumor volume quantification trend and individual lesion delineation trend will ultimately merge when lesion-wise classification becomes even better and is thus suited for tumor volume quantification.

There are some unsolved issues regarding the application of AI in the field of nuclear medicine and especially in oncological settings. As outlined, the quantification of the tumor volume comes into focus of many software tools that analyze PET-CT data. Yet, there is no consensus how to determine a reference standard for tumor volume quantification. It may be evident, that morphological information (e.g. obtained from the CT component) is not ideal as reference to assess the molecular volume. However, there are several strategies for the segmentation of PET volume as well, like applying a fixed threshold (e.g. every voxel >6 SUV is tumor), applying relative thresholding (e.g. 50% of local SUV_{max}), or others. Future studies have to evaluate which tumor segmentation method is closest to the actual tumor volume and should therefore be used as reference standard for AI algorithms. To this end, it might be warranted to employ the concept of probabilistic segmentations that addresses issues arising from inter- and intra-rater variance in tumor segmentations [5]. Finally, one has to bear in mind that it is at least as difficult to develop AI for a specific task as proving its incremental benefit for the patient and implementing it in the clinical routine [6, 7].

10.2 Brain

10.2.1 Glioma

The characterization of cerebral gliomas has moved from a morphological-based classification to molecular profiling, comprising of markers like IDH1 mutation status [8]. This is due to the heterogeneity of gliomas, which cannot sufficiently be differentiated by conventional imaging. Therefore, molecular imaging approaches together with machine learning methods have been proposed to enable an improved noninvasive glioma profiling. Kebir et al. could show that ^{11}C-MET PET and machine learning enabled the noninvasive diagnosis of the IDH1 status of gliomas; an area under the curve (AUC) of 0.79 was reached [9]. However, the analyzed patient collective was relatively small ($n = 39$) and future corroborating studies are needed.

Haubold et al. employed multiparametric ^{18}F-FET PET-MR to noninvasively estimate grading and molecular profiles of gliomas [10]. Interestingly, the integration of ^{18}F-FET features (like SUV_{max}) into the multiparametric MRI features has improved the estimation neither of grading nor of molecular profiling. For example, the estimation of IDH1 status had an AUC of 88% (excluding PET features). Yet again, the patient collective was relatively small ($n = 42$), especially given the large number of 19.284 features that were extracted for each patient.

10.3 Neck

10.3.1 Head and Neck Cancer

^{18}F-FDG PET-CT is a reference standard examination for the detection of cervical lymph node metastases of patients with head and neck cancer; especially, if subsequent radiotherapy is planned [11]. However, the differentiation between physiological lymph nodes and suspicious lymph node metastases in ^{18}F-FDG PET-CT might be challenging. To this end, Chen et al. have proposed a tool which combines both radiomics and 3D convolutional neuronal networks for the characterization of cervical lymph node metastases using PET-CT [12]. Unfortunately, the patient collective was small ($n = 59$) and the reference standard for nodal involvement was an expert rating.

Huang et al. proposed a method for the automated delineation of head and neck cancer using PET-CT data and demonstrated its feasibility [13]. Yet, despite the use of bicentric data, the generalizability of the presented approach still needs to be proven. Zhao et al. have followed a similar approach and aimed at the automated delineation of nasopharyngeal carcinoma on PET-CT data [14]. The authors adopted the U-Net design which used both PET and CT images as input and achieved a dice score (which is a measure of segmentation accuracy) of 87.5%.

10.3.2 Thyroid Cancer

Thyroid nodules are frequently seen on ultrasound examinations; however, only a small fraction of thyroid nodules is caused by thyroid cancer [15]. To facilitate the characterization of thyroid nodules as either malignancy suspicious or benign, the ACR TI-RADS system has been proposed [16]. ACR TI-RADS comprises five categories (like echogenicity or shape) and allocates a score for the degree of each category. The sum of all five category scores stratifies the likelihood of the presence of thyroid cancer. The likelihood of cancer is in turn graded in five categories (1-benign to 5-highly suspicious). Despite good reason for the individual categories, no study could corroborate a given score (e.g. in the echogenicity category, the hyperechoic criterium has a score of 1, whereas hyoechoic has a score of 2). Therefore, Wildman-Tobriner et al. used AI to evaluate, if the individual scores of ultrasound features were appropriate or if ACR TI-RADS could be simplified. Interestingly, the scores of their revised ACR TI-RADS called AI TI-RADS were indeed simplified (e.g. hyperechoic criterium got a score of 0 and was therefore neglectable, whereas hypoechoic remained with score of 2). Moreover, the authors could corroborate that the sensitivity of AI TI-RADS remained high compared to conventional ACR TI-RADS (93%), whereas the specificity of AI TI-RADS increased compared to ACR TI-RADS (65% vs. 47%). This interesting work could facilitate the use of this manual classification system and might be expanded to other classifications as well.

Instead of training a neuronal network to estimate an ACT TI-RADS score (or a similar classification), some groups directly used the histological classification as ground truth for training and evaluation. Ko et al. could show that a convolutional neuronal network obtained high AUC results (0.835–0.850) and was not statistically differed form radiologists (AUC: 0.805–0.860) [17]. Importantly, histological ground truth was present for all patients. There have also been reports on optimized network architectures dedicated to ultrasound images of thyroid cancer [18]. Li et al. presented a retrospective multicenter study evaluating the performance of a neuronal network in detecting thyroid cancer by ultrasound images, which comprised 45.644 patients [19]. Importantly, external validation cohorts were present as well. For the internal validation cohort, both sensitivity (93.4%) and specificity (86.1%) were remarkably high. The authors concluded that sensitivity was similar to a group of skilled radiologists, but the specificity was statistically significantly improved.

10.4 Thorax

10.4.1 Lung Cancer

Fluorodeoxyglucose (^{18}F-FDG) PET-CT is the standard diagnostic tool for the staging of patients with lung cancer [20]. Sibille et al. developed a software for the automated segmentation of suspicious FDG foci using acquisitions of 302 lung cancer patients amongst other patients [21]. The proposed software runs fully automatically and estimates not only the classification of each ^{18}F-FDG hot spot (suspicious i.e. metastasis vs. not suspicious i.e. physiologic) but also the anatomical location of each hot spot (e.g. lymph node level). The accuracies both of classification (AUC = 0.98) and of anatomical location (accuracy = 97% for body part, 84% for organ or tissue) were remarkably high. Interestingly, the proposed neuronal network did not segment the ^{18}F-FDG foci in the PET acquisition, but in contrast analyzed hotspots found by conventional thresholding. This procedure might lead to inaccuracies, as confluent lesions or confluence between a metastasis and an organ with physiological ^{18}F-FDG accumulation might not be separated properly by conventional thresholding. The neuronal networks used by this software require the input of coronal reformatted image data. Each tracer accumulation is analyzed separately and

only its immediate vicinity is present to the network. Because of that, the input of the entire PET as maximum intensity projection (MIP) significantly improved the accuracy. Similar to the human perception, the MIP and other reformations may facilitate the recognition of global uptake patterns, e.g. caused by brown adipose tissue activation. Additionally, CT information was used in conjunction with the PET as input for the neuronal network and significantly improved the accuracy compared to PET only inputs. Future studies have to evaluate the predictive potential of the automatically determined ^{18}F-FDG tumor volume.

10.5 Abdomen

10.5.1 Esophageal Cancer

Beukinga et al. used ^{18}F-FDG PET examinations before and after neoadjuvant radio chemotherapy to predict the outcome of patients suffering from esophageal cancer [22]. The authors extracted radiomic features, which combined with the T-stage could predict complete pathologic response with high accuracy (AUC = 0.81). However, only 73 patients were included in this study, which might limit the transferability to larger or inhomogeneous patient collectives.

10.5.2 Liver Tumor

Radioembolization with ^{90}Y spheres is a therapeutic option for patients with liver metastases or primary hepatic tumor and also known as selective internal radioembolization (SIRT). Due to impairment of uninvolved liver tissue and generally end stage disease, the prediction of overall survival prior to SIRT is clinically needed. Therefore, Ingirsch et al. had retrospectively analyzed electronic health records (e.g. blood level of bilirubin, age) of 366 patients that received ^{90}Y radioembolization by using machine learning methods [23]. The authors identified baseline cholinesterase and bilirubin levels as predictor for overall survival after SIRT.

10.5.3 Prostate Cancer

Prostate cancer is the leading cause of cancer-related death in men and has a remarkably early tendency to form metastases; already at time of prostatectomy, approximately 70% of men show prostate cancer cell in the bone marrow [24]. The sensitive detection of metastases as well as monitoring of the whole-body tumor load is of great clinical importance. To this end, prostate-specific membrane antigen (PSMA) targeting PET-CT has been widely employed and could demonstrate superior performance both in primary and recurrent prostate cancer [25, 26]. Several AI-based approaches have tried to analyze PSMA-PET examinations with regard to individual lesion classification and whole-body tumor volume.

Zhao et al. have developed a neuronal network for the delineation of PSMA avid metastases in the pelvic area [27]. The authors had adopted the U-Net architecture to include both PET and CT slices as input and aimed at a voxel wise segmentation of prostate cancer metastases [28]. The network employs axial, coronal and sagittal reformations as input to mimic the reading of a human expert. For training and evaluation, metastases were manually delineated by nuclear medicine experts in 193 PSMA PET acquisitions; their delineations were used as ground truth data. The limitation to the pelvic region was necessary due to proof of concept nature of the publication; however, extension to the whole body seems also feasible. The work of Zhao et al. is of great relevance, as it enables the fully automated segmentation of prostate cancer metastases with great precision (99%) and recall (99%). However, because of point spread artifacts, it could prove disadvantageous that the proposed neuronal network outputs the tumor segmentation.

Gafita et al. proposed an open source software (qPSMA) for the semi-automated quantification of the whole-body tumor burden in PSMA-PET CTs [29]. Despite the name prostate-specific membrane antigen, PSMA shows physiological accumulation in many organs, like in liver, spleen, bowel, kidneys, salivary glands and others. The qPSMA software assists the reading physician in segmenting all prostate cancer metastases by excluding some organs with physiological update from the analysis. To this end, a random forest-based algorithm is used by qPSMA to segment organs with physiological PSMA accumulation employing the CT component [30]. The qPSMA software not only masks out physiological PSMA uptake, but likewise segments PSMA foci with a patient specific SUV threshold. Each voxel exceeding this threshold is regarded as metastases, if it is not manually or automatically excluded. In addition, qPSMA enables the adjustment of predefined organ exclusion masks and facilitates the exclusion or inclusion of missed PSMA foci using brush tools. For example, liver metastases had to be added manually due to the heuristic logic that the liver uptake is physiologic, and the entire liver therefore be removed from the analysis. The inter-rater and intra-rater correlation of qPSMA is high for the segmentation of individual metastasis.

An approach similar to qPSMA was proposed by Seifert et al. [31]. Likewise, it facilitates the semiautomated quantification of the whole-body tumor volume by excluding physiologic PSMA foci from the analysis. Moreover, it automatically assigns the anatomical location to each PSMA focus. In contrast to qPSMA, the software employs a two-step approach for delineation of foci: first, voxels exceeding a patient-specific threshold are selected as candidate lesions. Second, these candidate lesions were segmented by thresholding with 50% of the local SUV_{max}. Thereby, no brush tools are needed for refinement; physiological candidate lesions can be deleted easily. The author could show that this procedure achieves a high inter-rater agreement. Interestingly, the authors also reported that semi-automatically quantified whole-body tumor volume stratified end-stage prostate cancer patients according to the overall survival.

10.6 Skeleton

10.6.1 Bone Metastases

Bone scans are primarily used for the detection and monitoring of bone metastases and one of the high throughput examinations of nuclear medicine. Especially for therapy monitoring of prostate cancer patients, bone scans are an established imaging method [32]. However, the interpretation of bone scans to calculate a quantitative biomarker, which is called bone scan index (BSI), is time-consuming [33, 34]. To calculate the BSI, at first, the fraction of metastatic involvement of each bone has to be calculated. Second, this fraction is multiplied with the fraction that the bone constitutes to the entire skeleton. By summation of all values, the BSI is obtained. Thereby, BSI represents the fraction of metastatically affected bone, i.e. a BSI of 3 means that 3% of the entire skeletal mass is affected by metastases.

Several solutions have been proposed to automatically quantify the BSI. Among them is the work of Ulmert et al., who proposed a method which uses neuronal networks for the automated segmentation and classification of hotspots in bone scans [35]. Interestingly, the development of the first prototype dates back to 2006, where AI was not the now established buzzword, which might be the reason why the authors called their work "computer-based decision support system" [36]. The automatically derived BSI could statistically significant stratify prostate cancer patients according to overall survival [37].

As mentioned above, PSMA-PET-CT has emerged as reference standard examination for patients with prostate cancer. Therefore, the quantification of the osseous tumor volume from PSMA-PET-CT, similar to the BSI, is of importance. To this end, Bieth et al. have proposed a software for the quantification of the osseous tumor burden using PSMA-PET-CT acquisitions [38]. Hammes et al. followed a similar approach (EBONI) and provided the source code of their software [39].

10.7 Hematopoietic System

10.7.1 Lymphoma

^{18}F-FDG -PET-CT is a standard diagnostic for staging and therapy monitoring of lymphoma patients. However, due to highly variable physiological ^{18}F-FDG uptake, the interpretation of ^{18}F-FDG PET acquisitions is challenging, especially for neuronal networks. The software proposed by Sibille et al. that was already presented above was not only trained using lung cancer patients, but with ^{18}F-FDG PET-CTs of lymphoma patients (n = 327) as well [21]. Therefore, the software obtained high accuracy in the classification (AUC = 0.95) and the determination of the anatomical location (Accuracy = 97% for body part and 84% for organ or tissue). Thereby, the automatic quantification of a whole-body tumor volume is feasible. Future studies have to elucidate if the automatically determined tumor volume can stratify patients according to their overall survival or other clinically relevant end points.

10.7.2 Multiple Myeloma

Multiple myeloma (MM) is a clonal plasma cell neoplasia and detection of bone lesions is crucial during diagnostic work-up. MM lesions not only display an important criterion for the initiation of treatment but moreover discriminate MM from pre-malignant diseases such as monoclonal gammopathy of undetermined significance. Whole body low-dose CT is the gold standard in MM, but MRI is attributed with a higher sensitivity in the detection of small MM lesions. CXCR4-directed PET imaging with ^{68}Ga-Pentixafor represents another imaging modality for the detection of active MM lesions.

Martínez-Martínez et al. have developed a fully automated method that identifies bone marrow infiltration in low-dose CT of MM patients [40]. Their method was validated on a dataset of

127 subjects where it was able to discriminate bone marrow infiltration in patients with MM from healthy controls with an AUC of 0.996. The limitation of their study is that their method is only validated for the bone marrow infiltration in the femur. However, lesion distribution in MM patients ranges from a single lesion to multiple lesions with a disseminated pattern and those lesions do not necessarily have to affect the femur.

An automated approach to determine whole-body bone lesions in MM patients was conducted by Xu et al. [41]. The combination of ^{68}Ga-Pentixafor PET that registers elevated CXCR4-expression within MM lesions with anatomical features from the CT-scan was used in this study. Two CNNs (V-Net and W-Net) were used for the segmentation and detection of MM lesions. Their study that was first verified in digital phantoms ($n = 120$) and further validated in a small patient cohort ($n = 12$) revealed that the W-Net architecture with the combination of PET and CT data was most accurate in lesion detection and achieved a dice-score of 73%. However, this study was mainly conducted on digital phantoms and further validation in a bigger patient cohort and correlation to clinical parameters such as treatment response or overall survival has to be evaluated.

References

1. Liu X, Faes L, Kale AU, et al. A comparison of deep learning performance against health-care professionals in detecting diseases from medical imaging: a systematic review and meta-analysis. Lancet Digit Heal. 2019;1:e271–97.
2. Nensa F, Demircioglu A, Rischpler C. Artificial intelligence in nuclear medicine. J Nucl Med. 2019;60:29S–37S.
3. Feld E, Harton J, Meropol NJ, et al. Effectiveness of first-line immune checkpoint blockade versus carboplatin-based chemotherapy for metastatic urothelial cancer. Eur Urol. 2019;76:524–32.
4. Cottereau AS, Becker S, Broussais F, et al. Prognostic value of baseline total metabolic tumor volume (TMTV0) measured on FDG-PET/CT in patients with peripheral T-cell lymphoma (PTCL)+. Ann Oncol. 2016;27:719–24.
5. Kohl SAA, Romera-Paredes B, Maier-Hein KH, Rezende DJ, Eslami SMA, Kohli P, Zisserman A,
Ronneberger O. A hierarchical probabilistic U-net for modeling multi-scale ambiguities. 2019. p. 1–25.
6. Rajkomar A, Dean J, Kohane I, et al. The practical implementation of artificial intelligence technologies in medicine. Nat Med. 2019;25:15–8.
7. Wiens J, Saria S, Sendak M, et al. Do no harm: a roadmap for responsible machine learning for health care. Nat Med. 2019;25:1337–40.
8. Louis DN, Perry A, Reifenberger G, von Deimling A, Figarella-Branger D, Cavenee WK, Ohgaki H, Wiestler OD, Kleihues P, Ellison DW. The 2016 World Health Organization classification of tumors of the central nervous system: a summary. Acta Neuropathol. 2016;131:803–20.
9. Kebir S, Weber M, Lazaridis L, et al. Hybrid 11 C-MET PET/MRI combined with "machine learning" in glioma diagnosis according to the revised glioma WHO classification 2016. Clin Nucl Med. 2019;44:214–20.
10. Haubold J, Demircioglu A, Gratz M, et al. Non-invasive tumor decoding and phenotyping of cerebral gliomas utilizing multiparametric 18F-FET PET-MRI and MR fingerprinting. Eur J Nucl Med Mol Imaging. 2019;47(6):1435–45. https://doi.org/10.1007/s00259-019-04602-2.
11. Grégoire V, Lefebvre JL, Licitra L, Felip E. Squamous cell carcinoma of the head and neck: EHNS-ESMO-ESTRO clinical practice guidelines for diagnosis, treatment and follow-up. Ann Oncol. 2010;21:184–6.
12. Chen L, Zhou Z, Sher D, Zhang Q, Shah J, Pham N-L, Jiang S, Wang J. Combining many-objective radiomics and 3D convolutional neural network through evidential reasoning to predict lymph node metastasis in head and neck cancer. Phys Med Biol. 2019;64:075011.
13. Huang B, Chen Z, Wu PM, et al. Fully automated delineation of gross tumor volume for head and neck cancer on PET-CT using deep learning: a dual-center study. Contrast Media Mol Imaging. 2018;2018:8923028. https://doi.org/10.1155/2018/8923028.
14. Zhao L, Lu Z, Jiang J, Zhou Y, Wu Y, Feng Q. Automatic nasopharyngeal carcinoma segmentation using fully convolutional networks with auxiliary paths on dual-modality PET-CT images. J Digit Imaging. 2019;32:462–70.
15. Smith-Bindman R, Lebda P, Feldstein VA, Sellami D, Goldstein RB, Brasic N, Jin C, Kornak J. Risk of thyroid cancer based on thyroid ultrasound imaging characteristics. JAMA Intern Med. 2013;173:1788.
16. Tessler FN, Middleton WD, Grant EG, et al. ACR thyroid imaging, reporting and data system (TI-RADS): white paper of the ACR TI-RADS committee. J Am Coll Radiol. 2017;14:587–95.
17. Ko SY, Lee JH, Yoon JH, et al. Deep convolutional neural network for the diagnosis of thyroid nodules on ultrasound. Head Neck. 2019;41:885–91.
18. Li H, Weng J, Shi Y, Gu W, Mao Y, Wang Y, Liu W, Zhang J. An improved deep learning approach for detection of thyroid papillary cancer in ultrasound images. Sci Rep. 2018;8:1–12.

19. Li X, Zhang S, Zhang Q, et al. Diagnosis of thyroid cancer using deep convolutional neural network models applied to sonographic images: a retrospective, multicohort, diagnostic study. Lancet Oncol. 2019;20:193–201.

20. Planchard D, Popat S, Kerr K, et al. Metastatic non-small cell lung cancer: ESMO Clinical Practice Guidelines for diagnosis, treatment and follow-up. Ann Oncol. 2018;29:iv192–237.

21. Sibille L, Seifert R, Avramovic N, Vehren T, Spottiswoode B, Zuehlsdorff S, Schäfers M. 18 F-FDG PET/CT uptake classification in lymphoma and lung cancer by using deep convolutional neural networks. Radiology. 2019;294(2):445–52.

22. Beukinga RJ, Hulshoff JB, Mul VEM, Noordzij W, Kats-Ugurlu G, Slart RHJA, Plukker JTM. Prediction of response to neoadjuvant chemotherapy and radiation therapy with baseline and restaging 18F-FDG PET imaging biomarkers in patients with esophageal cancer. Radiology. 2018;287:983–92.

23. Ingrisch M, Schöppe F, Paprottka K, Fabritius M, Strobl FF, De Toni EN, Ilhan H, Todica A, Michl M, Paprottka PM. Prediction of 90 Y radioembolization outcome from pretherapeutic factors with random survival forests. J Nucl Med. 2018;59:769–73.

24. Morgan TM, Lange PH, Porter MP, Lin DW, Ellis WJ, Gallaher IS, Vessella RL. Disseminated tumor cells in prostate cancer patients after radical prostatectomy and without evidence of disease predicts biochemical recurrence. Clin Cancer Res. 2009;15:677–83.

25. Hofman MS, Lawrentschuk N, Francis RJ, et al. Prostate-specific membrane antigen PET-CT in patients with high-risk prostate cancer before curative-intent surgery or radiotherapy (proPSMA): a prospective, randomised, multi-centre study. Lancet. 2020;395(10231):1208–16. https://doi.org/10.1016/S0140-6736(20)30314-7.

26. Fendler WP, Calais J, Eiber M, et al. Assessment of 68Ga-PSMA-11 PET accuracy in localizing recurrent prostate cancer: a prospective single-arm clinical trial. JAMA Oncol. 2019;5:856–63.

27. Zhao Y, Gafita A, Vollnberg B, Tetteh G, Haupt F, Afshar-Oromieh A, Menze B, Eiber M, Rominger A, Shi K. Deep neural network for automatic characterization of lesions on 68Ga-PSMA-11 PET/CT. Eur J Nucl Med Mol Imaging. 2020;47:603–13.

28. Ronneberger O, Fischer P, Brox T. U-Net: convolutional networks for biomedical image segmentation. In: Medical image computing and computer assisted intervention – MICCAI 2015, Lecture notes in computer science; 2015. p. 234–41.

29. Gafita A, Bieth M, Krönke M, Tetteh G, Navarro F, Wang H, Günther E, Menze B, Weber WA, Eiber M. qPSMA: semiautomatic software for whole-body tumor burden assessment in prostate cancer using 68 ga-PSMA11 PET/CT. J Nucl Med. 2019;60:1277–83.

30. Bieth M, Peter L, Nekolla SG, Eiber M, Langs G, Schwaiger M, Menze B. Segmentation of skeleton and organs in whole-body CT images via iterative trilateration. IEEE Trans Med Imaging. 2017;36:2276–86.

31. Seifert R, Herrmann K, Kleesiek J, Schafers MA, Shah V, Xu Z, Chabin G, Garbic S, Spottiswoode B, Rahbar K. Semi-automatically quantified tumor volume using Ga-68-PSMA-11-PET as biomarker for survival in patients with advanced prostate cancer. J Nucl Med. 2020;61(12):1786–92. https://doi.org/10.2967/jnumed.120.242057.

32. Armstrong AJ, Al-Adhami M, Lin P, et al. Association between new unconfirmed bone lesions and outcomes in men with metastatic castration-resistant prostate cancer treated with enzalutamide: secondary analysis of the PREVAIL and AFFIRM randomized clinical trials. JAMA Oncol. 2020;6:217–25.

33. Erdi YE, Humm JL, Imbriaco M, Yeung H, Larson SM. Quantitative bone metastases analysis based on image segmentation. J Nucl Med. 1997;38:1401–6.

34. Imbriaco M, Larson SM, Yeung HW, Mawlawi OR, Erdi Y, Venkatraman ES, Scher HI. A new parameter for measuring metastatic bone involvement by prostate cancer: the bone scan index. Clin Cancer Res. 1998;4:1765–72.

35. Ulmert D, Kaboteh R, Fox JJ, et al. A novel automated platform for quantifying the extent of skeletal tumour involvement in prostate cancer patients using the bone scan index. Eur Urol. 2012;62:78–84.

36. Sadik M, Jakobsson D, Olofsson F, Ohlsson M, Suurkula M, Edenbrandt L. A new computer-based decision-support system for the interpretation of bone scans. Nucl Med Commun. 2006;27:417–23.

37. Armstrong AJ, Anand A, Edenbrandt L, et al. Phase 3 assessment of the automated bone scan index as a prognostic imaging biomarker of overall survival in men with metastatic castration-resistant prostate cancer a secondary analysis of a randomized clinical trial. JAMA Oncol. 2018;4:944–51.

38. Bieth M, Krönke M, Tauber R, Dahlbender M, Retz M, Nekolla SG, Menze B, Maurer T, Eiber M, Schwaiger M. Exploring new multimodal quantitative imaging indices for the assessment of osseous tumor burden in prostate cancer using 68Ga-PSMA PET/CT. J Nucl Med. 2017;58:1632–7.

39. Hammes J, Täger P, Drzezga A. EBONI: a tool for automated quantification of bone metastasis load in PSMA PET/CT. J Nucl Med. 2017;59:1070–5.

40. Martínez-Martínez F, Kybic J, Lambert L, Mecková Z. Fully automated classification of bone marrow infiltration in low-dose CT of patients with multiple myeloma based on probabilistic density model and supervised learning. Comput Biol Med. 2016;71:57–66.

41. Xu L, Tetteh G, Lipkova J, Zhao Y, Li H, Christ P, Piraud M, Buck A, Shi K, Menze BH. Automated whole-body bone lesion detection for multiple myeloma on 68 Ga-Pentixafor PET/CT imaging using deep learning methods. Contrast Media Mol Imaging. 2018;2018:1–11.

Artificial Intelligence/Machine Learning in Nuclear Medicine and Hybrid Imaging

11

Robert J. H. Miller, Jacek Kwiecinski, Damini Dey, and Piotr J. Slomka

Contents

R. J. H. Miller
Department of Imaging (Division of Nuclear Medicine), Medicine (Division of Artificial Intelligence in Medicine), Cardiology, and Biomedical Sciences, Cedars-Sinai Medical Center, Los Angeles, CA, USA

Department of Cardiac Sciences, University of Calgary and Libin Cardiovascular Institute, Calgary, AB, USA

J. Kwiecinski
Department of Imaging (Division of Nuclear Medicine), Medicine (Division of Artificial Intelligence in Medicine), Cardiology, and Biomedical Sciences, Cedars-Sinai Medical Center, Los Angeles, CA, USA

Department of Interventional Cardiology and Angiology, Institute of Cardiology, Warsaw, Poland

D. Dey · P. J. Slomka (✉)
Department of Imaging (Division of Nuclear Medicine), Medicine (Division of Artificial Intelligence in Medicine), Cardiology, and Biomedical Sciences, Cedars-Sinai Medical Center, Los Angeles, CA, USA
e-mail: slomka@cshs.org

Coronary artery disease (CAD) remains the leading cause of mortality and morbidity worldwide. Recent statistics estimate that 18.2 million adults age 20 and older have CAD (~7% of the population) [1]. CAD is the number one cause of death and disability and accounts for healthcare expenditures which are projected to exceed $1 trillion by year 2035 [1]. Cardiac imaging with echocardiography, myocardial perfusion imaging (single photon emission tomography [SPECT] and positron emission tomography [PET]), computed tomography, and magnetic resonance imaging play a key role in the diagnosis and management of CAD [2, 3]. These advanced imaging modalities, along with other clinical tests, generate extensive amounts of data whose volume, heterogeneity, and complexity have made human-driven analysis increasingly impractical. Artificial intelligence (AI) methods such as machine learning (ML) are particularly well-suited to tackling the challenges of such complex "Big Data" and have shown great promise in addressing classification, clustering, and predictive modeling tasks in cardiovascular research [4]. In cardiac imaging, AI has the potential to reduce costs and improve value throughout the stages of image acquisition, interpretation, and clinical decision-making. Moreover, the precision of diagnosis or risk prediction—now possible with comprehensive advanced cardiovascular imaging—combined with "big data" from electronic health records and pathology, is likely to better characterize disease and enable personalized therapy.

In this chapter we present recent AI techniques developed for the analysis of hybrid cardiac imaging data (SPECT, PET, and computed tomography [CT]), including methods to optimally integrate associated clinical information. These AI techniques include emerging methods for image reconstruction, image segmentation, disease diagnosis, and outcome prediction. Additionally, we will review methods to automatically extract additional structural information from the associated CT scans obtained with hybrid scanners. Since cardiac nuclear emission scanning is increasingly being acquired in conjunction with CT, this valuable data regarding cardiac anatomy can complement the functional information provided by SPECT and PET.

11.1 Introduction to AI

Computer algorithms which perform tasks normally characteristic of human intelligence such as understanding language and recognizing images are referred to as AI [4, 5]. ML is a branch of AI which uses existing observations to determine which features best predict the outcome of interest to more accurately predict the outcomes of future observations. ML algorithms are well suited to integrate the diverse clinical, stress, and imaging information generated by a hybrid imaging scan.

Deep learning (DL) is a subset of ML which refers to algorithms with a multilayered learning approach. DL can be trained using either structured or unstructured data; however, the most common approach is a convolutional neural network (CNN)—especially suitable to be applied to images [4, 6]. CNNs differ from other artificial neural networks in that the neurons from adjacent layers are only connected to nearby neurons in the following layer. DL algorithms are well-suited to directly extract information from cardiovascular and hybrid images. For all AI approaches, it is critical to ensure that a large, diverse data set is used for training the algorithm and that predictions are tested using data that was not used in any way during model training.

11.2 AI to Improve Image Quality and Processing

11.2.1 Image Denoising

CNNs by their nature are suitable for image classification and image transformation. They have the potential to improve image quality, reduce radiation exposure and shorten image acquisition in cardiovascular nuclear medicine. This can be achieved by a process which can be thought of as specialized filtering. Such image enhancement is typically accomplished by architectures referred to as convolutional autoencoders, U-nets being a frequently used architecture [7, 8]. These techniques have been successfully applied to denoising of CT images [9]. Ramon et al. demonstrated in 1052 subjects that higher quality images could be generated from low-dose SPECT MPI using a 3D CNN [10]. The CNN was formed with stacked autoencoders designed to predict full-dose images from low-dose image reconstructions. In simulations, images denoised with the CNN using 1/16th of the standard dose achieved similar image quality to simulated images with 1/8th of the dose denoised with a standard filtering approach [10]. Song et al. demonstrated that spatial resolution can be improved by using a 3D convolutional residual network. The authors compared their predicted images with standard dose and Gaussian post-filtering, showing a reduction of the normalized mean square error by 6.13% and 11.05%, respectively [11]. Ladefoged et al. evaluated the potential of denoising ^{18}F-fluorodeoxyglucose cardiac PET images with a deep learning model, trained in 146 patients and tested in 20 patients, simulating dose reductions as low as 1% of the injected dose [12]. Their denoising models were able to recover the PET signal for both the static and gated images at these low doses, showing that a significant dose reduction can be achieved for myocardial ^{18}F-fluorodeoxyglucose PET images, used for viability testing in patients with ischemic heart disease, without significant loss of diagnostic accuracy. Both 1% and 10% dose reductions are possible and provide quantitative metrics clinically comparable to those obtained with a full dose [12]. Our group performed a preliminary study of image denoising in order to substantially reduce the length of coronary ^{18}F sodium fluoride acquisitions [13]. In this study we obtained similar quantitative metrics from the images reconstructed from 3 min of list mode data with CNN processing as those from traditional reconstruction with the original 30-min acquisitions. These kinds of postprocessing techniques are easy to implement clinically and can be rapidly applied to reconstructed data.

11.2.2 Image Reconstruction

The aforementioned approaches have utilized DL as a post-processing method; however, it is also possible to apply DL directly within iterative reconstruction framework. For example, Shiri et al. developed a DL model to achieve image quality comparable to standard SPECT images from incomplete datasets, namely counts obtained after reduction of the acquisition time per projection or a reduction of the number of angular projections [14]. They demonstrated in 363 patients that the DL model was able to effectively recover image quality and reduced the bias in quantification metrics as compared to a standard iterative ordered subsets expectation maximization approach. The resulting images provided similar automatic quantitation of perfusion (stress total perfusion deficit) and function (volume, eccentricity and shape index) compared to conventional full acquisition studies [14]. DL-based reconstructions are being researched extensively in general PET imaging [15–19]— and it is just a matter of time until they will be tested for cardiovascular applications. Given this encouraging data, it appears that DL algorithms will increasingly be used both during image reconstruction and as a post-processing technique to improve image quality and reduce radiation exposure and acquisition times.

11.2.3 AI Applications in Attenuation Correction

During image reconstruction of SPECT or PET, attenuation correction is a mechanism that enables adjustment for the amount of tissue between the source of radiation (myocardium) and the detectors of the scanner. This is typically achieved by CT on a hybrid PET/CT scanner or less commonly by segmented MR on a PET/MR system. Such patient-specific attenuation correction improves the specificity and the accuracy of myocardial perfusion imaging in the diagnosis of CAD. However, the attenuation maps on the hybrid PET/CT or SPECT/CT need to be properly registered to the emission data in order for the correction to be accurate. Misregistration between the perfusion and CT attenuation corrected images often results in artifacts that affect the diagnostic accuracy of PET/CT [20, 21]

Automatic co-registration of SPECT/PET and non-contrast CT is challenging because of the scant anatomical landmarks and possibly grossly abnormal perfusion images. AI-based techniques have been developed to improve registration of SPECT perfusion and CT attenuation correction maps. Ko et al. developed a CNN-based algorithm, trained to predict the extent of misregistration (rigid translations) between images in 3-dimensions compared to manually co-registered SPECT/CT images [22]. The algorithm was trained in 402 cases and tested in 100 cases, with residual misalignment between image pairs of 1.71 ± 1.32 mm during training and 2.38 ± 2.00 mm during testing as compared to experienced operators.

DL methods could be also utilized for generating attenuation maps from the emission data itself. The advantage of such an approach is the perfect registration of the emission data and generated pseudo-CT data, thus potentially avoiding misregistration artifacts on a hybrid system. Moreover, the use of CT for attenuation purposes increases radiation exposure to patients, thus simulated CT scan can lower the overall patient dose. The feasibility of AI-based alternate attenuation correction maps has been demonstrated for brain and whole body PET imaging on PET/MR systems, where CT is not available [23, 24]. These methods could also be applied to cardiovascular imaging. Recently Shi et al. trained a DL algorithm to predict CT-attenuation maps from myocardial perfusion SPECT projection data and showed that the synthetic attenuation maps (pseudo-CT) were qualitatively and quantitatively consistent with the CT-based attenuation maps [25]. The globally normalized mean absolute error between the pseudo-CT and standard CT-based attenuation maps was 3.60% ± 0.85% among the 25 testing subjects. Importantly the normalized mean absolute error between the reconstructed SPECT images that were corrected using the pseudo-CT and CT-based attenuation maps was 0.26% ± 0.15%, whereas the localized absolute percentage error was 1.33% ± 3.80% in the left ventricle myocardium and 1.07% ± 2.58% in the blood pool. In the future such perfectly registered pseudo-CT attenuation maps could be used to routinely apply attenuation correction to SPECT or PET images without additional radiation exposure, even if CT images are not available.

11.2.4 Image Segmentation

Accurate myocardial segmentation is necessary to ensure high precision of subsequent image quantitation and interpretation in cardiac SPECT and PET. While the vast majority of SPECT and PET myocardial perfusion quantification software packages perform this process automatically utilizing standard image processing approaches, AI-based algorithms can potentially further improve this task and significantly reduce the need for manual adjustments. For example, in cardiac SPECT and PET analysis, an accurate definition of the mitral valve plane remains a problematic area for automatic segmentation and this frequently requires manual correction. Betancur et al. developed a novel method for automatic valve plane localization [26] ML- and validated it with the anatomical information from contrast CT angiography -obtained on the hybrid SPECT/CT scanner (Fig. 11.1). ML allowed them to encapsulate expert knowledge and capture the complex pattern changes caused by valve plane variations. Using a support-vector machines (SVM) algorithm, they combined features such as intensity, shape, and information from gated images to localize the most likely valve plane position. The SVM algorithm demonstrated close agreement with expert interpreters (bias of 1 mm), with tighter limits of agreement compared to two independent experts (−7 to 10 mm vs. −10 to 10 mm). Wang et al. described an end-to-end CNN to segment left ventricular myocardium by delineating its endocardial and epicardial surface [27]. Their approach, which included a loss function which encouraged similarity and penalized discrepancies between the prediction and training dataset, demonstrated excellent precision for left ventricular myocardial volume (mean error − 1.1 ± 3.7%) [27].

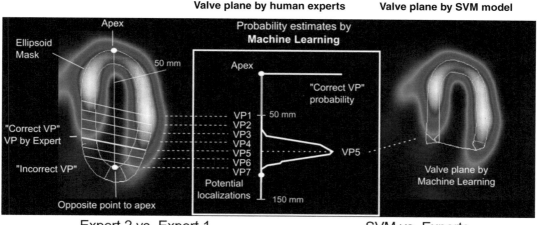

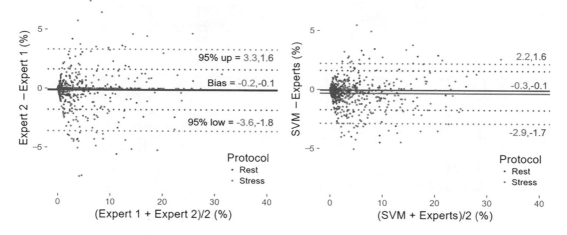

Fig. 11.1 Automatic valve plane localization (top). Bland-Altman difference plots show that global stress TPD (red) and rest TPD (blue) for valve plane positions were very similar between the results from two experts and automatic valve plan localization procedure (SVM) (bottom). This research was originally published in JNM. Betancur et al. Automatic Valve Plane Localization in Myocardial Perfusion SPECT/CT by Machine Learning: Anatomic and Clinical Validation. J Nucl Med. 2017;58:961–967. © SNMMI

11.2.5 CT Segmentation: Coronary Artery Calcium

Coronary artery calcium (CAC) is an unequivocal marker for atherosclerosis. Evidence to date has consistently shown that CAC accurately predicts cardiovascular events [28–36]. Non-contrast CT can reliably detect CAC [37, 38]—complementing MPI [39]. Hybrid PET/CT or SPECT/CT systems are capable of obtaining CAC CT scans. Quantification of CAC by CT provides an accurate measure of atherosclerotic burden [40].

We have shown the complementary role of CAC and PET scans (Fig. 11.2) and developed a combined PET+CAC score, which increased the diagnostic performance of PET [41, 42]. It has also been shown that myocardial flow reserve with PET and CAC provide complementary stratification of cardiac risk [43, 44]. CAC scan is low-cost and acquired without contrast, but does involve additional radiation and imaging time and therefore is not always performed. However, all current PET/CT MPI scans are acquired with ungated, low-dose CT scans for attenuation cor-

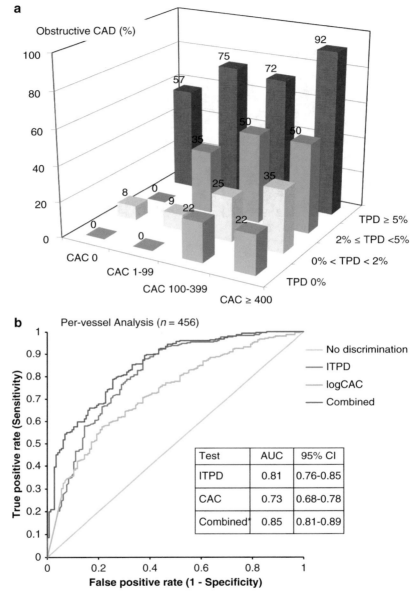

Fig. 11.2 (a) Prevalence of CAD as a function of CAC and total perfusion deficit (TPD) on a per-vessel basis (*n* = 456). Prevalence of obstructive coronary artery disease (CAD) across ischemic total perfusion deficit (ITPD) categories and coronary artery calcium (CAC) score categories (per-vessel analysis, *N* = 456). The "zero" risk of obstructive disease in vessels with either ITPD 0% or CAC score of 0, while the highest risk in vessels with either ITPD ≥5% or CAC score ≥400 was seen, *P* < 0.0001. (**b**) tenfold cross-validated receiver operating characteristics (ROC) analysis comparing combined per-formance of per-vessel ischemic total perfusion deficit (ITPD) and per-vessel coronary artery calcium score (CAC) versus ITPD alone in predicting obstructive CAD. * Asterisk indicates AUC of combined analysis—ITPD with per-vessel log CA. This research was originally published in JNM. Brodov et al. Combined Quantitative Assessment of Myocardial Perfusion and Coronary Artery Calcium Score by Hybrid 82Rb PET/CT Improves Detection of Coronary Artery Disease. J Nucl Med. 2015;56:1345–50. © SNMMI

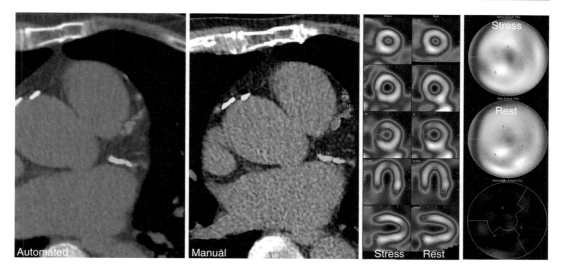

Fig. 11.3 Deep learning calcium detection on a CT attenuation scan from a hybrid scanner. Fully automated CNN (left) agrees with conventional manual calcium scoring (middle) of CTAC (red/green—coronary; yel- low—aorta) in a patient with high-risk multivessel disease (by invasive angiography) and a visually and quantitively normal SPECT MPI scan (right)

rection, which could also be used to estimate the CAC burden.

Currently CAC scoring is performed semi- automatically, where an operator selects areas of calcification, which are subsequently segmented automatically. AI was extensively used to develop automatic CAC scoring methods in diverse CT scans—beyond dedicated gated cardiac CAC scans. One approach involved a two-stage CNN developed to detect CAC [45], which was then evaluated in a large clinical study incorporating a wide range of CT scans [46]. Besides CAC scor- ing, DL methods have been used to detect cal- cium in the thoracic aorta and heart valves from low-dose, non-contrast chest CT [47]. Other methods have been proposed using DL with dual CNN to process scan rescan datasets simultane- ously, utilizing 5075 datasets for training and testing [48]. This approach achieved classifica- tion accuracy of 93% as compared with the expert interpretation. This method has also been applied to detect calcium from CT attenuation correc- tions scans obtained on hybrid scanners. In 133 consecutive patients undergoing myocardial per- fusion ^{82}Rubidium PET/CT, Isgum et al., showed good correlation between CAC scores derived from non-contrast CT attenuation maps obtained

on a hybrid PET/CT scanner and dedicated gated CAC scans [49]. Example of CAC segmentation performed by visual observer and DL is shown in Fig. 11.3. Such automatic segmentation of CT attenuation maps can provide valuable clinical information during reporting of hybrid imaging.

11.2.6 CT Segmentation: Epicardial Adipose Tissue

Beyond CAC, computed tomography also images the adipose (fat) tissue which surrounds the heart. While thoracic and epicardial adipose tissue (EAT) is currently not routinely measured or reported for cardiovascular risk assessment, EAT volume is emerging as an important predictor of adverse cardiovascular events and can therefore be used for risk stratification [50–54]. EAT can be obtained from routine non-contrast cardiac CT scans, but typically requires long manual pro- cessing times to measure. Fully automated meth- ods for segmentation of pericardial fat from cardiac CT have been proposed using DL meth- ods. Investigators developed fully automated CNN for EAT segmentation (QFAT) from non- contrast CT [55, 56]. This DL algorithm for EAT

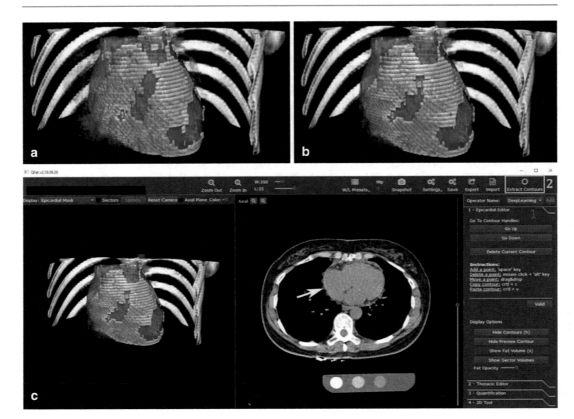

Fig. 11.4 Algorithm embedded in research software QFAT. Three-dimensional representations of epicardial adipose tissue (EAT) (EAT in pink overlaid on heart rendered in red), (**a**) as manually identified by the expert and, (**b**) as automatically identified by the algorithm. (**c**) Screenshot of QFAT software with the integrated deep learning approach. The pericardium is automatically identified (yellow arrow) by selecting a new operator (1, red) and by using the "extract contours" option (2, green). This research was originally published in Radiology: Artificial Intelligence. Commandeur et al. Fully Automated CT Quantification of Epicardial Adipose Tissue by Deep Learning: A Multicenter Study. Radiol Artif Intell. 2019;1 (6):e190045. © Radiological Society of North America

identification and quantification from non-contrast calcium scoring CT datasets was trained and validated with tenfold cross validation in 250 CT image sets by Commandeur et al. [56] The agreement between the proposed approach and an expert reader performing manual segmentation of EAT was high, with no bias and correlations of 0.945 and 0.926 in the training and validation datasets respectively [56]. Additionally, the variation of DL vs. expert interpretation was equivalent to the variation between two experienced observers. These results were further validated in a multicenter cohort with 850 cases. Automated segmentation of EAT was performed in a mean time of 1.57 ± 0.49 s, compared with approximately 15 min for experts (Fig. 11.4) [56]. Therefore, DL allowed for fast, robust, and fully automated quantification of EAT from non-contrast calcium scoring CT as well as an expert reader and could be integrated easily in clinical practice for cardiovascular risk assessment. DL algorithms for EAT quantification from CT have been implemented in the research tool QFAT at Cedars-Sinai and have been recently used in a novel combination of DL and classical ML for cardiovascular risk assessment. Such EAT measurements could potentially be integrated into comprehensive evaluations using hybrid imaging data on PET/CT or SPEC/CT hybrid scanners.

11.3 AI to Improve Physician Interpretation

11.3.1 Structured Reporting

One potential implementation of AI is for generating automated structured reports. This can be achieved with "expert systems"—a branch of AI in which algorithms utilize a combination of observed data and heuristic rules obtained from human experts to provide final predictions. Garcia et al. demonstrated that an expert system algorithm could generate an automated structured report for a SPECT myocardial perfusion exam which was non-inferior compared to nine expert readers [57]. The authors have employed 17-segment smart-scores which use a nonparametric normalized count distribution applied to information theory to generate a certainty of abnormality. This certainty for each segment is modified according to all the available perfusion and function information for that segment including rest, stress, changes between stress and rest, AC and non-AC images, and prone images [57]. The algorithm processes this information for all segments to generate the automated report. Such AI-generated automatic reports can be reviewed by physicians to expedite nuclear cardiology reporting or potentially improve accuracy.

11.3.2 Disease Diagnosis

AI can be trained to predict the likelihood of CAD, for example obstructive CAD, using either classical ML methods operating on quantified image features, or DL algorithms, which interrogate data directly. Arsanjani et al. demonstrated that an SVM model [58] which integrated numerical variables—total perfusion deficit (TPD), ischemic changes, and left ventricular ejection fraction—can significantly improve the diagnostic accuracy for obstructive CAD from MPI compared to standard quantitation with TPD (diagnostic accuracy 86% vs. 81%; $p < 0.01$) [59]. In a separate study including 957 scans from over 600 patients with correlating invasive coronary angiography data, it was also shown

that ML using the LogitBoost method outperforms two-position combined TPD for diagnosis of obstructive CAD [60].

A visual abnormal diagnosis could be used as a "gold standard" to train the AI methods for diagnosis from nuclear cardiology images. Spier et al. have developed a DL algorithm which achieved agreement of ~90% with expert visual interpretation of myocardial perfusion [61]. In a recent study, Liu et al. have shown that a CNN trained and internally cross-validated on over 37,000 stress-only SPECT perfusion scans can be reliably correlated with visual assessment of perfusion SPECT studies outperforming the quantitative assessment of stress only perfusion developed by the same group [62]. Using physician interpretation as an external gold standard for diagnosis may achieve better agreement than with the results of the invasive angiography. However, such training by definition cannot surpass the physicians' performance and can also be associated with potential training bias. It remains to be seen if such approaches are widely adopted.

Given the findings from the ISCHEMIA trial [63], which have raised questions over visual interpretation of regional perfusion for guiding decisions about revascularization, it is important to realize the importance of choosing an appropriate comparator for AI analysis. While matching or outperforming automatic software in detecting abnormal images is desirable, the patient needs to be central in all efforts in the medical field. Therefore, in view of the overall limitations of MPI and having in mind that the goal of noninvasive imaging in CAD is to distinguish patients who should proceed to invasive testing, it should be preferred to test the diagnostic accuracy of AI with invasive coronary angiography as the ground truth. Such a study design—testing whether DL algorithms can predict the likelihood of obstructive CAD directly from SPECT images—has been recently employed by Betancur et al. In a cohort that included 1638 patients from nine centers, the authors demonstrated that DL (using a combination of CNN and fully connected layers) improved detection of obstructive CAD compared to quantitation of perfusion with TPD on both a regional

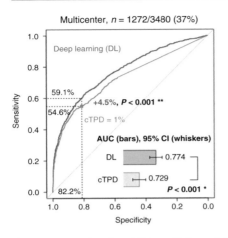

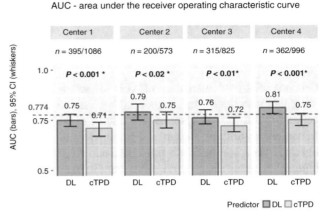

Fig. 11.5 Deep learning (DL) prediction of CAD from upright and supine MPS images (red) outperformed the current method—combined upright-supine TPD (cTPD) (blue). DL had an overall estimated per-vessel performance (left) externally validated (right) in four DL models (one per center)—each trained with data from the other three centers.

Red dotted line shows the overall multicenter AUC. This research was originally published in JNM. Betancur et al. Deep Learning Analysis of Upright-Supine High-Efficiency SPECT Myocardial Perfusion Imaging for Prediction of Obstructive Coronary Artery Disease: A Multicenter Study. J Nucl Med. 2019;60:664–670. © SNMMI

and per-patient basis [64]. With matched specificity, DL improved the per-vessel sensitivity to 69.8% from 64.4% with TPD ($p < 0.01$) [64]. Subsequently the same group demonstrated that a modified algorithm, utilizing both upright and supine imaging data from solid-state SPECT scanners, improved the diagnostic accuracy compared to combined upright-supine quantitative analysis developed previously by the same investigators in rigorous multisite external evaluation [65]. (Fig. 11.5) These CNN algorithms have been recently expanded to demonstrate the possibility of image-based explanation with image attention maps implemented in a clinical prototype for CAD diagnosis [66]. For example, this technique can be applied to SPECT MPI to highlight regions of perfusion polar maps which contribute most to the final DL predictions [67].

Apart from diagnosis of CAD, CNNs have also been applied to diagnose cardiac sarcoidosis from PET MPI, demonstrating improved sensitivity and specificity compared to two methods for quantification [68]. In a study based on a total of 85 patients (33 cardiac sarcoidosis patients and 52 patients without cardiac sarcoidosis) Togo et al. demonstrated that a deep CNN with

extracted high-level features from the polar maps (through the Inception-v3 network) achieved a high diagnostic accuracy for detecting cardiac sarcoidosis (sensitivity and specificity of 0.839, 0.870 respectively) [68]. This study focused on cardiac sarcoidosis but highlights how AI can benefit cardiac imaging beyond CAD.

11.3.3 Risk Prediction

AI algorithms also have a potential role in refining risk prediction for future adverse outcomes following nuclear cardiac imaging. The classical ML approach has a particular strength in its ability to combine large amounts of clinical, stress, and imaging data (with variables quantified by standard software) in an efficient and objective fashion. Arsanjani et al. trained an ML model to predict post-MPI revascularization in a cohort of 713 patients who underwent dual-isotope SPECT MPI and subsequent invasive angiography [69]. The ML model was compared to visual scoring of two expert readers. The ML approach had superior area under the receiver operating characteristic curve (AUC) (0.81 ± 0.2) for predicting revascularization compared to one of the readers (0.72 ± 0.02, $p < 0.01$) and quantitative assessment of perfusion (0.77 ± 0.2, $p < 0.01$). The study showed that the automatic ML approach, integrating a wide range of variables, is comparable or better than experienced readers in prediction of early revascularization and is significantly better than standalone measures of perfusion. In a subsequent multicenter study, Hu et al. demonstrated that a similar ML architecture could train a model which outperformed current methods for quantitative analysis of perfusion for prediction of revascularization on a per-patient and per-vessel basis [70]. In this study the overall feature importance graphs demonstrate that revascularization prediction can be obtained primarily from imaging variables. (Fig. 11.6) This study also proposed initial methods for explaining the prediction to the physicians by showing the relative importance of each feature.

AI models have also been developed to predict the risk for major adverse cardiovascular event (MACE). An ML model was developed using single-center SPECT MPI data ($n = 2619$) to determine the benefit of combining clinical, stress, and imaging features [71]. The ML model, trained and tested with tenfold cross-validation, had higher area under the receiver operating characteristic curve (AUC) for MACE compared to either stress TPD or ischemic TPD (AUC: 0.81 vs. 0.73 vs. 0.71, respectively; $p < 0.01$) [71]. Importantly, almost 20% of patients in the highest MACE risk (ninety-fifth or higher percentile) by the ML score had "normal" expert visual interpretation of myocardial perfusion highlighting an additional potential role of AI. Results from this study are shown in (Fig. 11.7). ML could potentially be used after expert interpretation to ensure that high-risk patients are not missed.

DL models have also been developed to predict MACE from rest and stress myocardial blood flow as well as myocardial flow reserve PET polar maps with high predictive accuracy [72]. In a study based on 1185 patients who underwent ^{13}N-ammonia PET, Juarez-Orozco et al. have shown that DL applied directly to polar-maps outperforms a comprehensive clinical model which includes: baseline characteristics (sex, age, body mass index, family CAD history, smoking, diabetes, dyslipidemia, and hypertension), the left ventricular systolic function (rest and stress left ventricular ejection fraction), and perfusion variables (regional rest and stress myocardial blood flow and myocardial perfusion reserve). AI-models could potentially be combined with a Cox proportional hazards model in order to provide time-to-event analyses. Such methods could provide more precise period-specific risk prediction.

Risk prediction can also be performed from CT scans automatically segmented using DL methods. In a study of 20,084 patients from several clinical trials, DL-derived automatic CAC score has been demonstrated to be a strong predictor of cardiovascular events, independent of other risk factors (multivariable-adjusted hazard ratios up to 4.3). Potentially DL can be applied to predicting cardiovascular mortality directly (without the need to derive calcium scores). In a set of 1583 participants of the National Lung Screening, this approach achieved good prognostic performance with AUC of 0.73. Both of these studies demonstrated the feasibility of obtaining important cardiovascular risk information from ungated chest CT scans, while CT scans obtained for the purpose of attenuation correction are typically lower radiation and ungated, which can reduce image quality. However, it has been demonstrated that CAC scores obtained automatically from PET CTAC correlate well with scores from separately obtained, same-day, ECG-gated CAC scans [49] and can be applied for risk prediction. Thus, it should be feasible to apply AI-based techniques to CT-attenuation maps of cardiac SPECT and PET to automatically extract useful diagnostic and prognostic information. The prognostic utility of such information was recently evaluated on a cohort of 747 patients with chest pain who underwent [82]Rubidium PET/CT. Dekker et al. showed that a DL model for quantification of CAC from non-contrast low-dose CT acquired for attenuation correction purposes predicts MACE independent of perfusion findings. Importantly, the addition of coronary calcium information resulted in a net reclassifica-

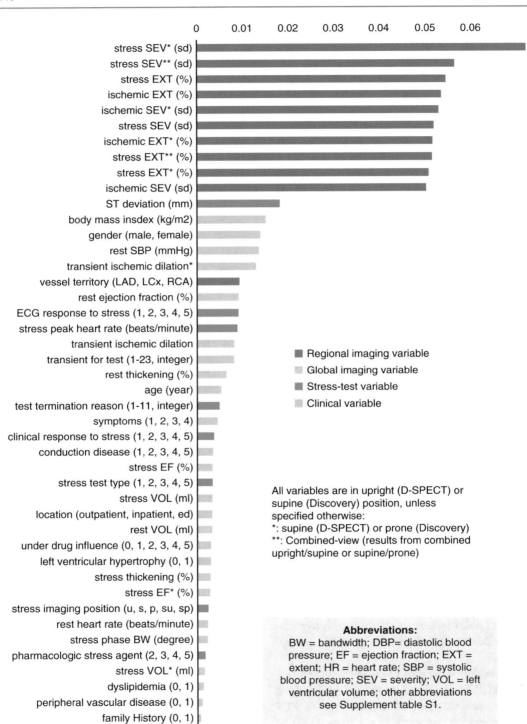

All variables are in upright (D-SPECT) or supine (Discovery) position, unless specified otherwise:
*: supine (D-SPECT) or prone (Discovery)
**: Combined-view (results from combined upright/supine or supine/prone)

Abbreviations:
BW = bandwidth; DBP= diastolic blood pressure; EF = ejection fraction; EXT = extent; HR = heart rate; SBP = systolic blood pressure; SEV = severity; VOL = left ventricular volume; other abbreviations see Supplement table S1.

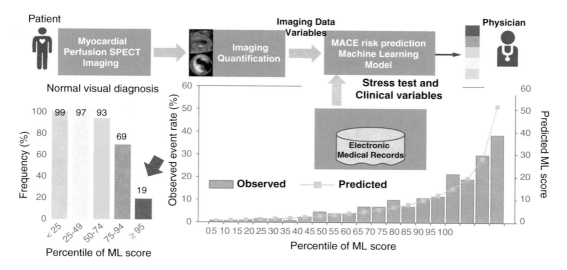

Fig. 11.7 Prediction of MACE by machine learning (ML). The composite ML risk score from imaging and clinical data can be presented to physicians as an annualized event risk. Frequency of patients with normal visual diagnosis versus ML score (left). 19% of patients with normal visual diagnosis (red arrow) were in the ≥95th percentile of MACE risk computed by ML. Observed (pink bars) and predicted (green curve) MACE rate according to percentile of ML score (right). Reprinted from JACC Cardiovascular Imaging, Vol 11, Betancur et al., Prognostic Value of Combined Clinical and Myocardial Perfusion Imaging Data Using Machine Learning, Pages 1000–1009, 2018, with permission from Elsevier

tion improvement of 0.13 (0.02–0.25) [73]. Routine implementation of deep learning for interrogating non-contrast CT data could provide clinicians with additional cardiovascular information with no processing overhead, when interpreting a nuclear cardiology scan.

The DL segmentation of EAT can be utilized for risk prediction models. These automatically derived EAT measures have demonstrated independent prognostic utility [55, 56, 74–77]. EAT may be particularly relevant for improving risk prediction in patients with cardiometabolic risk factors [78]. An ML risk score, integrating circulating biomarkers and computed tomography (CT) measures including CAC score end EAT

derived by deep learning, has been developed for the long-term prediction of hard cardiac events in 1069 asymptomatic subjects. The ML risk score (AUC 0.81) outperformed the CAC score (0.75) and ASCVD risk score (0.74; both $p = 0.02$) for the prediction of hard cardiac events [79]. (Fig. 11.8) With such tools, important prognostic data can be obtained from existing CT scans, which would not be obtained clinically due to the tedious manual task processing. This technique could potentially be used for hybrid (SPECT/CT and PET/CT) nuclear cardiology scans, where CT is obtained as an auxiliary scan for attenuation correction or with additional dedicated gated CT scans.

←

Fig. 11.6 The machine learning (ML) algorithm evaluated all 55 used variables independently to determine the IGR for each variable in each fold. 49 out of 55 variables had IGR > 0 and were selected. ML models were built with these selected variables. Most variables in the ranking are imaging variables (blue and light blue bars) with regional imaging variables (blue bars) leading, while clinical and stress-test variables also play roles in the prediction. Reprinted from EHJCI, Hu et al., Machine learning predicts per-vessel early coronary revascularization after fast myocardial perfusion SPECT: results from multicentre REFINE SPECT registry. European heart journal cardiovascular Imaging, 21:549–559, 2020, by permission of Oxford University Press

Fig. 11.8 Variable importance for the classification of hard cardiac events. (**a**) The top 25 variables are displayed: clinical risk factors in blue, quantitative imaging measures in grey, and serum biomarkers in red. The "gain" denotes how much a variable contributes to the prediction made by the XGBoost algorithm. (**b**) Receiver operator characteristic curves for the prediction of hard cardiac events. The machine learning model with serum biomarkers performed significantly better than the ASCVD risk score and CAC score (both $p = 0.02$). Reprinted from Atherosclerosis, Vol 318, Tamarappoo et al., Machine learning integration of circulating and imaging biomarkers for explainable patient-specific prediction of cardiac events: A prospective study, Pages 76–82, 2021, with permission from Elsevier

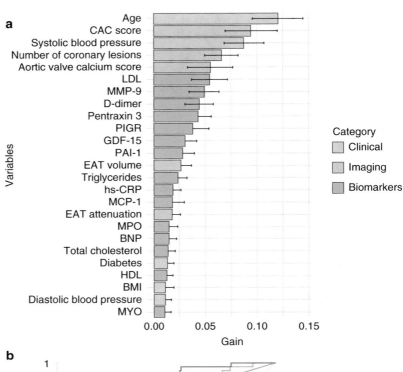

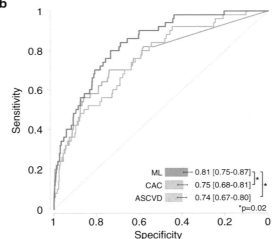

One issue in risk prediction with a large number of variables is the necessity to obtain these variables from health records—which is not always possible in real time during clinical interpretation. Therefore, it is important to establish if reduced variable models provide similar prognostic stratification. Haro Alonso et al. demonstrated that an ML model utiliz-ing only 6 variables provided superior risk prediction compared to a logistic regression model with 14 variables [80]. Such feature reduction would simplify the implementation of ML algorithms as modules in reporting software by limiting the additional work required by physicians or support staff to enable AI predictions.

11.4 Protocol Optimization: Application to Rest Scan Cancellation

While risk prediction may be important for treatment selection, potentially a more practical and simple application is to apply such technique for imaging protocol optimization. For example, in SPECT MPI stress-only imaging is associated with up to 60% reduction in effective radiation exposure compared to a standard one-day stress-rest exam [81] and shortening of examination time. Despite these substantial benefits, stress-only MPI protocols remain severely under-utilized (<12% worldwide <3% in the US) [82, 83]. It was recently demonstrated that ML models could also be used clinically to automatically identify patients for rest scan cancellation. These algorithms could potentially be used to identify patients with a low likelihood of having obstructive CAD [84] or those with a very low risk of MACE [85]. In a study of 20,414 patients using matched cancellation rates, subjects selected for rest scan cancellation with clinical methods had higher all-cause mortality (1.0% to 1.3%) compared to patients who were selected by corresponding ML thresholds (0.2% to 0.6%) [85]. The overall performance for risk prediction of 5-year risk of MACE was higher for AI-based approach than any of the previously proposed clinical approaches (Fig. 11.9a). This approach could potentially be implemented as a module in interpretation or reporting software to reduce the proportion of patients requiring rest imaging, obviating the need for an on-site physician and guaranteeing a high degree of safety. Such streamlined automated AI-selection of patients for stress-only protocols would lead to significant reductions in radiation exposure for patients and technical staff, as well as reduction in associated costs [86].

11.5 Explainable AI

Methods to improve the explainability of risk predictions are critical for clinical implementation. For traditional ML approaches, individual

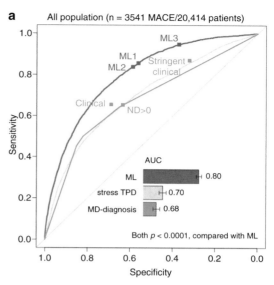

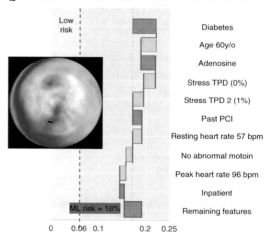

Fig. 11.9 (a) Machine learning (ML) with imaging and clinical data had higher area under operating curve (AUC) for MACE risk prediction compared to total perfusion deficit (TPD) and superior risk decision thresholds (ML1–3) vs. visual physician's reading with clinical data (MD, Clinical, Stringent clinical). (b) Personalized risk explanation. 60-y/o old male with normal stress perfusion (TPD)—decreasing risk (blue bars), but clinical features (diabetes, past revascularization [PCI]) increasing risk (red bars). AI-based 5-year MACE risk 18%. Reprinted from EHJCI, Hu et al., Prognostically safe stress-only single-photon emission computed tomography myocardial perfusion imaging guided by machine learning: report from REFINE SPECT, jeaa134, 2020, by permission of Oxford University Press

features contributing to the risk score for a given subject can be displayed. This approach was employed by Hu et al. to explain predictions regarding MACE risk and the safety of rest scan cancellation [70] (Fig. 11.9b). This information can be used by physicians to identify clinically actionable factors such as hypertension or diabetes mellitus. Additionally, these explanations could potentially improve the accuracy of combined reporting by allowing physicians to identify potential errors in ML risk predictions. Attention maps could be implemented to explain DL model predictions. Attention maps are heats maps which can be overlayed on the input images to highlight the image regions that triggered the final AI findings by backpropagating the finding through the CNN [87, 88]. Similarly attention maps can be applied to CT images. To reduce computational complexity, researchers have attempted direct scoring of CAC through regression of the calcium score, avoiding time-consuming intermediate CAC segmentation [89]. While there was no explicit segmentation, attention maps were used for visual explanation In direct CAC scoring, accomplished by a method termed deConvnet [88]—highlighting the image regions contributing to the calcium score.

11.6 Summary

AI has become an increasingly important tool, with rapidly expanding implications for nuclear cardiology and hybrid imaging. AI can significantly improve image processing, image reconstruction, potentially allowing reduction in radiation exposure or optimize image segmentation. Clinically, AI could potentially be implemented in order to provide structured reports, diagnose obstructive CAD, or optimally predict the likelihood of adverse events. AI shall undoubtedly play an increasing role in integrating the data acquired across imaging modalities in cardiology. Such areas are hybrid PET/MR, and SPECT/CT or PET/CT acquisitions which enable collecting a wealth of clinical variables which can guide patient management yet require careful analysis which could be enhanced with AI. Methods to improve the feasibility of implementing ML models and explain AI predictions are necessary for a more widespread uptake of this promising technology.

References

1. Virani SS, Alonso A, Benjamin EJ, Bittencourt MS, Callaway CW, Carson AP, Chamberlain AM, Chang AR, Cheng S, Delling FN, Djousse L, Elkind MSV, Ferguson JF, Fornage M, Khan SS, Kissela BM, Knutson KL, Kwan TW, Lackland DT, Lewis TT, Lichtman JH, Longenecker CT, Loop MS, Lutsey PL, Martin SS, Matsushita K, Moran AE, Mussolino ME, Perak AM, Rosamond WD, Roth GA, Sampson UKA, Satou GM, Schroeder EB, Shah SH, Shay CM, Spartano NL, Stokes A, Tirschwell DL, VanWagner LB, Tsao CW. American Heart Association Council on E, Prevention Statistics C and Stroke Statistics S. Heart Disease and Stroke Statistics-2020 Update: A Report From the American Heart Association. Circulation. 2020;141:e139–596.
2. Fihn SD, Blankenship JC, Alexander KP, Bittl JA, Byrne JG, Fletcher BJ, Fonarow GC, Lange RA, Levine GN, Maddox TM, Naidu SS, Ohman EM, Smith PK. 2014 ACC/AHA/AATS/PCNA/SCAI/STS focused update of the guideline for the diagnosis and management of patients with stable ischemic heart disease: a report of the American College of Cardiology/American Heart Association Task Force on Practice Guidelines, and the American Association for Thoracic Surgery, Preventive Cardiovascular Nurses Association, Society for Cardiovascular Angiography and Interventions, and Society of Thoracic Surgeons. J Am Coll Cardiol. 2014;64:1929–49.
3. Knuuti J, Wijns W, Saraste A, Capodanno D, Barbato E, Funck-Brentano C, Prescott E, Storey RF, Deaton C, Cuisset T, Agewall S, Dickstein K, Edvardsen T, Escaned J, Gersh BJ, Svitil P, Gilard M, Hasdai D, Hatala R, Mahfoud F, Masip J, Muneretto C, Valgimigli M, Achenbach S, Bax JJ. 2019 ESC Guidelines for the diagnosis and management of chronic coronary syndromes. Eur Heart J. 2020;41:407–77.
4. Dey D, Slomka PJ, Leeson P, Comaniciu D, Shrestha S, Sengupta PP, Marwick TH. Artificial intelligence in cardiovascular imaging: JACC state-of-the-art review. J Am Coll Cardiol. 2019;73:1317–35.
5. Slomka PJ, Miller RJ, Isgum I, Dey D. Application and translation of artificial intelligence to cardiovascular imaging in nuclear medicine and noncontrast CT. Semin Nucl Med. 2020;50:357–66.
6. Krittanawong C, Tunhasiriwet A, Zhang H, Wang Z, Aydar M, Kitai T. Deep learning with unsupervised feature in echocardiographic imaging. J Am Coll Cardiol. 2017;69:2100–1.
7. Çiçek Ö, Abdulkadir A, Lienkamp SS, Brox T, Ronneberger O. 3D U-Net: learning dense volumetric segmentation from sparse annotation. In:

International conference on medical image computing and computer-assisted intervention. 2016. p. 424–32.

8. Ronneberger O, Fischer P, Brox T. U-net: Convolutional networks for biomedical image segmentation. In: International conference on medical image computing and computer-assisted intervention. 2015. p. 234–41.

9. Chen H, Zhang Y, Kalra MK, Lin F, Chen Y, Liao P, Zhou J, Wang G. Low-dose CT with a residual encoder-decoder convolutional neural network. IEEE Trans Med Imaging. 2017;36:2524–35.

10. Ramon AJ, Yang Y, Pretorius PH, Johnson KL, King MA, Wernick MN. Initial investigation of low-dose SPECT-MPI via deep learning. In: 2018 IEEE nuclear science symposium and medical imaging conference proceedings (NSS/MIC). 2018. p. 1–3.

11. Song C, Yang Y, Wernick MN, Pretorius PH, King MA. Low-dose cardiac-gated spect studies using a residual convolutional neural network. In: 2019 IEEE 16th international symposium on biomedical imaging (ISBI 2019). 2019. p. 653–6.

12. Ladefoged C, Hasbak P, Hansen J, Kjer A, Hejgaard L, Andersen F. Low-dose PET reconstruction using deep learning: application to cardiac imaged with FDG. J Nucl Med. 2019;60:573.

13. Lassen ML, Commandeur F, Kwiecinski J, Dey D, Cadet S, Germano G, Berman D, Dweck M, Newby D, Slomka P. 10-fold reduction of scan time with deep learning reconstruction of coronary PET images. J Nucl Med. 2019;60:244.

14. Shiri I, AmirMozafari Sabet K, Arabi H, Pourkeshavarz M, Teimourian B, Ay MR, Zaidi H. Standard SPECT myocardial perfusion estimation from half-time acquisitions using deep convolutional residual neural networks. J Nucl Cardiol. 2021;28(6):2761–79.

15. Whiteley W, Luk WK, Gregor J. DirectPET: full-size neural network PET reconstruction from sinogram data. J Med Imag. 2020;7:032503.

16. Reader AJ, Corda G, Mehranian A, da Costa-Luis C, Ellis S, Schnabel JA. Deep learning for PET image reconstruction. IEEE Trans Radiat Plasma Med Sci. 2020;5:1–25.

17. Liu Z, Chen H, Liu H. Deep learning based framework for direct reconstruction of PET images. In: International conference on medical image computing and computer-assisted intervention. 2019. p. 48–56.

18. Häggström I, Schmidtlein CR, Campanella G, Fuchs TJ. DeepPET: a deep encoder–decoder network for directly solving the PET image reconstruction inverse problem. Med Image Anal. 2019;54:253–62.

19. Gong K, Catana C, Qi J, Li Q. PET image reconstruction using deep image prior. IEEE Trans Med Imaging. 2018;38:1655–65.

20. Slomka PJ, Diaz-Zamudio M, Dey D, Motwani M, Brodov Y, Choi D, Hayes S, Thomson L, Friedman J, Germano G, Berman D. Automatic registration of misaligned CT attenuation correction maps in Rb-82 PET/CT improves detection of angiographically significant coronary artery disease. J Nucl Cardiol. 2015;22:1285–95.

21. Gould KL, Pan T, Loghin C, Johnson NP, Guha A, Sdringola S. Frequent diagnostic errors in cardiac PET/CT due to misregistration of CT attenuation and emission PET images: a definitive analysis of causes, consequences, and corrections. J Nucl Med. 2007;48:1112–21.

22. Ko C-L, Cheng M-F, Yen R-F, Chen C-M, Lee W-J, Wang T-D. Automatic alignment of CZT myocardial perfusion SPECT and external non-contrast CT by deep-learning model and dynamic data generation. J Nucl Med. 2019;60:570.

23. Dong X, Lei Y, Wang T, Higgins K, Liu T, Curran WJ, Mao H, Nye JA, Yang X. Deep learning-based attenuation correction in the absence of structural information for whole-body positron emission tomography imaging. Phys Med Biol. 2020;65:055011.

24. Liu F, Jang H, Kijowski R, Bradshaw T, McMillan AB. Deep learning MR imaging-based attenuation correction for PET/MR imaging. Radiology. 2018;286:676–84.

25. Shi L, Onofrey JA, Liu H, Liu YH, Liu C. Deep learning-based attenuation map generation for myocardial perfusion SPECT. Eur J Nucl Med Mol Imaging. 2020;47:2383–95.

26. Betancur J, Rubeaux M, Fuchs TA, Otaki Y, Arnson Y, Slipczuk L, Benz DC, Germano G, Dey D, Lin CJ, Berman DS, Kaufmann PA, Slomka PJ. Automatic valve plane localization in myocardial perfusion SPECT/CT by machine learning: anatomic and clinical validation. J Nucl Med. 2017;58:961–7.

27. Wang T, Lei Y, Tang H, He Z, Castillo R, Wang C, Li D, Higgins K, Liu T, Curran WJ, Zhou W, Yang X. A learning-based automatic segmentation and quantification method on left ventricle in gated myocardial perfusion SPECT imaging: a feasibility study. Journal of nuclear cardiology: official publication of the American Society of Nuclear Cardiology. 2020;27(3):976–87.

28. Arad Y, Goodman KJ, Roth M, Newstein D, Guerci AD. Coronary calcification, coronary disease risk factors, C-reactive protein, and atherosclerotic cardiovascular disease events: the St. Francis Heart Study. J Am Coll Cardiol. 2005;46:158–65.

29. Shaw LJ, Raggi P, Schisterman E, Berman DS, Callister TQ. Prognostic value of cardiac risk factors and coronary artery calcium screening for all-cause mortality. Radiology. 2003;228:826–33.

30. Park R, Detrano R, Xiang M, Fu P, Ibrahim Y, LaBree L, Azen S. Combined use of computed tomography coronary calcium scores and C-reactive protein levels in predicting cardiovascular events in nondiabetic individuals. Circulation. 2002;106:2073–7.

31. Wong ND, Hsu JC, Detrano RC, Diamond G, Eisenberg H, Gardin JM. Coronary artery calcium evaluation by electron beam computed tomography and its relation to new cardiovascular events. Am J Cardiol. 2000;86:495–8.

32. Kondos GT, Hoff JA, Sevrukov A, Daviglus ML, Garside DB, Devries SS, Chomka EV, Liu K. Electron-beam tomography coronary artery cal-

cium and cardiac events: a 37-month follow-up of 5635 initially asymptomatic low- to intermediate-risk adults. Circulation. 2003;107:2571–6.

33. Greenland P, LaBree L, Azen SP, Doherty TM, Detrano RC. Coronary artery calcium score combined with Framingham score for risk prediction in asymptomatic individuals. JAMA. 2004;291:210–5.

34. Taylor AJ, Bindeman J, Feuerstein I, Cao F, Brazaitis M, O'Malley PG. Coronary calcium independently predicts incident premature coronary heart disease over measured cardiovascular risk factors: mean three-year outcomes in the Prospective Army Coronary Calcium (PACC) project. J Am Coll Cardiol. 2005;46:807–14.

35. Vliegenthart R, Oudkerk M, Hofman A, Oei HH, van Dijck W, van Rooij FJ, Witteman JC. Coronary calcification improves cardiovascular risk prediction in the elderly. Circulation. 2005;112:572–7.

36. Detrano R, Guerci AD, Carr JJ, Bild DE, Burke G, Folsom AR, Liu K, Shea S, Szklo M, Bluemke DA, O'Leary DH, Tracy R, Watson K, Wong ND, Kronmal RA. Coronary calcium as a predictor of coronary events in four racial or ethnic groups. N Engl J Med. 2008;358:1336–45.

37. Erbel R, Mohlenkamp S, Moebus S, Schmermund A, Lehmann N, Stang A, Dragano N, Gronemeyer D, Seibel R, Kalsch H, Brocker-Preuss M, Mann K, Siegrist J, Jockel KH, Heinz Nixdorf Recall Study Investigative Group. Coronary risk stratification, discrimination, and reclassification improvement based on quantification of subclinical coronary atherosclerosis: the Heinz Nixdorf Recall study. J Am Coll Cardiol. 2010;56:1397–406.

38. Greenland P, Blaha MJ, Budoff MJ, Erbel R, Watson KE. Coronary calcium score and cardiovascular risk. J Am Coll Cardiol. 2018;72:434–47.

39. Engbers EM, Timmer JR, Ottervanger JP, Mouden M, Knollema S, Jager PL. Prognostic value of coronary artery calcium scoring in addition to single-photon emission computed tomographic myocardial perfusion imaging in symptomatic patients. Circulation. Cardiovasc Imag. 2016;9:e003966.

40. Budoff MJ, Young R, Burke G, Jeffrey Carr J, Detrano RC, Folsom AR, Kronmal R, Lima JAC, Liu KJ, McClelland RL, Michos E, Post WS, Shea S, Watson KE, Wong ND. Ten-year association of coronary artery calcium with atherosclerotic cardiovascular disease (ASCVD) events: the multi-ethnic study of atherosclerosis (MESA). Eur Heart J. 2018;39:2401–8.

41. Brodov Y, Gransar H, Dey D, Shalev A, Germano G, Friedman JD, Hayes SW, Thomson LE, Rogatko A, Berman DS, Slomka PJ. Combined quantitative assessment of myocardial perfusion and coronary artery calcium score by hybrid 82Rb PET/CT improves detection of coronary artery disease. J Nucl Med. 2015;56:1345–50.

42. Zampella E, Acampa W, Assante R, Nappi C, Gaudieri V, Mainolfi CG, Green R, Cantoni V, Panico M, Klain M, Petretta M, Slomka PJ, Cuocolo A. Combined evaluation of regional coronary artery calcium and myocardial perfusion by (82)Rb PET/CT in the identification of obstructive coronary artery disease. Eur J Nucl Med Mol Imaging. 2018;45:521–9.

43. Naya M, Murthy VL, Foster CR, Gaber M, Klein J, Hainer J, Dorbala S, Blankstein R, Di Carli MF. Prognostic interplay of coronary artery calcification and underlying vascular dysfunction in patients with suspected coronary artery disease. J Am Coll Cardiol. 2013;61:2098–106.

44. Schenker MP, Dorbala S, Hong EC, Rybicki FJ, Hachamovitch R, Kwong RY, Di Carli MF. Interrelation of coronary calcification, myocardial ischemia, and outcomes in patients with intermediate likelihood of coronary artery disease: a combined positron emission tomography/computed tomography study. Circulation. 2008;117:1693–700.

45. Lessmann N, van Ginneken B, Zreik M, de Jong PA, de Vos BD, Viergever MA, Isgum I. Automatic calcium scoring in low-dose chest CT using deep neural networks with dilated convolutions. IEEE Trans Med Imaging. 2018;37:615–25.

46. van Velzen SG, Lessmann N, Velthuis BK, Bank IE, van den Bongard DH, Leiner T, de Jong PA, Veldhuis WB, Correa A, Terry JG. Deep learning for automatic calcium scoring in CT: validation using multiple cardiac CT and chest CT protocols. Radiology. 2020;295:66–79.

47. Šprem J, De Vos BD, Lessmann N, Van Hamersvelt RW, Greuter MJ, De Jong PA, Leiner T, Viergever MA, Išgum I. Coronary calcium scoring with partial volume correction in anthropomorphic thorax phantom and screening chest CT images. PLoS One. 2018;13:e0209318.

48. Huo Y, Terry JG, Wang J, Nath V, Bermudez C, Bao S, Parvathaneni P, Carr JJ, Landman BA. Coronary calcium detection using 3D attention identical dual deep network based on weakly supervised learning. Proc SPIE Int Soc Opt Eng. 2019;10949:1094917.

49. Isgum I, de Vos BD, Wolterink JM, Dey D, Berman DS, Rubeaux M, Leiner T, Slomka PJ. Automatic determination of cardiovascular risk by CT attenuation correction maps in Rb-82 PET/CT. J Nucl Cardiol. 2018;25:2133–42.

50. Iacobellis G, Pistilli D, Gucciardo M, Leonetti F, Miraldi F, Brancaccio G, Gallo P, di Gioia CR. Adiponectin expression in human epicardial adipose tissue in vivo is lower in patients with coronary artery disease. Cytokine. 2005;29:251–5.

51. Ding J, Kritchevsky SB, Harris TB, Burke GL, Detrano RC, Szklo M, Carr JJ. The association of pericardial fat with calcified coronary plaque. Obesity. 2008;16:1914–9.

52. Rosito GA, Massaro JM, Hoffmann U, Ruberg FL, Mahabadi AA, Vasan RS, O'Donnell CJ, Fox CS. Pericardial fat, visceral abdominal fat, cardiovascular disease risk factors, and vascular calcification in a community-based sample: the Framingham Heart Study. Circulation. 2008;117:605–13.

53. Mahabadi AA, Massaro JM, Rosito GA, Levy D, Murabito JM, Wolf PA, O'Donnell CJ, Fox CS,

Hoffmann U. Association of pericardial fat, intrathoracic fat, and visceral abdominal fat with cardiovascular disease burden: the Framingham Heart Study. Eur Heart J. 2009;30(7):850–6.

54. Mahabadi AA, Berg MH, Lehmann N, Kalsch H, Bauer M, Kara K, Dragano N, Moebus S, Jockel KH, Erbel R, Mohlenkamp S. Association of epicardial fat with cardiovascular risk factors and incident myocardial infarction in the general population: the Heinz Nixdorf Recall Study. J Am Coll Cardiol. 2013;61:1388–95.

55. Commandeur F, Goeller M, Razipour A, Cadet S, Hell MM, Kwiecinski J, Chen X, Chang HJ, Marwan M, Achenbach S, Berman DS, Slomka PJ, Tamarappoo BK, Dey D. Fully automated CT quantification of epicardial adipose tissue by deep learning: a multicenter study. Radiol Artif Intell. 2019;1:e190045.

56. Commandeur F, Goeller M, Betancur J, Cadet S, Doris M, Chen X, Berman DS, Slomka PJ, Tamarappoo BK, Dey D. Deep learning for quantification of epicardial and thoracic adipose tissue from non-contrast CT. IEEE Trans Med Imaging. 2018;37:1835–46.

57. Garcia EV, Klein JL, Moncayo V, Cooke CD, Del'Aune C, Folks R, Moreiras LV, Esteves F. Diagnostic performance of an artificial intelligence-driven cardiac-structured reporting system for myocardial perfusion SPECT imaging. J Nucl Cardiol. 2020;27:1652–64.

58. Chang CC, Lin CJ. LIBSVM: a library for support vector machines. ACM Trans Intell Syst Technol (TIST). 2011;2:27.

59. Arsanjani R, Xu Y, Dey D, Fish M, Dorbala S, Hayes S, Berman D, Germano G, Slomka P. Improved accuracy of myocardial perfusion SPECT for the detection of coronary artery disease using a support vector machine algorithm. J Nucl Med. 2013;54:549–55.

60. Arsanjani R, Xu Y, Dey D, Vahistha V, Shalev A, Nakanishi R, Hayes S, Fish M, Berman D, Germano G, Slomka PJ. Improved accuracy of myocardial perfusion SPECT for detection of coronary artery disease by machine learning in a large population. J Nucl Cardiol. 2013;20:553–62.

61. Spier N, Nekolla S, Rupprecht C, Mustafa M, Navab N, Baust M. Classification of polar maps from cardiac perfusion imaging with graph-convolutional neural networks. Sci Rep. 2019;9:7569.

62. Liu H, Wu J, Miller EJ, Liu C, Liu Y-H. Diagnostic accuracy of stress-only myocardial perfusion SPECT improved by deep learning. Eur J Nucl Med Mol Imaging. 2021:1–8.

63. Maron DJ, Hochman JS, Reynolds HR, Bangalore S, O'Brien SM, Boden WE, Chaitman BR, Senior R, Lopez-Sendon J, Alexander KP, Lopes RD, Shaw LJ, Berger JS, Newman JD, Sidhu MS, Goodman SG, Ruzyllo W, Gosselin G, Maggioni AP, White HD, Bhargava B, Min JK, GBJ M, Berman DS, Picard MH, Kwong RY, Ali ZA, Mark DB, Spertus JA, Krishnan MN, Elghamaz A, Moorthy N, Hueb WA, Demkow M, Mavromatis K, Bockeria O, Peteiro J, Miller TD, Szwed H, Doerr R, Keltai M, Selvanayagam JB, Steg PG, Held C, Kohsaka S, Mavromichalis S, Kirby R,

Jeffries NO, Harrell FE Jr, Rockhold FW, Broderick S, Ferguson TB Jr, Williams DO, Harrington RA, Stone GW, Rosenberg Y, ISCHEMIA Research Group. Initial invasive or conservative strategy for stable coronary disease. N Engl J Med. 2020;382:1395–407.

64. Betancur J, Commandeur F, Motlagh M, Sharir T, Einstein AJ, Bokhari S, Fish MB, Ruddy TD, Kaufmann P, Sinusas AJ, Miller EJ, Bateman TM, Dorbala S, Di Carli M, Germano G, Otaki Y, Tamarappoo BK, Dey D, Berman DS, Slomka PJ. Deep learning for prediction of obstructive disease from fast myocardial perfusion SPECT: a multicenter study. J Am Coll Cardiol Img. 2018;11:1654–63.

65. Betancur J, Hu LH, Commandeur F, Sharir T, Einstein AJ, Fish MB, Ruddy TD, Kaufmann PA, Sinusas AJ, Miller EJ, Bateman TM, Dorbala S, Di Carli M, Germano G, Otaki Y, Liang JX, Tamarappoo BK, Dey D, Berman DS, Slomka PJ. Deep learning analysis of upright-supine high-efficiency SPECT myocardial perfusion imaging for prediction of obstructive coronary artery disease: a multicenter study. J Nucl Med. 2019;60:664–70.

66. Otaki Y, Singh A, Kavanagh P, Miller RJ, Parekh T, Tamarappoo BK, Sharir T, Einstein AJ, Fish MB, Ruddy TD, Kaufmann PA, Sinusas AJ, Miller EJ, Bateman TM, Sharmila Dorbala M, Carli MD, Cadet S, Liang JX, Dey D, Berman DS, Slomka PJ. Clinical deployment of explainable artificial intelligence for diagnosis of coronary artery disease. JACC Cardiovas Imag. 2021. (In review).

67. Otaki Y, Tamarappoo B, Singh A, Sharir T, Hu LH, Gransar H, Einstein A, Fish M, Ruddy T, Kaufmann P, Sinusas A, Miller E, Bateman T, Dorbala S, Di Carli M, Liang J, Dey D, Berman D, Slomka P. Diagnostic accuracy of deep learning for myocardial perfusion imaging in men and women with a high-efficiency parallel-hole-collimated cadmium-zinc-telluride camera: multicenter study. J Nucl Med. 2020;61:92.

68. Togo R, Hirata K, Manabe O, Ohira H, Tsujino I, Magota K, Ogawa T, Haseyama M, Shiga T. Cardiac sarcoidosis classification with deep convolutional neural network-based features using polar maps. Comput Biol Med. 2019;104:81–6.

69. Arsanjani R, Dey D, Khachatryan T, Shalev A, Hayes SW, Fish M, Nakanishi R, Germano G, Berman DS, Slomka P. Prediction of revascularization after myocardial perfusion SPECT by machine learning in a large population. J Nucl Cardiol. 2015;22:877–84.

70. Hu LH, Betancur J, Sharir T, Einstein AJ, Bokhari S, Fish MB, Ruddy TD, Kaufmann PA, Sinusas AJ, Miller EJ, Bateman TM, Dorbala S, Di Carli M, Germano G, Commandeur F, Liang JX, Otaki Y, Tamarappoo BK, Dey D, Berman DS, Slomka PJ. Machine learning predicts per-vessel early coronary revascularization after fast myocardial perfusion SPECT: results from multicentre REFINE SPECT registry. Eur Heart J Cardiovasc Imaging. 2020;21:549–59.

71. Betancur J, Otaki Y, Motwani M, Fish MB, Lemley M, Dey D, Gransar H, Tamarappoo B, Germano G, Sharir T, Berman DS, Slomka PJ. Prognostic value of

combined clinical and myocardial perfusion imaging data using machine learning. J Am Coll Cardiol Img. 2018;11:1000–9.

72. Juarez-Orozco LE, Martinez-Manzanera O, van der Zant FM, Knol RJJ, Knuuti J. Deep learning in quantitative PET myocardial perfusion imaging: a study on cardiovascular event prediction. JACC Cardiovasc Imaging. 2020;13:180–2.

73. Dekker M, Waissi F, Bank IE, Isgum I, Scholtens AM, Velthuis BK, Pasterkamp G, de Winter RJ, Mosterd A, Timmers L. The prognostic value of automated coronary calcium derived by a deep learning approach on non-ECG gated CT images from ⁸²Rb-PET/CT myocardial perfusion imaging. Int J Cardiol. 2021;329:9–15. https://doi.org/10.1016/j.ijcard.2020.12.079.

74. Commandeur F, Slomka PJ, Goeller M, Chen X, Cadet S, Razipour A, McElhinney P, Gransar H, Cantu S, Miller RJH, Rozanski A, Achenbach S, Tamarappoo BK, Berman DS, Dey D. Machine learning to predict the long-term risk of myocardial infarction and cardiac death based on clinical risk, coronary calcium, and epicardial adipose tissue: a prospective study. Cardiovasc Res. 2020;116:2216–25.

75. Lin A, Wong ND, Razipour A, McElhinney PA, Commandeur F, Cadet SJ, Gransar H, Chen X, Cantu S, Miller RJH, Nerlekar N, Wong DTL, Slomka PJ, Rozanski A, Tamarappoo BK, Berman DS, Dey D. Metabolic syndrome, fatty liver, and artificial intelligence-based epicardial adipose tissue measures predict long-term risk of cardiac events: a prospective study. Cardiovasc Diabetol. 2021;20:27.

76. Tamarappoo B, Dey D, Shmilovich H, Nakazato R, Gransar H, Cheng VY, Friedman JD, Hayes SW, Thomson LE, Slomka PJ, Rozanski A, Berman DS. Increased pericardial fat volume measured from noncontrast CT predicts myocardial ischemia by SPECT. J Am Coll Cardiol Img. 2010;3:1104–12.

77. Goeller M, Achenbach S, Marwan M, Doris MK, Cadet S, Commandeur F, Chen X, Slomka PJ, Gransar H, Cao JJ, Wong ND, Albrecht MH, Rozanski A, Tamarappoo BK, Berman DS, Dey D. Epicardial adipose tissue density and volume are related to subclinical atherosclerosis, inflammation and major adverse cardiac events in asymptomatic subjects. J Cardiovasc Comput Tomogr. 2018;12:67–73.

78. Neeland IJ, Ross R, Despres JP, Matsuzawa Y, Yamashita S, Shai I, Seidell J, Magni P, Santos RD, Arsenault B, Cuevas A, Hu FB, Griffin B, Zambon A, Barter P, Fruchart JC, Eckel RH, International Atherosclerosis Society, International Chair on Cardiometabolic Risk Working Group on Visceral Obesity. Visceral and ectopic fat, atherosclerosis, and cardiometabolic disease: a position statement. Lancet Diabetes Endocrinol. 2019;7:715–25.

79. Tamarappoo BK, Lin A, Commandeur F, McElhinney PA, Cadet S, Goeller M, Razipour A, Chen X, Gransar H, Cantu S, Miller RJ, Achenbach S, Friedman J, Hayes S, Thomson L, Wong ND, Rozanski A, Slomka

PJ, Berman DS, Dey D. Machine learning integration of circulating and imaging biomarkers for explainable patient-specific prediction of cardiac events: a prospective study. Atherosclerosis. 2021;318:76–82.

80. Haro Alonso D, Wernick MN, Yang Y, Germano G, Berman DS, Slomka P. Prediction of cardiac death after adenosine myocardial perfusion SPECT based on machine learning. J Nucl Cardiol. 2019;26:1746–54.

81. Mercuri M, Pascual TNB, Mahmarian JJ, Shaw LJ, Dondi M, Paez D, Einstein AJ. Estimating the reduction in the radiation burden from nuclear cardiology through use of stress-only imaging in the United States and worldwide. JAMA Intern Med. 2016;176:269–73.

82. Einstein AJ, Pascual TN, Mercuri M, Karthikeyan G, Vitola JV, Mahmarian JJ, Better N, Bouyoucef SE, Hee-Seung Bom H, Lele V, Magboo VP, Alexanderson E, Allam AH, Al-Mallah MH, Flotats A, Jerome S, Kaufmann PA, Luxenburg O, Shaw LJ, Underwood SR, Rehani MM, Kashyap R, Paez D, Dondi M. Current worldwide nuclear cardiology practices and radiation exposure: results from the 65 country IAEA Nuclear Cardiology Protocols Cross-Sectional Study (INCAPS). Eur Heart J. 2015;36:1689–96.

83. Jerome SD, Tilkemeier PL, Farrell MB, Shaw LJ. Nationwide Laboratory adherence to myocardial perfusion imaging radiation dose reduction practices: a report from the intersocietal accreditation commission data repository. J Am Coll Cardiol Img. 2015;8:1170–6.

84. Eisenberg E, Betancur J, Hu LH, Sharir T, Einstein A, Ruddy T, Kaufmann P, Sinusas A, Miller E, Bateman T, Dorbala S, Di Carli M, Germano G, Otaki Y, Tamarappoo B, Dey D, Berman D, Slomka P. The diagnostic accuracy of machine learning from stress only fast-MPS. J Nucl Med. 2018;59:508.

85. Hu LH, Miller RJH, Sharir T, Commandeur F, Rios R, Einstein AJ, Fish MB, Ruddy TD, Kaufmann PA, Sinusas AJ, Miller EJ, Bateman TM, Dorbala S, Di Carli M, Liang JX, Eisenberg E, Dey D, Berman DS, Slomka PJ. Prognostically safe stress-only single-photon emission computed tomography myocardial perfusion imaging guided by machine learning: report from REFINE SPECT. European Heart Journal Cardiovascular Imaging. 2020;22(6):705–14.

86. Mearns BM. Stress-only SPECT reduces radiation exposure but does not affect mortality. Nat Rev Cardiol. 2010;7:178.

87. Selvaraju RR, Cogswell M, Das A, Vedantam R, Parikh D, Batra D. Grad-cam: visual explanations from deep networks via gradient-based localization. In: Proceedings of the IEEE international conference on computer vision. 2017. p. 618–26.

88. Zeiler MD, Fergus R. Visualizing and understanding convolutional networks. In: European conference on computer vision 2014. p. 818–833.

89. de Vos BD, Wolterink JM, Leiner T, de Jong PA, Lessmann N, Isgum I. Direct automatic coronary calcium scoring in cardiac and chest CT. IEEE Trans Med Imaging. 2019;38:2127–38.

Part III

Impact of AI and ML on Molecular Imaging and Theranostics

Artificial Intelligence Will Improve Molecular Imaging, Therapy and Theranostics. Which Are the Biggest Advantages for Therapy?

12

Georgios Kaissis and Rickmer Braren

Contents

12.1 Introduction

Artificial Intelligence (AI) approaches in medical imaging have witnessed significant evolution over the past years. The reasons for this are manifold: The field of computer vision has arguably seen the most drastic advance in its state of the art facilitated by the increasingly widespread application of deep learning [1], the introduction of large, curated data sets facilitating transfer learning approaches [2], the substantial research and industry interest in the domain and the availability of both hardware accelerators (mainly graphics processing units) and software frameworks providing pretrained algorithms and approachable application programming interfaces lowering the barrier to entry to the field. Furthermore, medical imaging represents an excellent target for machine learning applications as it is widely available in standardized data exchange formats and stored electronically [3]. Also, the availability of images alongside medical/radiological reports provide inbuilt human ground-truth assessments of relevant findings.

G. Kaissis (✉)
Technical University of Munich, Munich, Germany

Imperial College London, London, UK
e-mail: g.kaissis@tum.de

R. Braren
Technical University of Munich, Munich, Germany
e-mail: rbraren@tum.de

The trend of large dataset accrual has increasingly also manifested in the medical field, with large databases of medical imaging data being assembled as national efforts attempting to provide a cross-sectional assessment of large populations of both healthy volunteers and patients. The German National Cohort Health Study (*NAKO Gesundheitsstudie, www.nako.de*) and the United Kingdom Biobank [4] are examples of this development, providing access to thousands of imaging data sets to researchers and practitioners in the field, which can be used for the development of machine learning algorithms. These efforts supplement initiatives such as the [5], representing curated collections of oncology-specific material including medical imaging but also digital histopathology or genomic sequence data. The increasing roll-out of partially or fully electronic patient records signifies a further important step towards the collection of relevant metadata, which can be included in predictive models alongside image-based information. However, such data repositories are not without specific challenges: Large-scale data collection signifies an increased importance of privacy protection, for which next-generation methods have only recently been introduced [6]. Moreover, data quality is paramount for the development of predictive algorithms, thus care needs to be taken that images and clinical metadata are generated and expertly curated with high standards of quality assurance. Algorithms need to be trained and validated on diverse and representative patient collectives to ascertain not only their validity when applied to unseen data from new sources, but also to assert their fairness, control their bias and render them reproducible and interpretable. The deployment of machine learning algorithms to clinical routine poses great challenges of its own, necessitating interdisciplinary cooperation and continuous monitoring and improvements. Finally, the reimbursement of algorithm-based diagnostic services remains largely unresolved. Issues such as these represent but a limited subset of the parameters which need to be taken into account in the design of artificial intelligence algorithms for medical use and are discussed in other parts of this book, as well as touched upon later in this chapter.

Expectedly for a novel field, most of the literature published on the topic of artificial intelligence applications in medical imaging has focused on diagnostic applications in the field of oncology such as the prediction of tumor subtypes, genetic features, metastatic behavior or patient survival. Algorithms targeted at diagnosis often provide objectively verifiable outputs (e.g. by comparison of the algorithm's prediction to a histopathologic result), and can be compared to the performance of human experts (e.g. true/false positive/negative rates), facilitating their validation. The field of therapy monitoring and theranostics, that is, the image-based expression quantification of relevant therapeutic targets, has however not yet witnessed the same level of research activity. Several reasons emerge, such as the following:

1. Treatment represents a heterogenous clinical process characterized by the application of several therapeutic approaches, often simultaneously. For instance, oncologic therapy consists of surgical, pharmacologic, radiotherapeutic, and other supplemental interventions. Establishing causal relationships between a certain treatment and its effect is therefore often a difficult undertaking.

2. The interplay between treatment and disease is hard to accurately quantify. For example, tumors demonstrate therapy escape phenomena leading to treatment resistance, which can be hard to distinguish from inefficacy or primary failure of the treatment.

3. Cancer imaging is influenced by systemic effects such as individual toxicity or comorbidities that can have a modulating effect on local findings (e.g. perfusion effects of anti-vascular agents versus decrease in cardiovascular output causing tissue mal-perfusion) and which are hard to deconvolve from specific treatment outcomes.

4. Effects mediating treatment response are also functions of the complex genetic, transcriptomic, epigenetic, and environmental tumor

landscape in which causes and effects can be impossible to distinguish.

5. Novel treatments are continuously introduced, thus retrospectively collected data, often the bedrock of oncological machine learning applications, might not be applicable as algorithm training material.

6. Finally, cancer is insufficiently understood and represents a disease as individual as the patients themselves. Intra- and inter-tumoral heterogeneity thus pose hindrances to the applicability of algorithmic tools aimed foremost at generalization, drastically increasing the difficulty of training such algorithms.

In attempting to taxonomically classify the current literature about machine learning and artificial intelligence approaches for treatment response prediction and assessment as well as theranostics, two patterns emerge:

- The majority of studies focus on the prediction of therapy response from a single timepoint and single surrogate. Such studies attempt to capture information from a singular imaging study, often the baseline examination, to predict differences in treatment outcome by characterizing a specific tumor phenotype.
- Studies focusing on longitudinal/integrative monitoring of findings, for example, integrating the features of the tumor alongside relevant metadata and/or their evolution over the treatment period to predict the course of therapy.

With respect to the defining tumor features, research can be stratified into studies aiming at the quantification of tumor volume, either purely morphological or morphological and metabolic, for example, by the definition and automated tracking of metabolic tumor volume, and into studies concerned with higher-order descriptors of disease features or treatment targets. Such features can be derived from the tumor itself, for example, histogram metrics, texture features etc.

and/or incorporate other data, such as clinical record information.

Finally, from a methodological point of view, research can be divided into studies applying traditional computer vision techniques by utilizing predefined mathematical descriptors of the image (features) alongside machine learning-methods typically used for tabular data analysis such as regression models, tree-based algorithms etc. and studies applying deep neural networks directly to the imaging data. For the former, the term radiomics is often used. We would like to point out that this distinction is not formal, and the term radiomics is used for deep-neural-network-based algorithms as well. Due to its ill definition, we eschew the usage of this term altogether and refer instead to the techniques and algorithms in question by their technical description, which we believe to be more both clearer and more informative.

The methodological concerns applied to a study are also a function of the data used for algorithm development. Unlike pure anatomic imaging, which typically takes the form of a three-dimensional stack of images in black and white, hybrid and functional imaging usually provides at least two congruent images for the same anatomical location. In case of dynamic acquisitions, such as multiple contrast media phases, the dimensionality of the data further increases. This data is often heterogeneous with respect to its spatial resolution (e.g. the technical resolution of the scanner or the effects resulting from interactions of radionuclides with the tissue leading to, for example, the actual resolution of PET differing from the nominal resolution of the detector elements). These factors need to be taken into account and potentially corrected for in quantitative imaging studies.

In the following sections we will highlight and contrast relevant literature findings regarding the application of machine learning to therapy response evaluation with a focus on hybrid oncological imaging and provide recommendations and future directions for practitioners and researchers in the field.

12.2 Literature Review

12.2.1 Morphological and Metabolic Tumor Volume Tracking

12.2.1.1 Volumetry-Based Oncological Response Assessment Frameworks

The conceptually simplest automated therapy surveillance approaches rely on the quantification of the reduction in tumor volume using automated methods, thus mirroring human evaluation, for example, by application of the Response Evaluation Criteria in Solid Tumors (RECIST). RECIST was among the first attempts to quantify tumor response to treatment in imaging. However, it relies on two-dimensional evaluation and on the definition of so-called target lesions, which necessarily limits its scope and potential representativeness, since individual tumor manifestations are employed as surrogates of disease burden. RECIST evaluation suffers from further notable limitations, mainly in tumor entities with ill-defined margins (e.g. pancreatic cancer) and can be a poor correlate of therapy response due to phenomena such as pseudo-progression, whereby tumor volume initially increases in response to therapy due to inflammatory changes. The 2009 position paper by Wahl et al. introduced a systematic framework combining previous guidelines for incorporating metabolic and functional imaging-derived information into tumor response assessment called PERCIST (PET response criteria in solid tumors). The PERCIST framework stipulates the categories complete and partial metabolic response, stable metabolic disease, and progressive metabolic disease by measurement of lean body mass-adjusted standardized uptake value (SUL). Similar frameworks have been proposed by other working groups, such as the EORTC, as well as combined functional/morphologic criteria such as the Lugano criteria proposed in 2014, incorporating elements of both RECIST and radionuclide uptake information.

The quantitative nature of PET allows the calculation of absolute radionuclide activity per volume tissue, offering benefits over the standardized uptake value, which has been shown to depend on several extraneous parameters. Thus, more recently, parameters like the total lesion glycolysis (TLG) and metabolic tumor volume (MTV) have been proposed as more precise biomarkers of disease activity. These however require a definition of the tumor volume itself, also termed segmentation.

12.2.1.2 Automated Segmentation-Based Volumetry Techniques

The evolution of automated volumetry methods thus closely follows the evolution of automated tumor segmentation methods. Earlier studies [7–9] rely on legacy segmentation techniques such as region-growing, nearest-neighbor or probabilistic graphical methods [10]. Hybrid imaging provides a benefit in this regard by providing a form of pre-segmentation mask via the high-SUV tumor region, helping to guide algorithm behavior. Such iso-contour-based segmentation methods [11] have been demonstrated, for example, in sarcoma. Similar approaches can also be applied directly to metabolic tumor volume (MTV) tracking without the associated morphological imaging. This approach has shown promise in several tumor entities such as rectal cancer [12], lymphoma [13], gynecological tumors [14], or esophageal cancer [15]. However, it has been noted that MTV lacks standardization and large-scale external validation and thus cannot be assumed to be a universal gold standard for therapy surveillance in comparison to, for example, the standardized uptake value (SUV) [16].

12.2.1.3 Evolution of Automated Segmentation Using Neural Networks

Automated segmentation has witnessed a substantial evolution with the introduction of neural network-based segmentation methods. Earlier methods, based on fully convolutional neural networks [17] have more recently been superseded by encoder–decoder architectures with transverse short-circuits, such as the UNet architecture proposed by Ronneberger et al. in 2015 [18] and their conceptual evolutions such as Feature Pyramid Networks (FPNs) [19]. A common trait of these architectures is the utilization of image information captured at multiple scales and the transmission of high spatial frequency (i.e. high detail) image information from early to late parts of the network with corresponding feature map sizes. Encoder–decoder architectures have dominated the segmentation literature since ca. 2015, and can be applied both in two and three dimensions. Fully automatic segmentation has been proposed as a solution to the aforementioned standardization problem [20] and been successfully applied to both treatment response assessment, for example, in breast cancer [21], where it has been shown to outperform dynamic contrast-enhanced MRI, and treatment planning, for example, for brain tumor radiotherapy [22].

12.3   Quantitative Image and Texture Analysis in Oncological Therapy Response Monitoring

The advent of quantitative image analysis workflows within the past 5 years has generated significant interest in the utilization of image-derived data for tumor characterization. Such approaches rely on either the bulk extraction of tumor-related image features, their preprocessing and modeling using machine learning (also termed radiomics), or the end-to-end analysis of image data using neural networks. As discussed above, we will not terminologically differentiate between these approaches, believing them to not be mutually exclusive. However, it is expected that the numerous shortcomings of the so-called radiomics workflow will eventually lead to its replacement by algorithms and techniques based on more robust techniques and models, and not susceptible to the same technical limitations we will describe below. The typical workflow of quantitative image analysis studies is common to both approaches, consisting of a volume of interest definition step and a modeling step. For volume of interest definition i.e. segmentation, both manual and all above-mentioned automatic methods are applicable and commonly used. For details on the various techniques, we refer to the chapters in Part I of this book.

The research developments in the field of treatment supervision in hybrid imaging have closely followed the main oncologic application areas of PET.

12.3.1 Neuro-Oncology

In neuro-oncologic applications, for example, studies have focused on the identification of molecular phenotypes with relevance for therapy and prognosis, such as isocitrate dehydrogenase status [23] from amino acid (fluoroethyl tyrosine, FET) PET scans in gliomas. The authors found that the inclusion of radiomic parameters improved diagnostic accuracy compared to PET-derived metrics alone. Similarly, a recent study by Hotta et al. found image texture parameters derived from 11C-methionine PET to yield excellent discriminative performance between recurrence of malignant brain tumors and radiation necrosis [24], a topic of critical relevance for steering treatment decisions. A multitude of works (see e.g. overview in [25]) have focused on brain metastases, amongst others for differentiation of primary brain tumors from metastases, pinpointing the origin of metastatic lesions to the brain and for differentiating treatment-related changes from recurrence. Recent studies have also focused specifically on treatment, with studies by Cha et al. demonstrating strong performance of convolutional neural network ensembles in the prediction of metastatic lesion response to radiotherapy [26] from baseline imaging examinations.

12.3.2 Head and Neck Cancers

In head and neck cancers, several studies have demonstrated the benefits of integrating quantitative imaging features with morphological tumor descriptors for predictive modeling workflows. For instance, Fujima et al. showed that in patients who underwent chemoradiation treatment for pharyngeal cancer, tumor shape and texture features were highly predictive of progression-free and overall patient survival [27]. They note that clinical parameters alone were not sufficient for discriminating survival subgroups in their study. Feliciani et al. employed texture metrics derived from pretherapeutic FDG-PET and found these imaging biomarkers highly predictive of local chemoradiation therapy failure [28]. Crispin-Ortuzar and colleagues aimed at predicting head and neck tumor hypoxia, which is usually assessed, for example, with specific hypoxia radiotracers such as 18F-FMISO, using FDG-PET-derived texture parameters. They report substantial improvements over baseline FDG-PET performance alone and note that quantitative imaging biomarkers can provide an alternative to hypoxia-specific radiotracers where such are unavailable [29].

12.3.3 Lung Cancer

In lung cancer, the relevance of including FDG-PET into patient workup was shown in the 2002 PLUS trial [30], demonstrating a 20% reduction in unnecessary surgical interventions. Consequently, several studies have investigated quantitative imaging features, for example, in the prediction of histological subtypes [31] or post-treatment survival [32]. Oikonomou et al. studied the association of quantitative image features with several outcomes, including local and distant disease control, recurrence-free probability and survival metrics and found image-derived features to represent the only predictors of overall survival, disease-specific survival and regional disease control [33]. A recent multicenter trial by Dissaux et al. demonstrated that FDG-PET-derived texture features predict local disease control in patients undergoing stereotactic radiotherapy for early-stage non-small-cell lung cancer and highlighted the potential value of such algorithms for therapeutic decision-making. The large body of research into machine learning and quantitative imaging biomarker applications in lung cancer has also provided insight into key challenges associated with such applications. Yang et al. note that the widespread application of texture-derived image features as prognostic predictors is impeded by a lack of quality control

and robustness and proceed to demonstrate high inter-rater variability impacting the reproducibility of texture parameters [34]. Such challenges are of course not immanent to thoracic imaging workflows and have been repeatedly noted in previous studies irrespective of imaging modality applied [35, 36] with PET-specific solutions recently proposed [37].

12.3.4 Prostate Cancer

The role of hybrid imaging in prostate cancer is continuously evolving and expanding with the application of Gallium or Fluorine-labeled PSMA supported by recent meta-analyses [38, 39] and having been demonstrated to impact patient management in a majority of cases [40]. The first randomized prospective trial testing the influence of PSMA PET/CT on prostate patient outcome was announced in early 2019 [41]. Quantitative imaging feature studies have recently provided promising results applied to PSMA PET. For example, Zamboglou et al. demonstrate PSMA-PET-derived quantitative features to discriminate between cancer- and non-cancer-affected prostate tissue, as well as differentiate between Gleason scores of 7 and ≥ 8 and between patients with and without nodal involvement [42]. PSMA expression is an excellent example of a theranostic application, i.e. the specific expression monitoring of a therapy-relevant target: since Lutetium-PSMA can be used for radioligand treatment in advanced prostate cancer [43], machine-learning applications predicting response to such therapy directly from the images could hence represent a promising next step.

12.3.5 Breast Cancer

The field of breast cancer research has witnessed among the strongest advances in the utilization of quantitative imaging workflows and the application of machine intelligence, likely due to the high quality of image acquisition because of the lack of motion artifacts, the universal implementation of standardized reporting in the form of BIRADS and the high incidence. Hence, several studies have proposed image-derived features for the noninvasive characterization of breast cancer. For example, Antunovic et al. utilized pretreatment FDG-PET/CT of breast cancer and found histogram features to be associated with histopathological, molecular, and receptor expression subtypes [44]. Similarly, Huang et al. found image features derived from PET/MRI data to be associated with tumor grading, stage, subtype, recurrence, and survival [45]. Ou et al. utilize machine learning to differentiate between breast carcinoma and breast lymphoma based on texture features derived from FDG-PET/CT [46]. Focused on therapy response prediction, Antunovic and colleagues noted the association of molecular breast cancer subtypes with distinct responses to neoadjuvant chemotherapy and developed machine learning algorithms on FDG-PET/CT to predict pathological complete response in locally advanced breast cancer [47]. Ha et al. also utilized FDG-PET/CT to develop machine learning-derived metabolic signatures of breast cancer associated with Ki67 gene expression, pathological complete response to neoadjuvant chemotherapy and recurrence risk [48]. As noted above, however, such workflows are not without challenges and it was recently noted in the work by Sollini et al. that *most evidence on the utility [...] is at the feasibility level.* The authors recommend harmonization, validation on representative datasets and the establishment of guidelines for the application of quantitative imaging parameters in breast imaging [49].

12.3.6 Gastrointestinal Oncology

The largest body of work regarding therapy prediction using quantitative image-derived parameters in hybrid imaging has arguably been produced in the area of gastrointestinal oncology. In esophageal cancer for instance, several studies on radiomics workflows have highlighted the significance of heterogeneity-related image features and have derived models predictive of prognosis

and therapy response [50–52]. Yip et al. included longitudinally acquired datasets in their model and found a decrease in tumor heterogeneity-related texture and histogram features to be associated with tumor response and patient survival [53]. Ypsilantis et al. employed convolutional neural networks on PET scans and found them to outperform radiomics models in the prediction of therapy response in esophageal cancer [54]. Furthermore, sub-regional analyses, taking into account intra-tumoral heterogeneity are being assessed for their impact on the survival of esophageal cancer patients treated with chemoradiation, shown, for example, in the study by Xie et al. [55].

In pancreatic cancer, multiparametric imaging and machine learning have been investigated for differentiation of inflammatory and neoplastic processes [56]. The added utility of hybrid fusion imaging for the delineation of tumors has been noted by Belli et al. in a recent study [57] with applications in quantitative imaging workflows. In our own work, we note the importance and potential benefits of multiparametric data integration for accurate prognostic prediction in the field of pancreatic cancer [58]. Cui et al. identified quantitative parameters prognostic of stereotactic radiation therapy in pancreatic cancer from FDG-PET/CT imaging [59]. With the evolving role of hybrid imaging for therapy planning in pancreatic cancer [60, 61] especially with respect to neoadjuvant treatment regimens, as well as the advances in molecular subtyping including the distinction of differentially activated metabolic pathways, [62–64], it must be assumed that the scope of quantitative imaging workflows will soon expand further to hybrid imaging.

In rectal cancer, several studies have investigated the utility of pretreatment quantitative imaging biomarkers in the prediction of therapy response. The study by Lovinfosse and colleagues found texture parameters derived from pretreatment FDG-PET/CT predictive of survival in a cohort of patients with locally advanced rectal cancer treated with neoadjuvant chemoradiation, noting that these features outperformed volume-based parameters in predictive performance [65]. Amorim et al. compared FDG-PET- and diffusion-weighted MRI-derived parameters and observed the information gained from these modalities to be independent and complementary, underscoring the relevance of multiparametric hybrid imaging workflows in oncology [66]. The importance of tumor heterogeneity was noted by Bundschuh et al., who note that heterogeneity-related image features are relevant both early in the course of therapy and after its completion [67]. A similar dual timepoint study was performed by Jeon et al., who performed multiparametric modeling including clinical parameters and MRI-derived texture features and observed changes in these features to be associated with distinct risk phenotypes. The authors note that their results would be applicable to and benefit from the inclusion of functional imaging [68].

12.4   Discussion and Outlook

In this chapter, we review the applications of machine learning and artificial intelligence to therapy monitoring in the domain of molecular and hybrid imaging, as well as theranostics. Despite its somewhat earlier stage of evolution compared to applications purely focused on diagnosis, such as tumor detection or subtype classification, the multitude of studies presented showcase the intense research interest in the field and provide an outlook on the main objectives of techniques, algorithms, and applications aimed at therapy monitoring and response prediction. Evidently, diagnostic and theranostic applications are closely related. For example, specific tumor subtypes are associated with distinct therapy response, providing space for exploration of novel therapy targets and specific therapeutic agents. The clinical utilization of theranostic radiotracers is also expected to expand beyond the current main routine application of prostate imaging with PSMA: initial studies report successes, for example, in the application of texture analysis in neuroendocrine tumors [69]. The combined application of diagnostic and theranostic radiotracers has also been reported, with very recent results showcasing their complementary value in the outcome prediction of pancreatic

neuroendocrine neoplasms [70], expanding on previous studies reporting on combined radiotracer application [71]. We believe machine learning techniques to herald a transition towards integrated theranostic applications which will likely blur the current borders between diagnosis- and therapy-response-focused studies. This evolution will obviously not remain without challenges. Foremost, it will be predicated on the development and availability of emerging and novel theranostic radiotracers beyond the above-mentioned fields of prostate cancer and neuroendocrine tumors, as well as the understanding of their interaction with biological targets and their unique challenges and pitfalls [72], to enable their utilization in AI-guided and precision medicine applications [73].

Reviewing the current literature findings, a clear trend can be observed from tumor tissue and metabolic volume tracking applications towards image texture analysis which can be ascribed to the above-mentioned rise of quantitative imaging workflows [74] within the past few years. We however still observe specific challenges, several of which are unmet in current literature:

Nearly all of the studies outlined above utilize hybrid imaging-based texture analysis workflows. A more thorough investigation on the differential contribution of each modality to the predictive model, or an analysis of the added benefit of hybrid imaging over a single modality were not routinely performed. Anatomic and functional imaging have been shown to present specific and individual challenges with respect to texture analysis, rendering such a differentiated assessment necessary [75]. Furthermore, the difficulties of harmonizing quantitative imaging workflows and rendering them robust towards variances between diagnostic equipment vendors, differences in human performance and unstandardized texture feature specifications have been noted extensively in the literature [36], mostly aimed at anatomical imaging modalities. However, recent works have focused on harmonizing texture features specifically in functional imaging [37] alongside efforts for protocol standardization and guidelines aimed at hybrid imaging studies [76]. Ultimately, we believe handcrafted quantitative imaging features and the field of radiomics to represent an intermediate step in the evolution of machine learning application in medical imaging towards deep learning-based workflows. The latter offer greater representational flexibility and robustness, obviating post-processing and harmonization requirements in favor of data diversity and larger patient cohorts and rendering them inherently more suitable for multicentric studies [77–80]. The advent of deep learning and associated advances in image registration [81] will also signify greater facility in integrating additional information from studies acquired at multiple timepoints. Longitudinal imaging has been shown to offer deeper insight into therapy-related changes in tumor biology [82]; however, it was only performed in a small fraction of the studies presented above due to the difficulties of acquiring multi-timepoint imaging and the escalated requirements towards selection of time-stable and reproducible image features [83]. Lastly, many of the studies presented base their assessment of therapy response on surrogate measurements, for example, on tumor volume decrease or on associations between therapy response and a decrease in image heterogeneity believed to mirror biological phenomena, which cannot always be objectively validated. Furthermore, therapy response is a multifactorial process greatly dependent on clinical parameters, which should be included in the modeling process [58]. The introduction of algorithms enabling the direct prediction of patient survival from images and the associated clinical data [84] will thus improve the capabilities for pre-therapeutic risk stratification and provide higher confidence for guiding therapy decisions.

In conclusion, this chapter discusses the applications of machine learning-based medical image analysis workflows, their applications to therapy response monitoring and theranostics in a hybrid imaging setting, as well as current and future research directions. We believe that the concurrent evolution and innovations in the fields of oncologic hybrid imaging, theranostics, and computer vision will fuel scientific discovery in the field and provide the opportunity for clinical translation and improvements to patient care.

References

1. Sejnowski TJ. The unreasonable effectiveness of deep learning in artificial intelligence. Proc Natl Acad Sci. 2020;117(48):30033–8.
2. Deng J, Dong W, Socher R, Li L-J, Li K, Fei-Fei L. ImageNet: a large-scale hierarchical image database. In: CVPR09. 2009.
3. Gibaud B. The quest for standards in medical imaging. Eur J Radiol. 2011;78:190–8.
4. Sudlow C, Gallacher J, Allen N, Beral V, Burton P, Danesh J, et al. UK biobank: an open access resource for identifying the causes of a wide range of complex diseases of middle and old age. PLoS Med. 2015;12:e1001779.
5. Prior F, Smith K, Sharma A, Kirby J, Tarbox L, Clark K, et al. The public cancer radiology imaging collections of the cancer imaging archive. Scient Data. 2017;4:170124.
6. Kaissis GA, Makowski MR, Rückert D, Braren RF. Secure, privacy-preserving and federated machine learning in medical imaging. Nature Mach Intell. 2020;2:305–11.
7. Clark M, Hall L, Goldgof D, Velthuizen R, Murtagh F, Silbiger M. Automatic tumor segmentation using knowledge-based techniques. IEEE Trans Med Imaging. 1998;17:187–201.
8. Vokurka EA, Herwadkar A, Thacker NA, Ramsden RT, Jackson A. Using bayesian tissue classification to improve the accuracy of vestibular schwannoma volume and growth measurement. AJNR Am J Neuroradiol. 2002;23:459–67.
9. Haney SM, Thompson PM, Cloughesy TF, Alger JR, Toga AW. Tracking tumor growth rates in patients with malignant gliomas: a test of two algorithms. AJNR Am J Neuroradiol. 2001;22:73–82.
10. Zhao Z, Yang G, Lin Y, Pang H, Wang M. Automated glioma detection and segmentation using graphical models. PLoS One. 2018;13:e0200745.
11. Lee H, Paeng JC, Hong SH, Yoo HJ, Cheon GJ, Lee DS, et al. Appropriate margin thresholds for isocontour metabolic volumetry of fluorine-18 fluorodeoxyglucose PET in sarcoma. Nucl Med Commun. 2016;37:1088–94.
12. Bang J-I, Ha S, Kang S-B, Lee K-W, Lee H-S, Kim J-S, et al. Prediction of neoadjuvant radiation chemotherapy response and survival using pretreatment [18F] FDG PET/CT scans in locally advanced rectal cancer. Eur J Nucl Med Mol Imaging. 2015;43:422–31.
13. Kostakoglu L, Chauvie S. Metabolic tumor volume metrics in lymphoma. Semin Nucl Med. 2018;48:50–66.
14. Erdogan M, Erdemoglu E, Evrimler S, Hanedan C, Şengül SS. Prognostic value of metabolic tumor volume and total lesion glycolysis assessed by 18F-FDG PET/CT in endometrial cancer. Nucl Med Commun. 2019;40:1099–104.
15. Yildirim BA, Torun N, Guler OC, Onal C. Prognostic value of metabolic tumor volume and total lesion gly-

colysis in esophageal carcinoma patients treated with definitive chemoradiotherapy. Nucl Med Commun. 2018;39:553–63.

16. Gallamini A, Kostakoglu L. Metabolic tumor volume: we still need a platinum-standard metric. J Nucl Med. 2016;58:196–7.

17. Long J, Shelhamer E, Darrell T. Fully convolutional networks for semantic segmentation. arXiv e-prints [Internet]. 2014. Available from: http://arxiv.org/abs/1411.4038v2

18. Ronneberger O, Fischer P, Brox T. U-net: Convolutional networks for biomedical image segmentation. arXiv e-prints [Internet]. 2015. Available from: http://arxiv.org/abs/1505.04597v1

19. Wu X, Sahoo D, Zhang D, Zhu J, Hoi SC. Single-shot bidirectional pyramid networks for high-quality object detection. Neurocomputing. 2020;401:1–9.

20. Beichel RR, Smith BJ, Bauer C, Ulrich EJ, Ahmadvand P, Budzevich MM, et al. Multi-site quality and variability analysis of 3D FDG PET segmentations based on phantom and clinical image data. Med Phys. 2017;44:479–96.

21. Andreassen MMS, Goa PE, Sjøbakk TE, Hedayati R, Eikesdal HP, Deng C, et al. Semi-automatic segmentation from intrinsically-registered 18F-FDGPET/MRI for treatment response assessment in a breast cancer cohort: comparison to manual DCEMRI. MAGMA. 2019;33:317–28.

22. Rundo L, Stefano A, Militello C, Russo G, Sabini MG, D'Arrigo C, et al. A fully automatic approach for multimodal PET and MR image segmentation in gamma knife treatment planning. Comput Methods Prog Biomed. 2017;144:77–96.

23. Lohmann P, Lerche C, Bauer EK, Steger J, Stoffels G, Blau T, et al. Predicting IDH genotype in gliomas using FET PET radiomics. Sci Rep. 2018;8:13328.

24. Hotta M, Minamimoto R, Miwa K. 11C-methionine-PET for differentiating recurrent brain tumor from radiation necrosis: radiomics approach with random forest classifier. Sci Rep. 2019;9:15666.

25. Lohmann P, Kocher M, Ruge MI, Visser-Vandewalle V, Shah NJ, Fink GR, et al. PET/MRI radiomics in patients with brain metastases. Front Neurol. 2020;11:1.

26. Cha YJ, Jang WI, Kim M-S, Yoo HJ, Paik EK, Jeong HK, et al. Prediction of response to stereotactic radiosurgery for brain metastases using convolutional neural networks. Anticancer Res. 2018;38:5437–45.

27. Fujima N, Hirata K, Shiga T, Li R, Yasuda K, Onimaru R, et al. Integrating quantitative morphological and intratumoural textural characteristics in FDG-PET for the prediction of prognosis in pharynx squamous cell carcinoma patients. Clin Radiol. 2018;73(1059):e1–8.

28. Feliciani G, Fioroni F, Grassi E, Bertolini M, Rosca A, Timon G, et al. Radiomic profiling of head and neck cancer: 18F-FDG PET texture analysis as predictor of patient survival. Contrast Media Mol Imaging. 2018;2018:1–8.

29. Crispin-Ortuzar M, Apte A, Grkovski M, Oh JH, Lee NY, Schöder H, et al. Predicting hypoxia status

using a combination of contrast-enhanced computed tomography and [18F]-fluorodeoxyglucose positron emission tomography radiomics features. Radiother Oncol. 2018;127:36–42.

30. van Tinteren H, Hoekstra OS, Smit EF, van den Bergh JH, Schreurs AJ, Stallaert RA, et al. Effectiveness of positron emission tomography in the preoperative assessment of patients with suspected non-small-cell lung cancer: the PLUS multicentre randomised trial. Lancet. 2002;359:1388–92.

31. Hyun SH, Ahn MS, Koh YW, Lee SJ. A machine-learning approach using PET-based radiomics to predict the histological subtypes of lung cancer. Clin Nucl Med. 2019;44:956–60.

32. Ahn H, Lee H, Kim S, Hyun S. Pre-treatment 18F-FDG PET-based radiomics predict survival in resected non-small cell lung cancer. Clin Radiol. 2019;74:467–73.

33. Oikonomou A, Khalvati F, Tyrrell PN, Haider MA, Tarique U, Jimenez-Juan L, et al. Radiomics analysis at PET/CT contributes to prognosis of recurrence and survival in lung cancer treated with stereotactic body radiotherapy. Sci Rep. 2018;8:4003.

34. Yang F, Simpson G, Young L, Ford J, Dogan N, Wang L. Impact of contouring variability on oncological PET radiomics features in the lung. Sci Rep. 2020;10:369.

35. van Timmeren JE, Carvalho S, Leijenaar RTH, Troost EGC, van Elmpt W, de Ruysscher D, et al. Challenges and caveats of a multi-center retrospective radiomics study: an example of early treatment response assessment for NSCLC patients using FDG-PET/CT radiomics. PLoS One. 2019;14:e0217536.

36. Rizzo S, Botta F, Raimondi S, Origgi D, Fanciullo C, Morganti AG, et al. Radiomics: the facts and the challenges of image analysis. Eur Radiol Exp. 2018;2:36.

37. Orlhac F, Boughdad S, Philippe C, Stalla-Bourdillon H, Nioche C, Champion L, et al. A postreconstruction harmonization method for multicenter radiomic studies in PET. J Nucl Med. 2018;59:1321–8.

38. Hope TA, Goodman JZ, Allen IE, Calais J, Fendler WP, Carroll PR. Meta analysis of 68Ga-PSMA-11 PET accuracy for the detection of prostate cancer validated by histopathology. J Nucl Med. 2018;60:786–93.

39. Perera M, Papa N, Christidis D, Wetherell D, Hofman MS, Murphy DG, et al. Sensitivity, specificity, and predictors of positive 68 gaProstate-specific membrane antigen positron emission tomography in advanced prostate cancer: a systematic review and meta-analysis. Eur Urol. 2016;70:926–37.

40. Calais J, Fendler WP, Eiber M, Gartmann J, Chu F-I, Nickols NG, et al. Impact of 68Ga-PSMA-11 PET/CT on the management of prostate cancer patients with biochemical recurrence. J Nucl Med. 2017;59:434–41.

41. Calais J, Czernin J, Fendler WP, Elashoff D, Nickols NG. Randomized prospective phase III trial of 68Ga-PSMA-11 PET/CT molecular imaging for prostate cancer salvage radiotherapy planning [PSMA-SRT]. BMC Cancer. 2019;19:18.

42. Zamboglou C, Carles M, Fechter T, Kiefer S, Reichel K, Fassbender TF, et al. Radiomic features from PSMA PET for non-invasive intraprostatic tumor discrimination and characterization in patients with intermediate- and high-risk prostate cancer - a comparison study with histology reference. Theranostics. 2019;9:2595–605.

43. Hofman MS, Violet J, Hicks RJ, Ferdinandus J, Thang SP, Akhurst T, et al. [177 lu]-PSMA-617 radionuclide treatment in patients with metastatic castration-resistant prostate cancer (LuPSMA trial): A single-centre, single-arm, phase 2 study. Lancet Oncol. 2018;19:825–33.

44. Antunovic L, Gallivanone F, Sollini M, Sagona A, Invento A, Manfrinato G, et al. [18F]FDG PET/CT features for the molecular characterization of primary breast tumors. Eur J Nucl Med Mol Imaging. 2017;44:1945–54.

45. Huang S-y, Franc BL, Harnish RJ, Liu G, Mitra D, Copeland TP, et al. Exploration of PET and MRI radiomic features for decoding breast cancer phenotypes and prognosis. npj Breast Cancer. 2018;4:24.

46. Ou X, Zhang J, Wang J, Pang F, Wang Y, Wei X, et al. Radiomics based on 18 f-FDG PET/CT could differentiate breast carcinoma from breast lymphoma using machine-learning approach: a preliminary study. Cancer Med. 2019;9:496–506.

47. Antunovic L, Sanctis RD, Cozzi L, Kirienko M, Sagona A, Torrisi R, et al. PET/CT radiomics in breast cancer: promising tool for prediction of pathological response to neoadjuvant chemotherapy. Eur J Nucl Med Mol Imaging. 2019;46:1468–77.

48. Ha S, Park S, Bang J-I, Kim E-K, Lee H-Y. Metabolic radiomics for pretreatment 18F-FDG PET/CT to characterize locally advanced breast cancer: histopathologic characteristics, response to neoadjuvant chemotherapy, and prognosis. Sci Rep. 2017;7:1556.

49. Sollini M, Cozzi L, Ninatti G, Antunovic L, Cavinato L, Chiti A, et al. PET/CT radiomics in breast cancer: mind the step. Methods. 2021;188:122–32.

50. Yip C, Landau D, Kozarski R, Ganeshan B, Thomas R, Michaelidou A, et al. Primary esophageal cancer: heterogeneity as potential prognostic biomarker in patients treated with definitive chemotherapy and radiation therapy. Radiology. 2014;270:141–8.

51. van Rossum PSN, Fried DV, Zhang L, Hofstetter WL, van Vulpen M, Meijer GJ, et al. The incremental value of subjective and quantitative assessment of 18F-FDG PET for the prediction of pathologic complete response to preoperative chemoradiotherapy in esophageal cancer. J Nucl Med. 2016;57:691–700.

52. Xiong J, Yu W, Ma J, Ren Y, Fu X, Zhao J. The role of PET-based radiomic features in predicting local control of esophageal cancer treated with concurrent chemoradiotherapy. Sci Rep. 2018;8:9902.

53. Yip C, Davnall F, Kozarski R, Landau DB, Cook GJR, Ross P, et al. Assessment of changes in tumor heterogeneity following neoadjuvant chemotherapy in primary esophageal cancer. Dis Esophagus. 2014;28:172–9.

54. Ypsilantis P-P, Siddique M, Sohn H-M, Davies A, Cook G, Goh V, et al. Predicting response to neoadjuvant chemotherapy with PET imaging using convolutional neural networks. PLoS One. 2015;10:e0137036.

55. Xie C, Yang P, Zhang X, Xu L, Wang X, Li X, et al. Sub-region based radiomics analysis for survival prediction in oesophageal tumours treated by definitive concurrent chemoradiotherapy. EBioMedicine. 2019;44:289–97.

56. Zhang Y, Cheng C, Liu Z, Wang L, Pan G, Sun G, et al. Radiomics analysis for the differentiation of autoimmune pancreatitis and pancreatic ductal adenocarcinoma in 18 f-FDG PET/CT. Med Phys. 2019;46:4520–30.

57. Belli ML, Mori M, Broggi S, Cattaneo GM, Bettinardi V, Dell'Oca I, et al. Quantifying the robustness of [18 f]FDG-PET/CT radiomic features with respect to tumor delineation in head and neck and pancreatic cancer patients. Phys Med. 2018;49:105–11.

58. Kaissis GA, Jungmann F, Ziegelmayer S, Lohöfer FK, Harder FN, Schlitter AM, et al. Multiparametric modelling of survival in pancreatic ductal adenocarcinoma using clinical, histomorphological, genetic and image-derived parameters. J Clin Med. 2020;9:1250.

59. Cui Y, Song J, Pollom E, Shirato H, Chang D, Koong A, et al. Radiomic analysis of FDG-PET identifies novel prognostic imaging biomarkers in locally advanced pancreatic cancer patients treated with SBRT. Int J Radiat Oncol Biol Phys. 2015;93:S4–5.

60. Dholakia AS, Chaudhry M, Leal JP, Chang DT, Raman SP, Hacker-Prietz A, et al. Baseline metabolic tumor volume and total lesion glycolysis are associated with survival outcomes in patients with locally advanced pancreatic cancer receiving stereotactic body radiation therapy. Int J Radiat Oncol Biol Phys. 2014;89:539–46.

61. Mellon EA, Jin WH, Frakes JM, Centeno BA, Strom TJ, Springett GM, et al. Predictors and survival for pathologic tumor response grade in borderline resectable and locally advanced pancreatic cancer treated with induction chemotherapy and neoadjuvant stereotactic body radiotherapy. Acta Oncol. 2016;56:391–7.

62. Kaissis G, Ziegelmayer S, Lohöfer F, Steiger K, Algül H, Muckenhuber A, et al. A machine learning algorithm predicts molecular subtypes in pancreatic ductal adenocarcinoma with differential response to gemcitabine-based versus FOLFIRINOX chemotherapy. PLoS One. 2019;14:e0218642.

63. Kaissis GA, Ziegelmayer S, Lohöfer FK, Harder FN, Jungmann F, Sasse D, et al. Image-based molecular phenotyping of pancreatic ductal adenocarcinoma. J Clin Med. 2020;9:724.

64. Kaissis G, Ziegelmayer S, Lohöfer F, Algül H, Eiber M, Weichert W, et al. A machine learning model for the prediction of survival and tumor subtype in pancreatic ductal adenocarcinoma from preoperative diffusion-weighted imaging. Eur Radiol Exp. 2019;3:41.

65. Lovinfosse P, Polus M, Daele DV, Martinive P, Daenen F, Hatt M, et al. FDG PET/CT radiomics for predicting the outcome of locally advanced rectal

cancer. European Journal of Nuclear Medicine and Molecular Imaging. 2017;45:365–75.

66. Amorim BJ, Torrado-Carvajal A, Esfahani SA, Marcos SS, Vangel M, Stein D, et al. PET/MRI radiomics in rectal cancer: a pilot study on the correlation between PET- and MRI-derived image features with a clinical interpretation. Mol Imag Biol. 2020;22(5):1438–45.

67. Bundschuh RA, Dinges J, Neumann L, Seyfried M, Zsoter N, Papp L, et al. Textural parameters of tumor heterogeneity in 18F-FDG PET/CT for therapy response assessment and prognosis in patients with locally advanced rectal cancer. J Nucl Med. 2014;55:891–7.

68. Jeon SH, Song C, Chie EK, Kim B, Kim YH, Chang W, et al. Delta-radiomics signature predicts treatment outcomes after preoperative chemoradiotherapy and surgery in rectal cancer. Radiat Oncol. 2019;14:43.

69. Werner RA, Ilhan H, Lehner S, Papp L, Zsótér N, Schatka I, et al. Pre-therapy somatostatin receptor-based heterogeneity predicts overall survival in pancreatic neuroendocrine tumor patients undergoing peptide receptor radionuclide therapy. Mol Imaging Biol. 2018;21:582–90.

70. Mapelli P, Partelli S, Salgarello M, Doraku J, Pasetto S, Rancoita PM, et al. Dual tracer 68Ga-DOTATOC and 18F-FDG PET/computed tomography radiomics in pancreatic neuroendocrine neoplasms: an endearing tool for preoperative risk assessment. Nucl Med Commun. 2020;41(9):896–905.

71. Hindié E. The NETPET score: combining FDG and somatostatin receptor imaging for optimal management of patients with metastatic well-differentiated neuroendocrine tumors. Theranostics. 2017;7:1159–63.

72. Werner RA, Thackeray JT, Pomper MG, Bengel FM, Gorin MA, Derlin T, et al. Recent updates on molecular imaging reporting and data systems (MI-RADS) for theranostic radiotracersNavigating pitfalls of SSTR- and PSMA-targeted PET/CT. J Clin Med. 2019;8:1060.

73. van der Meel R, Sulheim E, Shi Y, Kiessling F, Mulder WJM, Lammers T. Smart cancer nanomedicine. Nat Nanotechnol. 2019;14:1007–17.

74. Gillies RJ, Kinahan PE, Hricak H. Radiomics: images are more than pictures, they are data. Radiology. 2016;278:563–77.

75. Cook GJ, Azad G, Owczarczyk K, Siddique M, Goh V. Challenges and promises of PET radiomics. Int J Radiat Oncol Biol Phys. 2018;102:1083–9.

76. Prenosil GA, Weitzel T, Fürstner M, Hentschel M, Krause T, Cumming P, et al. Towards guidelines to harmonize textural features in PET: Haralick textural features vary with image noise, but exposure-invariant domains enable comparable PET radiomics. PLoS One. 2020;15:e0229560.

77. Kuhl CK, Truhn D. The long route to standardized radiomics: unraveling the knot from the end. Radiology. 2020;295:339–41.

78. Truhn D, Schrading S, Haarburger C, Schneider H, Merhof D, Kuhl C. Radiomic versus convolutional neural networks analysis for classification of contrast-enhancing lesions at multiparametric breast MRI. Radiology. 2019;290:290–7.

79. Lou B, Doken S, Zhuang T, Wingerter D, Gidwani M, Mistry N, et al. An image-based deep learning framework for individualising radiotherapy dose: a retrospective analysis of outcome prediction. Lancet Digit Health. 2019;1:e136–47.

80. Sun Q, Lin X, Zhao Y, Li L, Yan K, Liang D, et al. Deep learning vs. radiomics for predicting axillary lymph node metastasis of breast cancer using ultrasound images: Don't forget the peritumoral region. Front Oncol. 2020;10:53.

81. Haskins G, Kruger U, Yan P. Deep learning in medical image registration: a survey. Mach Vis Appl. 2020;31:8.

82. Bak SH, Park H, Sohn I, Lee SH, Ahn M-J, Lee HY. Prognostic impact of longitudinal monitoring of radiomic features in patients with advanced non-small cell lung cancer. Sci Rep. 2019;9:8730.

83. Leijenaar RTH, Carvalho S, Velazquez ER, van Elmpt WJC, Parmar C, Hoekstra OS, et al. Stability of FDG-PET radiomics features: an integrated analysis of test-retest and inter-observer variability. Acta Oncol. 2013;52:1391–7.

84. Katzmann A, Mühlberg A, Sühling M, Nörenberg D, Maurus S, Holch JW, et al. Computed tomography image-based deep survival regression for metastatic colorectal cancer using a non-proportional hazards model. Predict Intell Med. 2019:73–80.

Integrative Computational Biology, AI, and Radiomics: Building Explainable Models by Integration of Imaging, Omics, and Clinical Data

13

I. Jurisica

Contents

Abbreviations

^{18}F-FDG	^{18}Fluoro-deoxy-glucose
AD	Alzheimer's disease
AI	Artificial intelligence
AUC	Area under the curve
cDNA	Complementary DNA
CNIL	National Commission on Informatics and Liberty
CPU	Central processing unit
CT	Computer tomography
DLBCL	Diffuse large B cell lymphoma
DNA	Deoxyribonucleic acid
ECG	Electrocardiography
EEG	Electroencephalography
EFS	Event-free survival
EIM	Electrical impedance myography
EOG	Electrooculography
EPR	Electronic patient record
FCSRT	Free and cued selective reminding test
fMRI	Functional magnetic resonance imaging
GLCM	Grey level co-occurrence matrix
GLNU	Grey-level non-uniformity
GLSZM	Grey-level size zone matrix
GPU	Graphical processing unit
HGZE	High grey-level zone emphasis
HT	High-throughput
ICD	International classification of diseases

I. Jurisica (✉)
Osteoarthritis Research Program, Division of
Orthopedic Surgery, Schroeder Arthritis Institute, and
Data Science Discovery Centre for Chronic Diseases,
Krembil Research Institute, University Health
Network, Toronto, ON, Canada
e-mail: juris@ai.utoronto.ca

IID	Integrated interactions database
IPIaa	Age-adjusted international prognostic index
LASSI-L	Loewenstein-Acevedo scale for semantic interference and learning
LGZE	Low grey-level zone emphasis
LUAD	Lung adenocarcinoma
LZE	Long-zone emphasis
LZHGE	Long-zone high grey-level emphasis
LZLGE	Long-zone low grey-level emphasis
mirDIP	microRNA data integration portal
miRNA	microRNA
ML	Machine learning
MRI	Magnetic resonance imaging
MSK	Musculoskeletal
MTV	Metabolic tumor volume
NDD	Neurodegenerative diseases
NHL	Non-Hodgkin's lymphoma
OS	Overall survival
OSEM	Ordered subset expectation maximisation
pathDIP	Pathway data integration portal
PET	Positron emission tomography
piRNA	Piwi-interacting RNA
PPI	Protein–protein interaction
PSF	Point spread function
RNA	Ribonucleic acid
RNAseq	RNA sequencing
ROC	Receiver operating characteristic
scRNAseq	Single-cell RNA sequencing
SD	Standard deviation
SNOMED CT	Standard nomenclature of medicine clinical terms
SUV	Standardised uptake value
SZE	Short-zone emphasis
SZHGE	Short-zone high grey-level emphasis
SZLGE	Short-zone low grey-level emphasis
TCGA	The cancer genome atlas
TILs	Tumor infiltrated lymphocytes
VOI	Volume of interest
ZLNU	Zone length non-uniformity
ZP	Zone percentage

13.1 Introduction

Technological advances and high-throughput (HT) assays are rapidly changing the way we formulate and test biological hypotheses. Advances in imaging modalities, RNA sequencing, and mass spectrometry analysis have enabled translational research and clinical applications to simultaneously view all genes expressed, identify proteome-wide changes, and assess interacting partners of each individual protein within a biological system. Such views are already having an impact on our understanding of human disease, particularly in the realm of cancer biology [1]. However, it may be challenging to identify useful information from these studies, ensure that signal is separated from noise, and provide hypotheses for further research, with the goal to deliver measurable clinical impact. Often we only have fragmented patient cohorts, small number of samples with large number of parameters, unknown or poorly understood biases of individual assays often lead to incorrect data processing which in turn leads to incorrect results. Diverse algorithms in analysis workflows produce different results, often further reducing signal from noise.

Addressing important clinical questions requires systematic knowledge management and analysis of the large volume of diverse information. Biomedical information is inherently multimodal, covering clinical parameters, images, gene expression, protein expression and protein interactions, metabolites, drugs and pathways. Analyzing these data and using it intelligently is a challenge because of their complexity, multiple interdependent factors, the uncertainty of these dependencies, and the continuous evolution of our understanding of the data. Proper data management and analysis will in turn impact prevention, early diagnosis, disease classification, prognostics, and treatment planning.

13.2 Artificial Intelligence and Data-Driven Science

Artificial intelligence (AI) research focuses on development of diverse algorithms, their application in multiple areas, and system performance and usability questions. AI algorithms fit into several broad categories, including representation and ontologies, search and retrieval, feature extraction, constraint optimization, and diverse learning strategies from classification and clustering, to decision trees, random forest, case-based reasoning, support vector machines, Naive Bayes, and neural networks.

Algorithms need to be properly trained and validated. This requires high-quality datasets, properly annotated, with sufficiently large number of samples for complex domains with high-dimensional parameters. Knowing the biases of individual assays used for data generation may help avoiding mistakes and reduce unwanted influences affecting AI system performance and

incorrect result interpretation. Evidence-based medicine and data-driven science rely on high-quality data and independently validated results. However, data correctness and truth may not always be straightforward to assess and quantify. It used to be true that we can rely on peer-reviewed, published literature. However, detailed analysis of over 2000 retracted articles in life science literature identified 67.4% of retractions as misconduct, with suspected fraud in over 43% of cases, and less than 22% identified as errors [2]. The number of retracted papers is growing alarmingly (Fig. 13.1), and many of the retracted papers are related to clinical studies, patient care, and treatment, and are published in high-impact

Fig. 13.1 (**a**) Adjusted to number of papers published in a given year, retractions have increased to over 10% a year since 2020. (**b**) The steady increase is especially alarming when one considers the trend over the last 70 years. The sharp jump starts at 2000, but the second drastic increase is shown during the pandemic

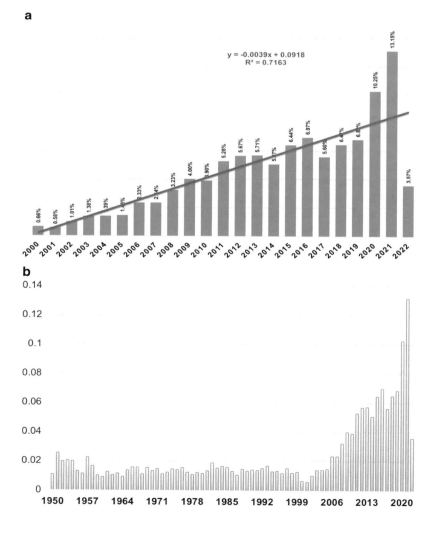

factor journals, and get hundreds or even thousands of citations. Some recent, COVID-research related paper retractions were dealt with fairly quickly [3, 4], but the process frequently takes months or even years [2] (not surprisingly, errors are usually identified twice as fast as fraud). This poses a substantial challenge for implementing evidence-based medicine, as it may take a few years before we realize the evidence is wrong, by which time we not only use the knowledge from these papers, but we use data to train and test AI algorithms. Training or validating AI systems on flawed data may not be obvious immediately. Open and reproducible science requires open publications as well as open data; without it it would hard or impossible to even identify papers with errors or suspected fraud. In addition, open data enables improved and richer curation efforts, such as IMEx consortium [5–9]. Well-organized, rich, curated portals ensure we can implement data-driven medicine, and analyze, model, validate and interpret results correctly.

Managing combined molecular, imaging, and patient data requires the support of the basic knowledge management functions:

1. *Knowledge acquisition*—identifying possible information sources (i.e., high-throughput platforms, instruments and their biases, wearable devices), and integrating such information into a knowledge base;
2. *Effective knowledge representation*—storing the knowledge in structures that support fast and accurate access, and provide multiple "networks" for linking semantics, relationships and guiding analysis, modeling and interepretation;
3. *Effective analysis, visualization, interpretation*—supporting scalable access to relevant knowledge, multi-dimensional analysis with diverse tools, and scalable, intuitive, and interactive visualization to support visual data mining and interpretation.

Successful integration of such algorithms into efficient and effective workflows must consider specifics of individual application areas. Medical AI applications range from computer vision and robotics in computer-assisted surgeries, through planning and scheduling of radiology and other treatments, data mining and machine learning from omics and imaging data, natural language understanding for patient records and reports and for conversational systems, knowledge representation and reasoning, planning, scheduling, and modeling. Requirements of specific areas introduce additional constraints for AI systems.

Usability questions are important especially in critical application such as medicine, but they are frequently ignored or handled only as an afterthought, and not planned from the initial design. This is one of the main reasons why despite many published papers in this area, real applications in medicine are not frequent. The most important issues, especially in biomedical applications, include privacy and security [10–15], trust and robustness [16], ethics and fairness [17], uncertainty and reliability [18, 19], reproducibility [20–22] and explainability [23–27], and effective human computer interaction interfaces [25].

Completely replacing human experts from the biomedical workflow is not feasible due to legal considerations, but AI-based optimization of the workflow can improve quality and reduce costs [28]. Human-in-the-loop ensures that cases substantially different from the training data or complex cases will be handled properly by human experts. In addition, future innovation and progress also requires human-in-the-loop [25]. While efforts in democratization of AI enables broader application of successful algorithms, it can also lead to their suboptimal or completely incorrect use and overinterpretation of results, if the users are not properly trained and understand required assumptions and existing biases, constraints, and proper use of such tools.

It is critical to know the end-user of the AI system; not only because of appropriate interface, but also because of the need to tailore false positives and false negatives towards the application use case. For example, a phone-based classifier skin lesions would likely be used by general public as a first step in screening, and thus false negatives need to be low, at an expense of higher false positives. The workflow would need to account for this bias, and the second level assessment would need to reduce false positives with additional assessments. However, useful system built for the expert radiologists should perfectly classify "simpler" cases automatically, and characterize complex cases for "discussion" with human experts (as in clinical rounds) by using an ensemble AI-system that combines multiple algorithms (with diverse biases) and is trained on different data sets (to increase diversity). Thus, properly using such systems in the more complex pipeline could optimize the cost, reduce false negatives and false positives, and in turn improve patient outtcomes.

Explainability, while often neglected, is growing in its importance in AI research [29]. Creating explainable models is essential in medical applications to ensure trust in recommendations and decision support [24, 30]. It is also vital for ensuring system evolution, due to cohort drift, change of data and equipment over time, as explanations and models help address false positives, false negatives, identify possible trends and patterns or outliers. Explainable models help prioritize validation and identify signal from noise [31].

13.3 Multimodal Imaging and Radiomics

Different imaging modalities offer new insights [32–36]. Multimodal imaging thus provides more accurate and robust biomarkers [36–42]. However, computed tomography (CT), ultrasound, magnetic resonance imaging (MRI), MR spectroscopy, positron emission tomography (PET) or optical imaging have varied availability, reproducibility, cost-efficiency, acquisition time, and resolution, and thus their applications need to be tailored to a specific workflow. Regardless of the imaging modality, extracting useful features by signal processing [43–51] can be enhanced by using AI algorithms, which in turn can substantially improve data interpretation and patient care [32, 52–68]. In both cases, one can focus on global or local features and implement (semi)manual or fully automated image segmentation. Important characteristics to extract and characterize include intensity (histogram, skewness, kurtosis), texture (gray level co-occurrence matrix (GLCM), fractal

analysis, wavelet, quad tree decomposition), and shape (sphericity, compactness).

Same as for AI algorithms discussed above, reproducibility and robustness of radiomic features are essential for generating useful results [69]. Standardizing acquisition protocols and "normalizing" instruments by using phantoms [70–76] are essential for integrating larger datasets, validating signatures and models on independent datasets, and in turn leading to improving clinical outcomes and results.

While the applications cover diverse medical areas, predominant focus is on cancer, as determined by word frequency analysis in the published radiomics-related papers (Fig. 13.2). Imaging features/biomarkers can be used individually or in combination with other clinical information to diagnose and characterize tumors and metastasis [77–81], and predict immunotherapy targets [45, 64, 82–87]. For example, frequently used imaging biomarkers in lung cancer include radiomic features, followed by CT features, and neural network-analyzed PET parameters [88]. While many papers show benefits of fully automated AI-imaging systems [89–95], there is an advantage of using human-in-the-loop to handle complex cases [96].

Combining ultrasound imaging with RNA sequencing data helped to identify and characterize at a gene and pathway levels three sub-phenotypes in patients with active psoriatic arthritis. Considering the sub-phenotypes show distinct clinical features, the characterization at biological pathway level helps identify possible mechanisms leading to clinical differences and potential prevention and treatment [97]. Integration can improve confidence in findings [98–100], and reduce both type I and II errors. For example, in Alzheimer's disease (AD) different studies provide individual insight into early diagnosis but also disease progression and treatment strategies, such as, imaging [101–108], electroencephalography (EEG) [109], circulating RNA [110] or miRNA [111], psychological tests [112, 113], and sleep pattern (using wearables) [114]. Combining individual data sets leads to improved diagnostics, e.g., different imaging modalities and early diagnosis [115–118], integrated miRNA and piRNA [119], combined genetic and biochemical

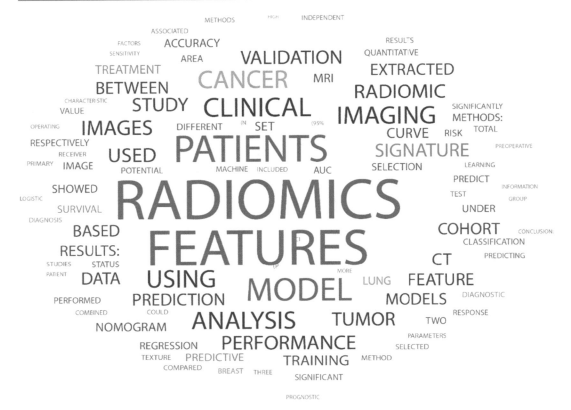

Fig. 13.2 Analyzing the frequency of words in radiomics literature published so far highlights that clinical application focus mostly on cancer (lung and breast), with the goal to predict treatment and survival, as highlighted by word cloud analysis. Large font size corresponds to more frequent terms. Paper titles were obtained from PubMed and data was processed using Matlab R2019b wordcloud package

markers [120–124], and combined biochemical and cognitive markers [125].

Further integration of omics methods and algorithms could lead to an ensemble system, confirming some findings and thus increasing confidence and reducing false positives and false negatives. Omics-based biomarkers may also provide a less-invasive and cheaper alternative to imaging for early detection of AD [126].

13.4 Integrative Computational Biology

In systems biology research, we must ensure that discovered patterns and proposed models are both statistically sound, and biologically and clinically meaningful. When analyzing data and building predictive models, it is essential to critically evaluate and interpret the prediction and create plausible and explainable models. This will help to ensure that seemingly important patterns in data are not artifacts of, for example, literature or data collection bias. To achieve this, one has to carefully design what data is being used to compute background distribution, how to handle missing values, how to preprocess and normalize data, and how to adjust parameters for confounding variables. Systems biology research uses methods from multiple disciplines, including variety of biochemical assays for omics platforms, diverse statistical, signal processing and AI-based algorithms. As outlined in Fig. 13.3, on the one hand, translational research influences what methods are needed, but on the other hand, new method development drives progress in the clinical research.

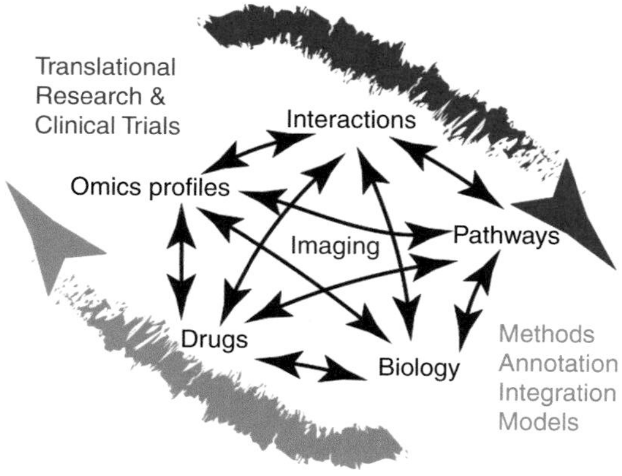

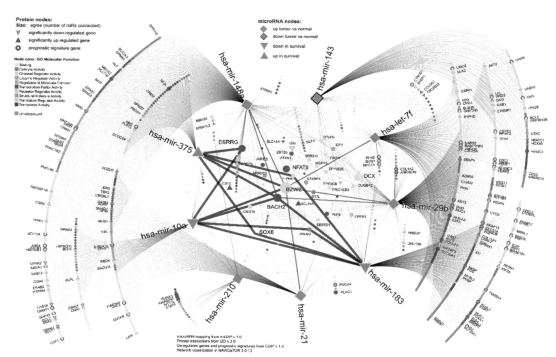

Fig. 13.3 Translational research and clinical trials both generate data for analytic pipelines and provide validation platforms for novel hypotheses and models. Combining diverse data from multiple imaging modalities with diverse omics platforms, biology assays, drug information, pathways, and rich interaction networks creates the comprehensive platform for hypotheses generation, leading to formation and validation of explainable models for disease and healthy states. Importantly, the relationships across data modalities help reduce biases and errors in each individual platform, by *de facto* reinforcement modeling

While individual analyses provide useful results, integrating them across different modalities—imaging, genomics, proteomics, metabolomics, clinical—may provide superior performance and ability to generate explainable models, providing improved mechanistic insight. Such integration provides a platform for reinforcement modeling—validating and enhancing individual models through multiple layers of integration. This can be achieved by using fusion [127–129] and networks that link individual layers of data with relationships, such as transcription factor or microRNA regulatory networks, physical protein interactions, signaling and metabolic pathways [130–132]. These relationships enable us to identify and explain unexpected patterns observed in data [132], identify broader patterns by moving from gene/protein-centric to complex/pathway-centric features [133], and identify broad deregulated signaling cascades [130]. Such integration helps reducing noise from individual data sets and increases confidence in the result, as highlighted in Fig. 13.4. Here, data from the Cancer Genome

Fig. 13.4 Data from TCGA LUAD integrated using microRNA-gene [135] and protein–protein interaction [136] networks. Highlighted are known up−/downregulated and prognostic genes. Network was visualized in NAViGaTOR 3.0.13 [137], and the SVG output file was processed in Adobe Illustrator 2020 to produce the final PNG image

Atlas and lung adenocarcinoma (LUAD) data set [134] were integrated using protein interaction networks, microRNA-gene networks, and gene ontology annotation. While there are almost 400 shared gene targets of the nine differential microRNAs, too many to interpret or validate, only those highlighted have multiple support, and thus higher confidence for further functional studies and validation. Importantly, substantial fraction of microRNA targets has been shown as deregulated and prognostic in LUAD, as highlighted by node outline and protein names. This not only confirms the importance of identified deregulated microRNAs in LUAD but also provides a possible mechanism and explainable model on how they relate to clinically relevant targets. A more comprehensive analysis later showed that integrating copy number aberrations, gene expression, and microRNAs with networks not only explains paradoxical expression patterns but also identifies and validates prognostic genes in LUAD [132].

Analogously, even if all the markers and features from radiomics would be sufficient for

diagnosis or prognosis, molecular profiles, AI algorithms, and integrative computational biology are needed to identify possible new drug targets, combination therapies, and select the right patient for the right treatment at the right time. Recently, a pathway-based patient model combined with multi-scale Bayesian network model TransPRECISE provided useful information on predicting specific treatment options [138].

Additional benefits can be achieved by combining imaging and network analysis algorithms. For example, fMRI data analysis can be represented as graphs, such as structural brain networks [139], neuro-connectivity after brain injury [140, 141], or functional connectivity in Schizophrenia [142]. Once constructed, these networks can be analyzed by the graph theory algorithms (e.g., [143–150]) to identify network structure–function relationships. As an example, focusing on a possible connection between AKT and BTK1 (Fig. 13.5), the network highlights the link between musculoskeletal (MSK; red edges and red node outlines) and neurodegenerative (NDD)

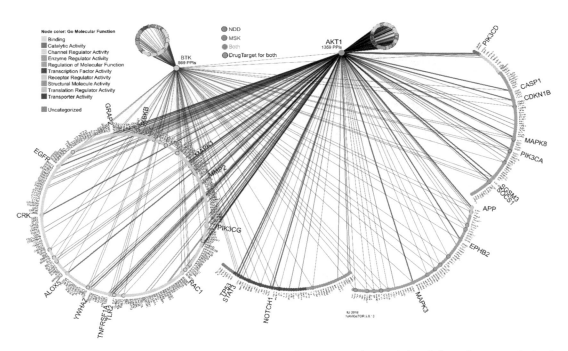

Fig. 13.5 Exploring the connection between BTK and AKT1, highlighting unique and common disease relationships (neurodegenerative (NDD) and musculoskeletal (MSK) diseases) and drug targets, as highlighted by the color and font size, as per legend. Protein interactions, disease annotation, and drug information were obtained from IID v.2018 [152]. Network was created in NAViGaTOR 3.0.13 [137], and the SVG output file was processed in Adobe Illustrator 2020 to produce the final PNG file

diseases (blue lines and blue node outlines), in addition to identifying know drug targets (large font).

13.5 Patient-Centric Medicine: Preventive and Data-Driven

Understanding and successfully treating multi-genic diseases requires systems-oriented research focused on the implication of disease-perturbed molecular interaction networks and pathways. These networks represent crucial relationships among genes and proteins, their mutations, chromosomal aberrations, microRNA deregulation, and other epigenetic and metabolic changes.

Decision support systems in medicine need to be robust across assays, instruments, and patient cohorts, handling uncertainty and missing data gracefully. However, quality of data and literature-based evidence may be questionable [2], leading to low reproducibility and errors. Due to mistakes and fraud in data and literature, these systems must also be able to handle incorrect information and data, again highlighting the value of integrative approach and explainable models that help separate signal from noise by combining evidence or exploring explanatory relationships.

Genomic medicine enhanced with cognitive analytics provides the necessary platform for precision patient care. Expanding genomic medicine with network biology, quantified patient assessment and computational modeling leads to new opportunities for translational research and provide patient-centric treatment strategies. Characterizing patient's life style is vital for assessing predisposition, prognosis, and treatment outcome. Providing measurable feedback on life style change may alter risk, increase compliance, and improve treatment effect. Importantly, we need to also understand the implication of the environment, by studying and quantifying effects of exposome on human condition [151].

In precision medicine, achieving high accuracy/precision evaluated on a specific patient cohort is the minimal required condition; ideally, the predictor is validated on multiple independent cohorts, and there is a clear understanding of the boundaries of the model, i.e., where it can be safely applied, and where standard of care should be used instead. To ensure patient-centric medicine and increase the level of trust in the AI systems, they must be able to determine confidence of prediction for a given patient despite uncertainties. Optimal use of the system would also require to know what are the costs and consequences of false positives and false negatives, and adjust training, validation, and performance accordingly.

While many papers have been published and multiple AI approaches passed diverse validations, their translation to medical practice in general remains low. Some of the reasons stem from the strict privacy issues that limit access to samples and thus prevent broad (and proper) training and validation. The system has to also integrate into the existing workflows, and thus it is important to determine what is the baseline performance we strive to achieve, and who and how will use the system. Are we striving to build systems that are superior to general practitioners or systems that improve performance of experts, by automatically solving simpler cases and augmenting human expert performance in solving complex cases by providing multiple views, classifications and annotations? For example, as shown in [153], an AI system is on par with human experts in the UK (also because the UK system uses two radiologists to make a decision), and the same AI system is superior to a radiology reader in the US, where single expert is sufficient to make a decision.

One size does not fit all. Unusually complex or rare cases are often discussed at clinical rounds, to ensure best possible treatment and continuous learning. Thus, using an ensemble of AI systems would help ensure high accuracy and lower false positive and false negative rates. The systems should have clear boundaries based on training/validation cohort characteristics, defer the analysis to human experts when dealing with outliers, and provide confidence in and explanation of the decision suggested. Considering risks and costs of care path, such ensemble systems would further enable to prioritize and optimize decision recommendations.

While we characterize diseases with the latest molecular technologies, e.g., (single cell) RNA sequencing and proteomic and metabolomic platforms, we continue collecting other patient data unreliably and sporadically, much of it using questionnaires or snapshots of sampled measures. We know that tobesity correlates with the risk of many diseases, including heart condition, diabetes, and cancer. Just one example of many; we know that body mass index (BMI) is an imprecise and limited estimate of overall fat percentage and fitness, especially when estimated from the weight and height, yet it remains to be used in clinical studies, and linked to disease risk. It has been introduced 200 years ago for tracking obesity, but its value is diminished when measuring health on an individual level. Alternative approaches could be as simple as measuring tape (for assessing waist or neck circumference), or more advanced with wearable devices. Molecular profiles from omics datasets provide detailed information about complex diseases on gene, protein, and metabolite level. If we add rich and temporal data streams from wearable devices to each patient's record, we will create unprecedented opportunities for better understanding how life style affects disease and healthy states. Devices such as Skulpt (http://www.skulpt.me) will provide details about fat deposition and overall fitness, replacing the two-century-old BMI. Based on electrical impedance myography (EIM) measurements, it provides more detailed and accurate measurement of fat and muscle quality, and thus overall fitness level for an individual, and quantitative change over time.

We need more precise measures of fitness and body mass—we need to move from evidence-based medicine to data-driven medicine. Knowing the heart rate, real-time electro cardio gram (ECG), breathing rate and volume, sleeping pattern and quality, and overall activity may also provide valuable insights into our health, yet, measuring them in the clinic, or for a few days using holster, provides only a limited (often biased) snapshot, not delivering sufficient value for the new data-driven medicine.

Even simple devices, such as bracelets and trackers, provide more detailed information about sleep patterns, steps, or overall activity, replacing vague statements about "150 minutes of moderate activity a week is beneficial" with more precise measure of duration, intensity, type and frequency of activities, and most importantly, tracking and adjusting it for each individual patient. The challenges are to provide "simple" recommendations, empower the user and health provider, but that can also create unforeseen problems such as depression or eating disorders [154]. Increasingly, even with appropriate measures taken [155], hacker attacks and misuse of such personal information have been growing. Despite this, there is a steady increase in companies providing developing such devices and delivering their potential for scientific use (Fig. 13.6). However, having precise measure-

Fig. 13.6 The trend in PubMed papers with "wearable" is growing steadily since 2000. The trend continues, as in the first half year of 2022 more articles have been published on the topic compared to the first 10 years combined

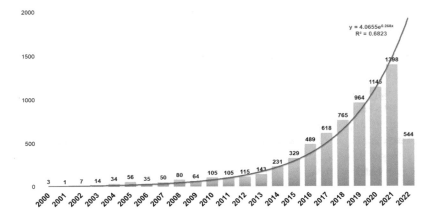

ments is not sufficient. Humans are known to ignore recommendations and follow their bad habits. To fully and maximally engage most individuals, we need to create smart social networking that will motivate and empower patients and increase compliance [156–158].

At present, the data collected by wearable devices focuses the consumer market; however, it is inevitable that after necessary approvals, applications in medical settings will prevail. Taking frequency of words in PubMed titles related to wearable devices already suggest trends, as highlighted in Fig. 13.7.

We will need to adapt the computing infrastructure to handle such streams of data, and to find ways to integrate it with imaging and omics platforms, and by using AI to analyze and interpret it wisely and effectively. This will enable a transformative change to move from *reactive* to *preventive* and *predictive* medicine.

However, as proper knowledge management is essential in AI and omics, it is crucial withfor wearable data streams, to ensure that translational research does not chase *statistically significant patterns* that are biologically and clinically useless. Since such data are challenging to share, and may be easily altered by mistake or fraud, ensuring reproducible science and reducing errors in data handling will be paramount. Privacy issues cannot be stressed enough, as they help to build trust in using such devices, and thus principles of privacy by design have to be integral to product development and data management [11].

The role of exercise within the scope of cancer rehabilitation has been studied in the last decade [159–188]. The combination of aerobic exercise and resistance training has been shown to provide many physiological and psychological health benefits for cancer prevention, concurrent treatment, and prevention of recurrence, such as maintaining and improving muscle mass, strength, cardiorespiratory fitness, body function, physical activity levels and capacity, increased immune function, less psychological and emotional stress and improved mood, reduced depression and anxiety, increased quality of life, less severe and less frequent symptoms or side effects to other treatments, shortened hospitalization, reduced likelihood of cardiovascular disease and diabetes, and lowers chance of cancer relapse.

Combined, these approaches will change the way we consider disease. We will start moving from diagnosing and treating disease to preventing it. Importantly, we could transform healthcare to care about health, and not just sick and disease, and to move from cohort to patient-centric medicine. Wearable devices will be monitoring individuals precisely and longitudinally, and they will assess an increasing number of features, similarly as we moved from cDNA arrays

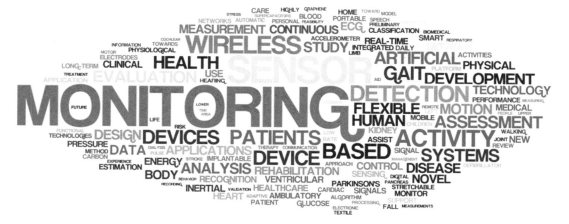

Fig. 13.7 Word clouds from PubMed titles on relevant wearable articles (the more frequent the word in the title, the larger it is). Created using Wordle (http://www.wordle. net). While "monitoring" is the main focus at present, "patients," "disease," and "health" are clearly gaining on importance

to Affymetrix platforms, to RNAseq and scRNA-seq. This will lead to 24/7 model of data collection—precisely and continuously tracking our activity, sleep, inactivity, food, and calorie intake, and pollutants in the environment. Data mining and machine learning algorithms will identify trends and interesting patterns both at the population level and for each individual, with personalized, calibrated trends generated and used as preventive measures for each patient. The data-driven aspect will change how we consider evidence, recommendations, and belief in guidelines. No longer will imprecise guidelines with "one size fits all" suffice—we need to provide customized "dose" prescribed for individuals, moving towards person-driven approaches. Clearly, "the future is connected", and through the collective data handling and analysis [163], we will manage even the most complex diseases, eventually.

As highlighted before though, patient-centric, data-driven medicine requires high quality, comprehensive data, and multiple levels of independent validation, with explainable models helping to increase trust and usability of such systems. Importantly, it is also essential to determine who and how will use the system and optimize it accordingly, as even useful applications may result in negative outcomes when used improperly or suboptimally [154].

References

1. Andrea D, Xueqing Z, Tauanne DA, Andrea M-M, Gene Ching CK, João MLD, et al. Substitution mutational signatures in whole-genome sequenced cancers in the UK population. Science. 2022;376(6591):ab19283.
2. Fang FC, Steen RG, Casadevall A. Misconduct accounts for the majority of retracted scientific publications. Proc Natl Acad Sci U S A. 2012;109(42):17028–33.
3. Mehra MR, Desai SS, Kuy S, Henry TD, Patel AN. Retraction: cardiovascular disease, drug therapy, and mortality in Covid-19. N Engl J Med [Letter Retraction of Publication]. 2020;382(26):2582. https://doi.org/10.1056/NEJMoa2007621.
4. Mehra MR, Ruschitzka F, Patel AN. Retraction-hydroxychloroquine or chloroquine with or without a macrolide for treatment of COVID-19: a multi-

national registry analysis. Lancet [Retraction of Publication]. 2020;395(10240):1820.
5. Hermjakob H, Montecchi-Palazzi L, Bader G, Wojcik J, Salwinski L, Ceol A, et al. The HUPO PSI's molecular interaction format—a community standard for the representation of protein interaction data. Nat Biotechnol. 2004;22(2):177–83.
6. Orchard S, Kerrien S, Abbani S, Aranda B, Bhate J, Bidwell S, et al. Protein interaction data curation: the International Molecular Exchange (IMEx) consortium. Nat Methods [Research Support, NIH, Extramural Research Support, Non-US Gov't]. 2012;9(4):345–50.
7. Del-Toro N, Duesbury M, Koch M, Perfetto L, Shrivastava A, Ochoa D, et al. Capturing variation impact on molecular interactions in the IMEx Consortium mutations data set. Nat Commun [Dataset Research Support, NIH, Extramural Research Support, Non-US Gov't]. 2019;10(1):10.
8. Perfetto L, Pastrello C, Del-Toro N, Duesbury M, Iannuccelli M, Kotlyar M, et al. The IMEx coronavirus interactome: an evolving map of Coronaviridae-host molecular interactions. Database (Oxford). 2020:baaa096.
9. Porras P, Barrera E, Bridge A, Del-Toro N, Cesareni G, Duesbury M, et al. Towards a unified open access dataset of molecular interactions. Nat Commun. 2020;11(1):6144.
10. Barth-Jones D, El Emam K, Bambauer J, Cavoukian A, Malin B. Assessing data intrusion threats. Science [Letter Comment]. 2015;348(6231):194–5.
11. Cavoukian A. Safeguarding health information. Health Law Can. 1998;18(4):115–7.
12. Moore W, Frye S. Review of HIPAA, Part 1: history, protected health information, and privacy and security rules. J Nucl Med Technol [Review]. 2019;47(4):269–72.
13. Torkzadehmahani R, Nasirigerdeh R, Blumenthal DB, Kacprowski T, List M, Matschinske J, et al. Privacy-preserving artificial intelligence techniques in biomedicine. arXiv:2007.11621. 2020.
14. Zerka F, Barakat S, Walsh S, Bogowicz M, Leijenaar RTH, Jochems A, et al. Systematic review of privacy-preserving distributed machine learning from federated databases in health care. JCO Clin Cancer Inform [Research Support, Non-US Gov't]. 2020;4:184–200.
15. Kaissis GA, Makowski MR, Rückert D, Braren RF. Secure, privacy-preserving and federated machine learning in medical imaging. Nat Mach Intell. 2020;2:305–11.
16. Zwanenburg A. Radiomics in nuclear medicine: robustness, reproducibility, standardization, and how to avoid data analysis traps and replication crisis. Eur J Nucl Med Mol Imaging. 2019;46(13):2638–55.
17. Lavery JV, IJsselmuiden C. The research fairness initiative: filling a critical gap in global research ethics. Gates Open Res. 2018;2:58.

18. Krynski TR, Tenenbaum JB. The role of causality in judgment under uncertainty. J Exp Psychol Gen. 2007;136(3):430–50.
19. Begley CG, Ellis LM. Drug development: raise standards for preclinical cancer research. Nature. 2012;483(7391):531–3.
20. Prinz F, Schlange T, Asadullah K. Believe it or not: how much can we rely on published data on potential drug targets? Nat Rev Drug Discov [Letter Comment]. 2011;10(9):712.
21. Clements JC. Is the reproducibility crisis fuelling poor mental health in science? Nature [News Comment]. 2020;582(7811):300.
22. Collins FS, Tabak LA. Policy: NIH plans to enhance reproducibility. Nature. 2014;505(7485):612–3.
23. Yang Z, Zhang A, Sudjianto A. Enhancing explainability of neural networks through architecture constraints. IEEE Trans Neural Netw Learn Syst. 2021;32(6):2610–21.
24. Windisch P, Weber P, Furweger C, Ehret F, Kufeld M, Zwahlen D, et al. Implementation of model explainability for a basic brain tumor detection using convolutional neural networks on MRI slices. Neuroradiology. 2020;62(11):1515–8.
25. Holzinger A, Langs G, Denk H, Zatloukal K, Muller H. Causability and explainability of artificial intelligence in medicine. Wiley Interdiscip Rev Data Min Knowl Discov [Review]. 2019;9(4):e1312.
26. Coeckelbergh M. Artificial intelligence, responsibility attribution, and a relational justification of explainability. Sci Eng Ethics. 2020;26(4):2051–68.
27. Petkovic D, Altman R, Wong M, Vigil A. Improving the explainability of random forest classifier—user centered approach. In: Pacific symposium on biocomputing pacific symposium on biocomputing. [Research Support, NIH, Extramural Research Support, Non-US Gov't]. 2018;23:204–15.
28. Kalra A, Chakraborty A, Fine B, Reicher J. Machine learning for automation of radiology protocols for quality and efficiency improvement. J Am Coll Radiol. 2020;17(9):1149–58.
29. Montani S, Striani M. Artificial intelligence in clinical decision support: a focused literature survey. Yearbook of medical informatics. Review. 2019;28(1):120–7.
30. Diprose WK, Buist N, Hua N, Thurier Q, Shand G, Robinson R. Physician understanding, explainability, and trust in a hypothetical machine learning risk calculator. J Am Med Inform Assoc. 2020;27(4):592–600.
31. Lohmann P, Kocher M, Ruge MI, Visser-Vandewalle V, Shah NJ, Fink GR, et al. PET/MRI radiomics in patients with brain metastases. Front Neurol [Review]. 2020;11:1.
32. Sollini M, Antunovic L, Chiti A, Kirienko M. Towards clinical application of image mining: a systematic review on artificial intelligence and radiomics. Eur J Nucl Med Mol Imaging. 2019;46(13):2656–72.
33. Ibrahim A, Vallieres M, Woodruff H, Primakov S, Beheshti M, Keek S, et al. Radiomics analysis for clinical decision support in nuclear medicine. Semin Nucl Med [Review]. 2019;49(5):438–49.
34. Lee G, Lee HY, Park H, Schiebler ML, van Beek EJR, Ohno Y, et al. Radiomics and its emerging role in lung cancer research, imaging biomarkers and clinical management: state of the art. Eur J Radiol [Review]. 2017;86:297–307.
35. Anthony GJ, Cunliffe A, Castillo R, Pham N, Guerrero T, Armato SG 3rd, et al. Incorporation of pre-therapy (18) F-FDG uptake data with CT texture features into a radiomics model for radiation pneumonitis diagnosis. Med Phys. 2017;44(7):3686–94.
36. Yin Q, Hung SC, Rathmell WK, Shen L, Wang L, Lin W, et al. Integrative radiomics expression predicts molecular subtypes of primary clear cell renal cell carcinoma. Clin Radiol. 2018;73(9):782–91.
37. Li ZY, Wang XD, Li M, Liu XJ, Ye Z, Song B, et al. Multi-modal radiomics model to predict treatment response to neoadjuvant chemotherapy for locally advanced rectal cancer. World J Gastroenterol. 2020;26(19):2388–402.
38. Zhuo EH, Zhang WJ, Li HJ, Zhang GY, Jing BZ, Zhou J, et al. Radiomics on multi-modalities MR sequences can subtype patients with non-metastatic nasopharyngeal carcinoma (NPC) into distinct survival subgroups. Eur Radiol. 2019;29(10):5590–9.
39. Zhuo EH, Zhang WJ, Li HJ, Zhang GY, Jing BZ, Zhou J, et al. Correction to: Radiomics on multi-modalities MR sequences can subtype patients with non-metastatic nasopharyngeal carcinoma (NPC) into distinct survival subgroups. Eur Radiol [Published Erratum]. 2019;29(7):3957.
40. Lv W, Ashrafinia S, Ma J, Lu L, Rahmim A. Multi-level multi-modality fusion radiomics: application to PET and CT imaging for prognostication of head and neck cancer. IEEE J Biomed Health Inform. 2020;24(8):2268–77.
41. Bagher-Ebadian H, Janic B, Liu C, Pantelic M, Hearshen D, Elshaikh M, et al. Detection of dominant intra-prostatic lesions in patients with prostate cancer using an artificial neural network and MR multi-modal radiomics analysis. Front Oncol. 2019;9:1313.
42. Zhong QZ, Long LH, Liu A, Li CM, Xiu X, Hou XY, et al. Radiomics of multiparametric MRI to predict biochemical recurrence of localized prostate cancer after radiation therapy. Front Oncol. 2020;10:731.
43. Wagner MW, Bilbily A, Beheshti M, Shammas A, Vali R. Artificial intelligence and radiomics in pediatric molecular imaging. Methods [Review]. 2021;188:37–43.
44. Dercle L, Lu L, Schwartz LH, Qian M, Tejpar S, Eggleton P, et al. Radiomics response signature for identification of metastatic colorectal cancer sensitive to therapies targeting EGFR pathway. J Natl Cancer Inst. 2020;112(9):902–12.

45. Ha S. Perspectives in radiomics for personalized medicine and theranostics. Nucl Med Mol Imaging. 2019;53(3):164–6.

46. Chen C, Guo X, Wang J, Guo W, Ma X, Xu J. The diagnostic value of radiomics-based machine learning in predicting the grade of meningiomas using conventional magnetic resonance imaging: a preliminary study. Front Oncol. 2019;9:1338.

47. Leijenaar RT, Carvalho S, Velazquez ER, van Elmpt WJ, Parmar C, Hoekstra OS, et al. Stability of FDG-PET radiomics features: an integrated analysis of test-retest and inter-observer variability. Acta Oncol [Research Support, Non-US Gov't]. 2013;52(7):1391–7.

48. Jack CR Jr, Barkhof F, Bernstein MA, Cantillon M, Cole PE, Decarli C, et al. Steps to standardization and validation of hippocampal volumetry as a biomarker in clinical trials and diagnostic criterion for Alzheimer's disease. Alzheimers Dement. [Research Support, N.I.H., Extramural Research Support, Non-U.S. Gov't]. 2011;7(4):474–85e4.

49. Rizzo S, Botta F, Raimondi S, Origgi D, Buscarino V, Colarieti A, et al. Radiomics of high-grade serous ovarian cancer: association between quantitative CT features, residual tumour and disease progression within 12 months. Eur Radiol. 2018;28(11):4849–59.

50. Sala E, Mema E, Himoto Y, Veeraraghavan H, Brenton JD, Snyder A, et al. Unravelling tumour heterogeneity using next-generation imaging: radiomics, radiogenomics, and habitat imaging. Clin Radiol [Review]. 2017;72(1):3–10.

51. Vargas HA, Veeraraghavan H, Micco M, Nougaret S, Lakhman Y, Meier AA, et al. A novel representation of inter-site tumour heterogeneity from pretreatment computed tomography textures classifies ovarian cancers by clinical outcome. Eur Radiol [Evaluation Studies]. 2017;27(9):3991–4001.

52. Xie C, Du R, Ho JW, Pang HH, Chiu KW, Lee EY, et al. Effect of machine learning re-sampling techniques for imbalanced datasets in (18)F-FDG PET-based radiomics model on prognostication performance in cohorts of head and neck cancer patients. Eur J Nucl Med Mol Imaging. 2020;47(12):2826–35.

53. Wildeboer RR, Mannaerts CK, van Sloun RJG, Budaus L, Tilki D, Wijkstra H, et al. Automated multiparametric localization of prostate cancer based on B-mode, shear-wave elastography, and contrast-enhanced ultrasound radiomics. Eur Radiol. 2020;30(2):806–15.

54. Wang X, Wan Q, Chen H, Li Y, Li X. Classification of pulmonary lesion based on multiparametric MRI: utility of radiomics and comparison of machine learning methods. Eur Radiol. 2020;30(8):4595–605.

55. Wang H, Song B, Ye N, Ren J, Sun X, Dai Z, et al. Machine learning-based multiparametric MRI radiomics for predicting the aggressiveness of papillary thyroid carcinoma. Eur J Radiol [Evaluation Study]. 2020;122:108755.

56. Wang H, Chen H, Duan S, Hao D, Liu J. Radiomics and machine learning with multiparametric preoperative MRI may accurately predict the histopathological grades of soft tissue sarcomas. J Magn Reson Imaging. 2020;51(3):791–7.

57. Song J, Yin Y, Wang H, Chang Z, Liu Z, Cui L. A review of original articles published in the emerging field of radiomics. Eur J Radiol [Review]. 2020;127:108991.

58. Rogers W, Thulasi Seetha S, Refaee TAG, Lieverse RIY, Granzier RWY, Ibrahim A, et al. Radiomics: from qualitative to quantitative imaging. Br J Radiol [Review]. 2020;93(1108):20190948.

59. Peng A, Dai H, Duan H, Chen Y, Huang J, Zhou L, et al. A machine learning model to precisely immunohistochemically classify pituitary adenoma subtypes with radiomics based on preoperative magnetic resonance imaging. Eur J Radiol. 2020;125:108892.

60. Mokrane FZ, Lu L, Vavasseur A, Otal P, Peron JM, Luk L, et al. Radiomics machine-learning signature for diagnosis of hepatocellular carcinoma in cirrhotic patients with indeterminate liver nodules. Eur Radiol. 2020;30(1):558–70.

61. Haider SP, Mahajan A, Zeevi T, Baumeister P, Reichel C, Sharaf K, et al. PET/CT radiomics signature of human papilloma virus association in oropharyngeal squamous cell carcinoma. Eur J Nucl Med Mol Imaging. 2020;47(13):2978–91.

62. Varghese B, Chen F, Hwang D, Palmer SL, De Castro Abreu AL, Ukimura O, et al. Objective risk stratification of prostate cancer using machine learning and radiomics applied to multiparametric magnetic resonance images. Sci Rep [Research Support, NIH, Extramural Research Support, US Gov't, Non-PHS Research Support, Non-US Gov't]. 2019;9(1):1570.

63. Oyama A, Hiraoka Y, Obayashi I, Saikawa Y, Furui S, Shiraishi K, et al. Hepatic tumor classification using texture and topology analysis of non-contrast-enhanced three-dimensional T1-weighted MR images with a radiomics approach. Sci Rep [Research Support, Non-US Gov't]. 2019;9(1):8764.

64. Sun R, Limkin EJ, Vakalopoulou M, Dercle L, Champiat S, Han SR, et al. A radiomics approach to assess tumour-infiltrating CD8 cells and response to anti-PD-1 or anti-PD-L1 immunotherapy: an imaging biomarker, retrospective multicohort study. Lancet Oncol [Research Support, Non-US Gov't]. 2018;19(9):1180–91.

65. Oakden-Rayner L, Carneiro G, Bessen T, Nascimento JC, Bradley AP, Palmer LJ. Precision radiology: predicting longevity using feature engineering and deep learning methods in a radiomics framework. Sci Rep. 2017;7(1):1648.

66. Stone JR, Wilde EA, Taylor BA, Tate DF, Levin H, Bigler ED, et al. Supervised learning technique for the automated identification of white matter hyperintensities in traumatic brain injury. Brain Inj. 2016;30(12):1458–68.

67. Aerts H. Data science in radiology: a path forward. Clin Cancer Res [Letter Research Support, NIH, Extramural]. 2018;24(3):532–4.

68. Vukicevic AM, Milic V, Zabotti A, Hocevar A, De Lucia O, Filippou G, et al. Radiomics-based assessment of primary Sjogren's syndrome from salivary gland ultrasonography images. IEEE J Biomed Health Inform. 2020;24(3):835–43.

69. Berenguer R, Pastor-Juan MDR, Canales-Vazquez J, Castro-Garcia M, Villas MV, Mansilla Legorburo F, et al. Radiomics of CT features may be nonreproducible and redundant: influence of CT acquisition parameters. Radiology. 2018;288(2):407–15.

70. Zwanenburg A, Vallieres M, Abdalah MA, Aerts H, Andrearczyk V, Apte A, et al. The image biomarker standardization initiative: standardized quantitative radiomics for high-throughput image-based phenotyping. Radiology. 2020;295(2):328–38.

71. Nardone V, Reginelli A, Guida C, Belfiore MP, Biondi M, Mormile M, et al. Delta-radiomics increases multicentre reproducibility: a phantom study. Med Oncol. 2020;37(5):38.

72. Zhovannik I, Bussink J, Traverso A, Shi Z, Kalendralis P, Wee L, et al. Learning from scanners: bias reduction and feature correction in radiomics. Clin Transl Radiat Oncol. 2019;19:33–8.

73. Saeedi E, Dezhkam A, Beigi J, Rastegar S, Yousefi Z, Mehdipour LA, et al. Radiomic feature robustness and reproducibility in quantitative bone radiography: a study on radiologic parameter changes. J Clin Densitom. 2019;22(2):203–13.

74. Orlhac F, Frouin F, Nioche C, Ayache N, Buvat I. Validation of a method to compensate multicenter effects affecting CT Radiomics. Radiology [Multicenter Study Validation Study]. 2019;291(1):53–9.

75. Kalendralis P, Traverso A, Shi Z, Zhovannik I, Monshouwer R, Starmans MPA, et al. Multicenter CT phantoms public dataset for radiomics reproducibility tests. Med Phys. 2019;46(3):1512–8.

76. Baessler B, Weiss K, Pinto Dos Santos D. Robustness and reproducibility of radiomics in magnetic resonance imaging: a phantom study. Investig Radiol. 2019;54(4):221–8.

77. Shofty B, Artzi M, Shtrozberg S, Fanizzi C, DiMeco F, Haim O, et al. Virtual biopsy using MRI radiomics for prediction of BRAF status in melanoma brain metastasis. Sci Rep. 2020;10(1):6623.

78. Huang CY, Lee CC, Yang HC, Lin CJ, Wu HM, Chung WY, et al. Radiomics as prognostic factor in brain metastases treated with gamma knife radiosurgery. J Neuro-Oncol. 2020;146(3):439–49.

79. Wu G, Chen Y, Wang Y, Yu J, Lv X, Ju X, et al. Sparse representation-based radiomics for the diagnosis of brain tumors. IEEE Trans Med Imaging. 2018;37(4):893–905.

80. Peng L, Parekh V, Huang P, Lin DD, Sheikh K, Baker B, et al. Distinguishing true progression from radionecrosis after stereotactic radiation therapy for brain metastases with machine learning and radiomics. Int J Radiat Oncol Biol Phys. 2018;102(4):1236–43.

81. Kang D, Park JE, Kim YH, Kim JH, Oh JY, Kim J, et al. Diffusion radiomics as a diagnostic model for atypical manifestation of primary central nervous system lymphoma: development and multicenter external validation. Neuro-Oncology. 2018;20(9):1251–61.

82. Yu H, Meng X, Chen H, Han X, Fan J, Gao W, et al. Correlation between mammographic radiomics features and the level of tumor-infiltrating lymphocytes in patients with triple-negative breast cancer. Front Oncol. 2020;10:412.

83. Park KJ, Lee JL, Yoon SK, Heo C, Park BW, Kim JK. Radiomics-based prediction model for outcomes of PD-1/PD-L1 immunotherapy in metastatic urothelial carcinoma. Eur Radiol. 2020;30(10):5392–403.

84. Mu W, Tunali I, Gray JE, Qi J, Schabath MB, Gillies RJ. Radiomics of (18)F-FDG PET/CT images predicts clinical benefit of advanced NSCLC patients to checkpoint blockade immunotherapy. Eur J Nucl Med Mol Imaging. 2020;47(5):1168–82.

85. Hectors SJ, Lewis S, Besa C, King MJ, Said D, Putra J, et al. MRI radiomics features predict immuno-oncological characteristics of hepatocellular carcinoma. Eur Radiol. 2020;30(7):3759–69.

86. Avanzo M, Stancanello J, Pirrone G, Sartor G. Radiomics and deep learning in lung cancer. Strahlenther Onkol [Review]. 2020;196(10): 879–87.

87. Tang C, Hobbs B, Amer A, Li X, Behrens C, Canales JR, et al. Development of an immune-pathology informed radiomics model for non-small cell lung cancer. Sci Rep. 2018;8(1):1922.

88. Ninatti G, Kirienko M, Neri E, Sollini M, Chiti A. Imaging-based prediction of molecular therapy targets in NSCLC by radiogenomics and AI approaches: a systematic review. Diagnostics (Basel) [Review]. 2020;10(6):359.

89. Wang X, Zhang L, Yang X, Tang L, Zhao J, Chen G, et al. Deep learning combined with radiomics may optimize the prediction in differentiating high-grade lung adenocarcinomas in ground glass opacity lesions on CT scans. Eur J Radiol. 2020;129:109150.

90. Kakileti ST, Madhu HJ, Manjunath G, Wee L, Dekker A, Sampangi S. Personalized risk prediction for breast cancer pre-screening using artificial intelligence and thermal radiomics. Artif Intell Med. 2020;105:101854.

91. Wang K, Qiao Z, Zhao X, Li X, Wang X, Wu T, et al. Individualized discrimination of tumor recurrence from radiation necrosis in glioma patients using an integrated radiomics-based model. Eur J Nucl Med Mol Imaging. 2020;47(6):1400–11.

92. Currie G, Hawk KE, Rohren E, Vial A, Klein R. Machine learning and deep learning in medical imaging: intelligent imaging. J Med Imaging Radiat Sci. 2019;50(4):477–87.

93. Sheth D, Giger ML. Artificial intelligence in the interpretation of breast cancer on MRI. J Magn Reson Imaging [Review]. 2020;51(5):1310–24.

94. Castiglioni I, Gallivanone F, Soda P, Avanzo M, Stancanello J, Aiello M, et al. AI-based applications in hybrid imaging: how to build smart and truly

multi-parametric decision models for radiomics. Eur J Nucl Med Mol Imaging. 2019;46(13):2673–99.

95. Veit-Haibach P, Buvat I, Herrmann K. EJNMMI supplement: bringing AI and radiomics to nuclear medicine. Eur J Nucl Med Mol Imaging [Editorial]. 2019;46(13):2627–9.

96. Bejnordi BE, Litjens G, van der Laak JA. Machine learning compared with pathologist assessment-reply. JAMA [Letter Comment]. 2018;319(16):1726.

97. Eder L, Li Q, Rahmati S, Rahman P, Jurisica I, Chandran V. Defining imaging subphenotypes of psoriatic arthritis: integrative analysis of imaging data and gene expression in a PsA patient cohort. Rheumatology (Oxford). 2022: keac078.

98. Viswanath SE, Tiwari P, Lee G, Madabhushi A. Dimensionality reduction-based fusion approaches for imaging and non-imaging biomedical data: concepts, workflow, and use-cases. BMC Med Imaging [Research Support, Non-US Gov't Research Support, NIH, Extramural Research Support, US Gov't, Non-PHS]. 2017;17(1):2.

99. Joaquim HPG, Costa AC, Talib LL, Dethloff F, Serpa MH, Zanetti MV, et al. Plasma metabolite profiles in first episode psychosis: exploring symptoms heterogeneity/severity in schizophrenia and bipolar disorder cohorts. Front Psych. 2020;11:496.

100. Lee E, Choi JS, Kim M, Suk HI. Toward an interpretable Alzheimer's disease diagnostic model with regional abnormality representation via deep learning. Neuroimage [Research Support, Non-US Gov't]. 2019;202:116113.

101. Hamelin L, Lagarde J, Dorothee G, Leroy C, Labit M, Comley RA, et al. Early and protective microglial activation in Alzheimer's disease: a prospective study using 18F-DPA-714 PET imaging. Brain [Research Support, Non-US Gov't]. 2016;139(Pt 4):1252–64.

102. Scheltens P. Imaging in Alzheimer's disease. Dialogues Clin Neurosci [Review]. 2009;11(2):191–9.

103. Magnin B, Mesrob L, Kinkingnehun S, Pelegrini-Issac M, Colliot O, Sarazin M, et al. Support vector machine-based classification of Alzheimer's disease from whole-brain anatomical MRI. Neuroradiology. 2009;51(2):73–83.

104. Gauthier S, Dubois B, Feldman H, Scheltens P. Revised research diagnostic criteria for Alzheimer's disease. Lancet Neurol [Comment Letter]. 2008;7(8):668–70.

105. Dubois B, Feldman HH, Jacova C, Dekosky ST, Barberger-Gateau P, Cummings J, et al. Research criteria for the diagnosis of Alzheimer's disease: revising the NINCDS-ADRDA criteria. Lancet Neurol [Research Support, Non-US Gov't Review]. 2007;6(8):734–46.

106. Claus JJ, Dubois EA, Booij J, Habraken J, de Munck JC, van Herk M, et al. Demonstration of a reduction in muscarinic receptor binding in early Alzheimer's disease using iodine-123 dexetimide

single-photon emission tomography. Eur J Nucl Med. 1997;24(6):602–8.

107. Deweer B, Lehericy S, Pillon B, Baulac M, Chiras J, Marsault C, et al. Memory disorders in probable Alzheimer's disease: the role of hippocampal atrophy as shown with MRI. J Neurol Neurosurg Psychiatry [Research Support, Non-US Gov't]. 1995;58(5):590–7.

108. Blin J, Baron JC, Dubois B, Crouzel C, Fiorelli M, Attar-Levy D, et al. Loss of brain 5-HT2 receptors in Alzheimer's disease. In vivo assessment with positron emission tomography and [18F]setoperone. Brain. 1993;116(Pt 3):497–510.

109. Rossini PM, Di Iorio R, Vecchio F, Anfossi M, Babiloni C, Bozzali M, et al. Early diagnosis of Alzheimer's disease: the role of biomarkers including advanced EEG signal analysis. Report from the IFCN-sponsored panel of experts. Clin Neurophysiol [Review]. 2020;131(6):1287–310.

110. Ludwig N, Fehlmann T, Kern F, Gogol M, Maetzler W, Deutscher S, et al. Machine learning to detect Alzheimer's disease from circulating non-coding RNAs. Genom Proteom Bioinform [Research Support, Non-US Gov't]. 2019;17(4):430–40.

111. McKeever PM, Schneider R, Taghdiri F, Weichert A, Multani N, Brown RA, et al. MicroRNA expression levels are altered in the cerebrospinal fluid of patients with young-onset Alzheimer's disease. Mol Neurobiol. 2018 Dec;55(12):8826–41.

112. Matias-Guiu JA, Cabrera-Martin MN, Curiel RE, Valles-Salgado M, Rognoni T, Moreno-Ramos T, et al. Comparison between FCSRT and LASSI-L to detect early stage Alzheimer's disease. J Alzheimers Dis. 2018;61(1):103–11.

113. Bechard LE, Beaton D, McGilton K, Tartaglia MC, Black S. Physical activity perceptions, experiences, and beliefs of older adults with mild cognitive impairment or Alzheimer's disease and their care partners. Appl Physiol Nutr Metab. 2020;45(11):1216–24.

114. Ettore E, Bakardjian H, Sole M, Levy Nogueira M, Habert MO, Gabelle A, et al. Relationships between objectives sleep parameters and brain amyloid load in subjects at risk for Alzheimer's disease: the INSIGHT-preAD study. Sleep [Research Support, Non-US Gov't]. 2019;42(9):zsz137.

115. Ortner M, Drost R, Hedderich D, Goldhardt O, Muller-Sarnowski F, Diehl-Schmid J, et al. Amyloid PET, FDG-PET or MRI?—the power of different imaging biomarkers to detect progression of early Alzheimer's disease. BMC Neurol. 2019;19(1):264.

116. Oliveira PP Jr, Nitrini R, Busatto G, Buchpiguel C, Sato JR, Amaro E Jr. Use of SVM methods with surface-based cortical and volumetric subcortical measurements to detect Alzheimer's disease. J Alzheimers Dis. 2010;19(4):1263–72.

117. Ebrahimighahnavieh MA, Luo S, Chiong R. Deep learning to detect Alzheimer's disease from neuroimaging: a systematic literature review. Comput Methods Prog Biomed. 2020;187:105242.

118. Sabri O, Sabbagh MN, Seibyl J, Barthel H, Akatsu H, Ouchi Y, et al. Florbetaben PET imaging to detect amyloid beta plaques in Alzheimer's disease: phase 3 study. Alzheimers Dement. [Clinical Trial, Phase III Multicenter Study Research Support, Non-U.S. Gov't]. 2015;11(8):964–74.

119. Jain G, Stuendl A, Rao P, Berulava T, Pena Centeno T, Kaurani L, et al. A combined miRNA-piRNA signature to detect Alzheimer's disease. Transl Psychiatry [Multicenter Study Research Support, Non-US Gov't]. 2019;9(1):250.

120. Lannfelt L. Biochemical diagnostic markers to detect early Alzheimer's disease. Neurobiol Aging [Review]. 1998;19(2):165–7.

121. Hampel H, Toschi N, Baldacci F, Zetterberg H, Blennow K, Kilimann I, et al. Alzheimer's disease biomarker-guided diagnostic workflow using the added value of six combined cerebrospinal fluid candidates: Abeta1-42, total-tau, phosphorylated-tau, NFL, neurogranin, and YKL-40. Alzheimers Dement [Multicenter Study Research Support, Non-U.S. Gov't]. 2018;14(4):492–501.

122. Kunkle BW, Grenier-Boley B, Sims R, Bis JC, Damotte V, Naj AC, et al. Genetic meta-analysis of diagnosed Alzheimer's disease identifies new risk loci and implicates Abeta, tau, immunity and lipid processing. Nat Genet [Meta-Analysis Research Support, Non-US Gov't]. 2019;51(3):414–30.

123. Lambert JC, Ibrahim-Verbaas CA, Harold D, Naj AC, Sims R, Bellenguez C, et al. Meta-analysis of 74,046 individuals identifies 11 new susceptibility loci for Alzheimer's disease. Nat Genet [Meta-Analysis Research Support, NIH, Extramural Research Support, Non-US Gov't]. 2013;45(12):1452–8.

124. Thijssen EH, La Joie R, Wolf A, Strom A, Wang P, Iaccarino L, et al. Diagnostic value of plasma phosphorylated tau181 in Alzheimer's disease and frontotemporal lobar degeneration. Nat Med [Research Support, NIH, Extramural Research Support, Non-US Gov't]. 2020;26(3):387–97.

125. Edwards M, Balldin VH, Hall J, O'Bryant S. Combining select neuropsychological assessment with blood-based biomarkers to detect mild Alzheimer's disease: a molecular neuropsychology approach. J Alzheimers Dis [Research Support, NIH, Extramural]. 2014;42(2):635–40.

126. Xicota L, Ichou F, Lejeune FX, Colsch B, Tenenhaus A, Leroy I, et al. Multi-omics signature of brain amyloid deposition in asymptomatic individuals at-risk for Alzheimer's disease: the INSIGHT-preAD study. EBioMedicine. 2019;47: 518–28.

127. Leung CK, Braun P, Cuzzocrea A. AI-based sensor information fusion for supporting deep supervised learning. Sensors (Basel). 2019;19(6):1345.

128. Zizzo AN, Erdman L, Feldman BM, Goldenberg A. Similarity network fusion: a novel application to making clinical diagnoses. Rheum Dis Clin North Am [Review]. 2018;44(2):285–93.

129. Wang B, Mezlini AM, Demir F, Fiume M, Tu Z, Brudno M, et al. Similarity network fusion for aggregating data types on a genomic scale. Nat Methods [Research Support, Non-US Gov't Research Support, US Gov't, Non-PHS]. 2014;11(3):333–7.

130. Kennedy SA, Jarboui MA, Srihari S, Raso C, Bryan K, Dernayka L, et al. Extensive rewiring of the EGFR network in colorectal cancer cells expressing transforming levels of KRAS(G13D). Nat Commun [Research Support, Non-U.S. Gov't]. 2020;11(1):499.

131. Enfield KSS, Marshall EA, Anderson C, Ng KW, Rahmati S, Xu Z, et al. Epithelial tumor suppressor ELF3 is a lineage-specific amplified oncogene in lung adenocarcinoma. Nat Commun [Research Support, Non-US Gov't]. 2019;10(1):5438.

132. Tokar T, Pastrello C, Ramnarine VR, Zhu CQ, Craddock KJ, Pikor LA, et al. Differentially expressed microRNAs in lung adenocarcinoma invert effects of copy number aberrations of prognostic genes. Oncotarget. 2018;9(10):9137–55.

133. Martinez VD, Vucic EA, Thu KL, Pikor LA, Lam S, Lam WL. Disruption of KEAP1/CUL3/RBX1 E3-ubiquitin ligase complex components by multiple genetic mechanisms: association with poor prognosis in head and neck cancer. Head Neck [Research Support, NIH, Extramural Research Support, Non-US Gov't]. 2015;37(5):727–34.

134. Cancer Genome Atlas Research Network. Comprehensive molecular profiling of lung adenocarcinoma. Nature. [Research Support, N.I.H., Extramural Research Support, Non-U.S. Gov't]. 2014;511(7511):543–50.

135. Shirdel EA, Xie W, Mak TW, Jurisica I. NAViGaTing the micronome—using multiple microRNA prediction databases to identify signalling pathway-associated microRNAs. PLoS One [Comparative Study Evaluation Studies Research Support, Non-US Gov't]. 2011;6(2):e17429.

136. Brown KR, Jurisica I. Unequal evolutionary conservation of human protein interactions in interologous networks. Genome Biol. 2007;8(5):R95.

137. Brown KR, Otasek D, Ali M, McGuffin MJ, Xie W, Devani B, et al. NAViGaTOR: network analysis, visualization and graphing Toronto. Bioinformatics. 2009;25(24):3327–9.

138. Bhattacharyya R, Ha MJ, Liu Q, Akbani R, Liang H, Baladandayuthapani V. Personalized network modeling of the pan-cancer patient and cell line interactome. JCO Clin Cancer Inform. 2020;4:399–411.

139. Ingalhalikar M, Smith A, Parker D, Satterthwaite TD, Elliott MA, Ruparel K, et al. Sex differences in the structural connectome of the human brain. Proc Natl Acad Sci U S A [Comparative Study Research Support, NIH, Extramural Research Support, Non-US Gov't]. 2014;111(2):823–8.

140. Bigler ED. Default mode network, connectivity, traumatic brain injury and post-traumatic amnesia. Brain [Research Support, N.I.H., Extramural Research

Support, U.S. Gov't, Non-P.H.S. Comment]. 2016;139(Pt 12):3054–7.

141. Bigler ED, Abildskov TJ, Goodrich-Hunsaker NJ, Black G, Christensen ZP, Huff T, et al. Structural neuroimaging findings in mild traumatic brain injury. Sports Med Arthrosc Rev [Review]. 2016;24(3):e42–52.

142. Cui LB, Liu L, Wang HN, Wang LX, Guo F, Xi YB, et al. Disease definition for schizophrenia by functional connectivity using radiomics strategy. Schizophr Bull. 2018;44(5):1053–9.

143. Milo R, Shen-Orr S, Itzkovitz S, Kashtan N, Chklovskii D, Alon U. Network motifs: simple building blocks of complex networks. Science. 2002;298:824–7.

144. Shen-Orr SS, Milo R, Mangan S, Alon U. Network motifs in the transcriptional regulation network of Escherichia coli. Nat Genet. 2002;31(1):64–8.

145. Mangan S, Alon U. Structure and function of the feed-forward loop network motif. Proc Natl Acad Sci U S A. 2003;100(21):11980–5.

146. Alon U. Network motifs: theory and experimental approaches. Nat Rev Genet. 2007;8(6):450–61.

147. Milenkovic T, Lai J, Przulj N. GraphCrunch: a tool for large network analyses. BMC Bioinform. 2008;9:70.

148. Geraci J, Liu G, Jurisica I. Algorithms for systematic identification of small subgraphs. Methods Mol Biol [Research Support, Non-US Gov't]. 2012;804:219–44.

149. Przulj N, Wigle DA, Jurisica I. Functional topology in a network of protein interactions. Bioinformatics. 2004;20(3):340–8.

150. Barrios-Rodiles M, Brown KR, Ozdamar B, Bose R, Liu Z, Donovan RS, et al. High-throughput mapping of a dynamic signaling network in mammalian cells. Science. 2005;307(5715):1621–5.

151. Zhang X, Gao P, Snyder MP. The Exposome in the era of the quantified self. Annu Rev Biomed Data Sci. 2021;4:255–77.

152. Kotlyar M, Pastrello C, Malik Z, Jurisica I. IID 2018 update: context-specific physical protein-protein interactions in human, model organisms and domesticated species. Nucleic Acids Res. 2019;47(D1):D581–9.

153. McKinney SM, Sieniek M, Godbole V, Godwin J, Antropova N, Ashrafian H, et al. International evaluation of an AI system for breast cancer screening. Nature [Evaluation Study Research Support, NIH, Extramural]. 2020;577(7788):89–94.

154. Rich E, Lewis S, Lupton D, Miah A, Piwek L. Digital health generation?: young People's use of 'healthy lifestyle. Technologies. Bath: University of Bath; 2020.

155. Cilliers L. Wearable devices in healthcare: privacy and information security issues. Health Inf Manag. 2020;49(2–3):150–6.

156. Rejeski WJ, Brawley LR, Ettinger W, Morgan T, Thompson C. Compliance to exercise therapy in older participants with knee osteoarthritis: implica-

tions for treating disability. Med Sci Sports Exerc [Clinical Trial Randomized Controlled Trial]. 1997;29(8):977–85.

157. Bonato P. Advances in wearable technology for rehabilitation. Stud Health Technol Inform. 2009;145:145–59.

158. Shallwani S, Dalzell MA, Sateren W, O'Brien S. Exercise compliance among patients with multiple myeloma undergoing chemotherapy: a retrospective study. Supportive Care Cancer. 2015;23(10):3081–8.

159. Davies NJ, Batehup L, Thomas R. The role of diet and physical activity in breast, colorectal, and prostate cancer survivorship: a review of the literature. Br J Cancer [Research Support, Non-US Gov't Review]. 2011;105(Suppl 1):S52–73.

160. Norman A, Moradi T, Gridley G, Dosemeci M, Rydh B, Nyren O, et al. Occupational physical activity and risk for prostate cancer in a nationwide cohort study in Sweden. Br J Cancer. 2002;86(1):70–5.

161. Wannamethee SG, Shaper AG, Walker M. Physical activity and risk of cancer in middle-aged men. Br J Cancer. 2001;85(9):1311–6.

162. Abioye AI, Odesanya MO, Ibrahim NA. Physical activity and risk of gastric cancer: a meta-analysis of observational studies. Br J Sports Med. 2015;49(4):224–9.

163. Contrepois K, Wu S, Moneghetti KJ, Hornburg D, Ahadi S, Tsai MS, et al. Molecular choreography of acute exercise. Cell. 2020;181(5):1112–30 e16.

164. McTiernan A, Stanford JL, Weiss NS, Daling JR, Voigt LF. Occurrence of breast cancer in relation to recreational exercise in women age 50–64 years. Epidemiology [Research Support, Non-US Gov't Research Support, US Gov't, PHS]. 1996;7(6):598–604.

165. Goh J, Kirk EA, Lee SX, Ladiges WC. Exercise, physical activity and breast cancer: the role of tumor-associated macrophages. Exerc Immunol Rev [Review]. 2012;18:158–76.

166. Basen-Engquist K, Carmack C, Brown J, Jhingran A, Baum G, Song J, et al. Response to an exercise intervention after endometrial cancer: differences between obese and non-obese survivors. Gynecol Oncol [Comparative Study Observational Study Research Support, NIH, Extramural Research Support, Non-US Gov't]. 2014;133(1): 48–55.

167. Cannioto RA, Moysich KB. Epithelial ovarian cancer and recreational physical activity: a review of the epidemiological literature and implications for exercise prescription. Gynecol Oncol Rev. 2015;137(3):559–73.

168. Spector D, Deal AM, Amos KD, Yang H, Battaglini CL. A pilot study of a home-based motivational exercise program for African American breast cancer survivors: clinical and quality-of-life outcomes. Integr Cancer Ther [Research Support, NIH, Extramural]. 2014;13(2):121–32.

169. Gil-Rey E, Quevedo-Jerez K, Maldonado-Martin S, Herrero-Roman F. Exercise intensity guidelines for

cancer survivors: a comparison with reference values. Int J Sports Med. 2014;35(14):e1–9.

170. Irwin ML, McTiernan A, Baumgartner RN, Baumgartner KB, Bernstein L, Gilliland FD, et al. Changes in body fat and weight after a breast cancer diagnosis: influence of demographic, prognostic, and lifestyle factors. J Clin Oncol. 2005;23(4):774–82.

171. Granger CL, McDonald CF, Berney S, Chao C, Denehy L. Exercise intervention to improve exercise capacity and health related quality of life for patients with non-small cell lung cancer: a systematic review. Lung Cancer [Review]. 2011;72(2):139–53.

172. Pettapiece-Phillips R, Narod SA, Kotsopoulos J. The role of body size and physical activity on the risk of breast cancer in BRCA mutation carriers. Cancer Causes Control. 2015;26(3):333–44.

173. Friedenreich CM, McGregor SE, Courneya KS, Angyalfi SJ, Elliott FG. Case-control study of lifetime total physical activity and prostate cancer risk. Am J Epidemiol. 2004;159(8):740–9.

174. Buffart LM, Galvao DA, Chinapaw MJ, Brug J, Taaffe DR, Spry N, et al. Mediators of the resistance and aerobic exercise intervention effect on physical and general health in men undergoing androgen deprivation therapy for prostate cancer. Cancer [Randomized Controlled Trial Research Support, Non-US Gov't]. 2014;120(2):294–301.

175. Moore SC, Peters TM, Ahn J, Park Y, Schatzkin A, Albanes D, et al. Age-specific physical activity and prostate cancer risk among white men and black men. Cancer [Research Support, NIH, Extramural]. 2009;115(21):5060–70.

176. Singh AA, Jones LW, Antonelli JA, Gerber L, Calloway EE, Shuler KH, et al. Association between exercise and primary incidence of prostate cancer: does race matter? Cancer. 2013;119(7):1338–43.

177. Magbanua MJ, Richman EL, Sosa EV, Jones LW, Simko J, Shinohara K, et al. Physical activity and prostate gene expression in men with low-risk prostate cancer. Cancer Causes Control [Research Support, NIH, Extramural Research Support, Non-US Gov't]. 2014;25(4):515–23.

178. Richman EL, Kenfield SA, Stampfer MJ, Paciorek A, Carroll PR, Chan JM. Physical activity after diagnosis and risk of prostate cancer progression: data from the cancer of the prostate strategic urologic research endeavor. Cancer Res. [Research Support, N.I.H., Extramural Research Support, U.S. Gov't Research Support, U.S. Gov't, Non-P.H.S.]. 2011;71(11):3889–95.

179. Sprod LK, Palesh OG, Janelsins MC, Peppone LJ, Heckler CE, Adams MJ, et al. Exercise, sleep quality, and mediators of sleep in breast and prostate cancer patients receiving radiation therapy. Community Oncol. 2010;7(10):463–71.

180. Galvao DA, Taaffe DR, Spry N, Joseph D, Newton RU. Combined resistance and aerobic exercise program reverses muscle loss in men undergoing androgen suppression therapy for prostate cancer without bone metastases: a randomized controlled trial. J Clin Oncol. 2010;28(2):340–7.

181. Lakoski SG, Willis BL, Barlow CE, et al. Midlife cardiorespiratory fitness, incident cancer, and survival after cancer in men: the cooper center longitudinal study. JAMA Oncol. 2015;1(2):231–7.

182. Santa Mina D, Alibhai SM, Matthew AG, Guglietti CL, Pirbaglou M, Trachtenberg J, et al. A randomized trial of aerobic versus resistance exercise in prostate cancer survivors. J Aging Phys Act. 2013;21(4):455–78.

183. Demark-Wahnefried W, Clipp EC, Lipkus IM, Lobach D, Snyder DC, Sloane R, et al. Main outcomes of the FRESH START trial: a sequentially tailored, diet and exercise mailed print intervention among breast and prostate cancer survivors. J Clin Oncol [Clinical Trial, Phase II Multicenter Study Randomized Controlled Trial Research Support, N.I.H., Extramural Research Support, Non-U.S. Gov't]. 2007;25(19):2709–18.

184. Gardner JR, Livingston PM, Fraser SF. Effects of exercise on treatment-related adverse effects for patients with prostate cancer receiving androgen-deprivation therapy: a systematic review. J Clin Oncol Review. 2014;32(4):335–46.

185. Parsons JK. Prostate cancer and the therapeutic benefits of structured exercise. J Clin Oncol [Comment Editorial]. 2014;32(4):271–2.

186. Winters-Stone KM, Beer TM. Review of exercise studies in prostate cancer survivors receiving androgen deprivation therapy calls for an aggressive research agenda to generate high-quality evidence and guidance for exercise as standard of care. J Clin Oncol [Comment Letter]. 2014;32(23):2518–9.

187. Mennen-Winchell LJ, Grigoriev V, Alpert P, Dos Santos H, Tonstad S. Self-reported exercise and bone mineral density in prostate cancer patients receiving androgen deprivation therapy. J Am Assoc Nurse Pract [Research Support, Non-US Gov't]. 2014;26(1):40–8.

188. Antonelli JA, Jones LW, Banez LL, Thomas JA, Anderson K, Taylor LA, et al. Exercise and prostate cancer risk in a cohort of veterans undergoing prostate needle biopsy. J Urol [Research Support, Non-US Gov't]. 2009;182(5):2226–31.

Legal and Ethical Aspects of Machine Learning: Who Owns the Data?

14

Barbara Prainsack and Elisabeth Steindl

Contents

14.1 Introduction

It is no exaggeration to say that we are in the midst of an "AI ethics bubble". The ethics of artificial intelligence makes headlines in public media and the topic of major international conferences. Technology corporations in particular are channeling funding into the creation of AI ethics institutes and endowed chairs, such as recently seen at universities in Oxford, Munich, and Cambridge, MA (e.g. [1, 2]). While corporations have collaborated with academia for many decades, if not centuries, what is new here is the strong focus on ethics.

Perhaps this is not surprising, given that AI—used here as an umbrella term for various technologies that mimic human intelligence—has become a symbol for societal concerns about the mastery of machines over people. It is seen as posing various challenges to society, ranging from voter manipulation to other threats to democracy [3], to the technological replacement of human labour [4]. The replacement of human labour is an aspect that is particularly pertinent to medicine as well: Some studies predict that up to half of all the existing jobs in the United States are at risk of automation [5]. Among medical professionals, radiologists and pathologists are seen as particularly vulnerable to technological replacement [6–8]. Against this backdrop, it could be argued, technology companies have a particularly great need to ensure that their devel-

B. Prainsack (✉)
Department of Political Science, University of Vienna, Vienna, Austria
e-mail: barbara.prainsack@univie.ac.at

E. Steindl
Department of Innovation and Digitalisation in Law, University of Vienna, Vienna, Austria

opment and use of AI complies with ethical standards.

But there is also a more sinister reason for the current ethics bubble. Corporations that use AI to develop new services, increase market shares, and expand their global reach, are currently pitching "ethics" against "regulation". Strict regulation of AI, and in particular, machine learning, they argue, puts Europe, North America and other world regions at risk of falling further behind the AI capabilities of China, and is thus problematic. They suggest that rather than putting up "red tape" for technology, societies should ensure the creation of good ethics guidelines that ensure that AI is "trustworthy" ([9], and in reference to [10]). Such playing out of ethics against regulation is, of course, not only politically problematic but also factually flawed: Ethics and regulation take different forms and are issued by different institutions, but they mutually influence and enable each other. Ethical considerations are always part of regulatory processes and guidelines, and regulation, in turn, is necessary to enforce ethical norms and commitments. Also in this chapter, ethical and regulatory and legal aspects are treated as closely intertwined, and not as something that can, or should be, strictly separated.

Before we look at the legal and regulatory aspects of AI in imaging—and zoom into the question of who owns the data that is used for this purpose—let us first look at what the issues are the ethics scholarship has identified in this context.

14.2 Opening the "Ethics Bubble": What Are the Concerns?

There has recently been a terminological shift in discussions of the ethics of AI. Until about mid-2019, the term "artificial intelligence" was widely used as an umbrella term for all computational processes that mimic human intelligence. More recently, following criticism of the unduly vague and wide use of the term in ethical and regulatory discussions, the terms that are used have become more specific: Policy and academic papers alike increasingly use the term "machine learning" to denote applications of AI that improve with only very little, or even no, input from humans. Also in this chapter, the term machine learning is used to refer to processes and technologies whereby machines discern patterns in data with only little steering from humans, while "AI" is used to denote instances in which debates refer to even wider areas of machine "intelligence", or to the attempt to make machines act like humans.

Although AI has a history of many decades (e.g. [11]), there has been an increase in AI technologies in recent years. This is mostly due to increasing computational power and increasing opportunities for automation and digitisation. These, in turn, have been made possible by "datafication", which means the capturing and storing of information about people's lives, their bodies, and about their environments, that were previously unrecorded. For example, even a decade ago, the only way to learn about people's exercise levels was by asking them what type of exercise they had done within a specific period of time, and how much of it. Today, this information is, for many of us, automatically captured by activity trackers built into our smartphones, or measured in other, often remote and unobtrusive ways. The legal scholar Harry Surden called this the end of structural privacy [12], meaning that the domains of our lives and bodies that remain unseen and "uncounted" are becoming smaller and smaller. There is ever less of us and our lives that is not datafied.

For healthcare, the availability of data about various aspects of the lives and bodies of patients, often over a long period of time, is seen as an unprecedented opportunity. Here, AI is portrayed as an answer to the problem of data interpretation: While the production of data has become relatively cheap, and greater amounts of data are being produced each day, making sense of these data has remained expensive [13]. To bridge this "interpretation gap", machine learning in particular has been suggested as a solution. Moreover, in many aspects of healthcare, AI is already in use: from telemedicine to supporting communication with patients to billing and insurance. In medical imaging, molecular imaging is expected to benefit significantly from machine learning; and deep-learning based interpretation is hoped to help reduce interobserver variability in nuclear imaging (e.g. [14]; see also [15]).

What are the key ethical challenges related to AI? Over the last years, ethicists and other experts have raised a range of concerns related to AI that can be largely grouped in three clusters: Fairness, accountability, and transparency (FAT). The paradigmatic challenge for fairness is biased training data (see [16, p. 176]): This is the case when a specific population group, such as elderly people, members of minorities, or the uninsured, are underrepresented, or entirely missing, from a data set. It is not always straightforward to know, however, when bias exists, or when it is problematic [17]. For example, in the context of the training of an algorithm to classify pulmonary tuberculosis (e.g. [18]), what constitutes a non-biased dataset: A dataset that is representative of people who typically suffer from TB? One that reflects the demographic composition of the patient population treated in a specific hospital? Or a dataset that represents the demographic composition of the city? Of the entire nation even? Moreover, if it is known, for example, that minority populations have been underrepresented in training data for machine learning for years, would it be mandated for ethical reasons to oversample members of the minority populations in question to make up for previous discrimination? There are no definitive answers to these questions; instead, they illustrate the intricacies of knowing when a bias exists, and when a bias is problematic, that is, when it has a negative impact on equity.[1]

While fairness ultimately pertains to questions about equity, the second criterion within the FAT paradigm, accountability, relates to the question of who can be held responsible for outcomes. Here, also legal questions about liability come into play. Very broadly speaking (and without consideration of specific configurations in particular jurisdictions; for more details on these, see [16, 19]), liability for harm caused by machine learning applications can only kick in when someone has been negligent, either a physician or a company. Negligence on the side of physicians or healthcare workers, in turn, requires that there is a duty of care towards patients that was breached. As Schönberger emphasises, not all erroneous predictions by an AI system that caused harm to a patient mean that physicians or healthcare organisations they work for are liable; they can only be held accountable if they used the AI in a way that they should not have [16, p. 197].

The other type of liability besides that of physicians and healthcare providers is product liability. This becomes relevant when patients suffer harm from products that were defective in their design, manufacturing, or warning—in other words, products that did not operate as they should have. The legal concept of liability was developed with the idea in mind that those held liable would be people, not machines. They were written for people who have a sense of responsibility, which machines do not have. Moreover, machines would not be affected by any of the conventional sanctions (e.g. fines) that our law system applies. Algorithms, in contrast to book titles that suggest otherwise (e.g. [20]), do not "want" things—they are not human. This raises a few issues when liability laws are applied to machines: First, if AI works in the form of non-embedded software (meaning that the software is not built into other machines such as phones, cars, or pacemakers) then it is not clear whether it is covered by existing liability legislation such as

---

[1]It is mandated here to clarify the difference between inequality and inequity. The two terms are often conflated in common parlance, but they mean different things. Inequality means that resources or benefits are distributed unequally over different groups. Using the example of health outcomes, if women and men have different life expectancies, that is an inequality. Not all inequalities, however, are also unfair: if the different outcome can be explained by voluntary actions, for example. If Laura and Amir, who are married, and who grew up in similar social strata and in the same town, have different health status because Amir likes to tend to the garden in his spare time while Laura goes paragliding, and due to multiple sport-ing accidents she now suffers chronic pain, then the difference in health status between them is not an inequity. As a rule of thumb, if we cannot find any factor that justifies different outcomes, then we should treat different outcomes as inequities.

the European Union's Product Liability Directive, for example. Second, current approaches bypass the problem that the legal concept of liability was designed to apply to humans by holding the people who build or use the machines liable for the actions of the machines. As Schönberger argues [16], the more "autonomous" machines become, that is, the less their actions can be traced back to decisions taken by humans, the more difficult it becomes to hold the humans "behind" the machines accountable. Scholars are discussing a number of ways to address these problems. These include giving some kind of personhood status to intelligent machines (e.g. [21])[2]; another solution that is discussed is to hold the healthcare professionals that are using AI even more strictly accountable for the "decisions" of the machine than at present. For example, doctors would then be responsible for harm if they did not take adequate measures to evaluate how accurate the algorithm is that they are using [16].

The last notion in the FAT-paradigm is transparency. At times, transparency is a precondition of liability, and at other times, it goes beyond it. While liability refers to the consequences for someone who bears responsibility for something in the case of harm (i.e. in the case of negligence or even intentional wrongdoing), a certain level of transparency is required for the assessment of whether any wrongdoing took place. Especially in the context of unsupervised machine learning, where no function is associated with the input,[3] it is often difficult, if not impossible, to know how the software arrived at a specific outcome because the path to achieving the outcome was not designed into the system, and is impossible

Table 14.1 A graded scale ethical scrutiny of machine learning in healthcare

Level of ethical sensitivity	Use of AI
Low	AI to support non-medical aspects (e.g. scheduling, video-conferencing)
Intermediate	AI to support diagnosis or treatment choice ("thinking AI")
High	AI to make decisions ("acting AI")

for observers to understand. It is because of this lack of transparency that some ethicists have argued that the use of unsupervised machine learning in healthcare is ethically more problematic than supervised machine learning [22]. Such proposals, however, neglect the question of where in healthcare machine learning is put to use. If it is used in core medical contexts, such as for diagnosis and treatment decisions, then the lack of transparency seems much more concerning than if unsupervised machine learning is used within an application to enable video consultations. For this reason, we propose a graded scale ethical scrutiny of machine learning in healthcare (Table 14.1) that distinguishes between three levels of ethical sensitivity: At the lowest level of concern are uses of machine learning (and other AI) for non-medical aspects, such as appointment scheduling or videoconferencing. At the intermediate level are applications of machine learning in key medical activities such as the establishment of a diagnosis or treatment decision, but where machine learning is only aiding human decision making without suggesting a final decision ("thinking AI"). At the highest level of ethical sensitivity is the use of machine learning for key medical activities where the software makes the decision, e.g. if a machine that automatically classified a disease and gave a treatment decision that was binding ("acting AI"), which is so far not part of routine clinical care.

Other factors that are to be considered include whether or not machine learning is supervised (which is less ethically problematic because of higher level of transparency) or unsupervised (more ethically sensitive due to lower levels of

---

[2]The European Parliament has adopted a resolution in 2017 with recommendations to the Commission on Civil Law Rules on Robotics suggesting to prompt a legal status for robots (https://www.europarl.europa.eu/doceo/document/TA-8-2017-0051_EN.html?redirect#BKMD-12). The Commission, however, did not follow this recommendation in its recent strategies addressing AI.

[3]Within supervised machine learning, the machine is told by a human what to look for: e.g. it is shown pictures of dogs and then asked to look for dogs in other images. Within unsupervised machine learning, the machine is not told what to look for, but just commanded to look for patterns.

transparency), whether the tool has been validated, and whether the people using the tool are conscious of the possibility and consequences of potential bias ("fairness through awareness", [23]).

14.3   Going Beyond FAT: Beyond Medical Ethics

Ethics guidelines, ethics codes, as well as papers addressing ethical concerns in connection with AI in healthcare regularly discuss phenomena that map against the FAT paradigm—even if they discuss these issues under different labels. But there are also contributions that raise bigger questions. A statement by the European Group on Ethics on AI, robotics and "autonomous" systems" (2018), for example, draws attention to the need for AI to be put in the service of broader societal and ethical values, including human dignity, responsibility, democracy, justice, equity, solidarity, sustainability, and deliberation. Moreover, scholars such as Karen Yeung use the term "ethics washing" to refer to situations where AI ethics serves mostly as an empty vessel that can be filled with any content that seems suitable, and where ethics lacks the necessary tools to enforce its own claims [9]. Taken together, these points of critique call for an ethics that does not accept current institutional arrangements and configurations of power as they are, and within these, try to make AI "more ethical". Instead, they call for a political ethics that is concerned also with how new technological practices affect the distribution of entitlements, duties, and resources within and across populations. The FAT paradigm goes some way in that direction, but not far enough.

An important underpinning of such a more political ethics of AI is to leave the specificities of medical ethics behind, and instead treat AI ethics as a form of data ethics. A key argument in favour of the latter is that many ethical issues in connection with machine learning emerge due to the integration and use of large amounts of personal data. But such a move from medical to data ethics may not be as easy to do as it may seem. It would require a fundamental shift in the points of refer-

ence used by ethics frameworks—most prominently the focus only on individual rights. As many scholars have argued, most of the risks in connection with data use are personal and collective, and they cannot be broken down into individual bits (e.g. [24]). Moreover, many of the scholars and approaches that are populating the rapidly growing field of AI ethics were trained in medical ethics or bioethics. It will be difficult to expand (and, in some cases, change) the reference points and institutional structures that these experts are operating with and within.

What is the problem with the categories and focus points of medical ethics—why can they not be transposed to AI ethics? The main reason is that the key reference point of medical ethics is the human body; the early codifications of medical ethics established that people have a right to be informed about, and consent to, what happens to their bodies. This framework emerged partly in response to the horrific human rights infringements of the Nazi period and other instances when harmful or even torturous "experiments" were imposed on people under the guise of science. Data ethics, on the other hand, does not take the physical body as its reference point, but the "data body"—which is of a very different nature. First of all, the data body does not have clear borders and boundaries; the data that represents a person, namely, the data capturing her behaviour, her diseases, etc., is spread over many places and can be accessed by many people at the same time. This means, also, that the frame of an intervention that medical ethics operates with does not work for data ethics. An intervention into a person's data is not comparable to a body that is operated on to take out a gallbladder, or to test a new drug. There is often no clear beginning and no clear end to an "operation" on a dataset—data is interrogated continuously [25]. In addition, in traditional medical ethics, it is normally clearly apparent who carries out the procedure and who is at risk: The latter is normally the patient. In data ethics, "procedures" can be carried out by many different people in different places at the same time—primary and secondary data users (the latter are researchers, for example, who reuse datasets from other research teams, or even from the clinic), commercial enterprises, etc. The people at risk from these procedures can be totally unrelated from those who have given their data. In other words, risks in data ethics are not limited to specific individuals, but they are collective.

Understanding AI ethics as a kind of data ethics, and not as a field of application for medical ethics, also affects how we think about data ownership.

14.4   Who Owns Patient Data?

This simple question is not easy to answer. It will concern us for the rest of this chapter. The problem starts with defining ownership. While the related term "property" has clearly definable legal meaning, ownership can relate to legal entitlements, but it can also refer to a moral claim on something. People who say that they own their personal data do not always mean to express a legal opinion. Rather than implying that they have the right to destroy or sell their data, which are some of the key characteristics that distinguish property rights from other entitlements, what they often mean to say is: "I should have a say in who uses my data, what they do with it, and who benefits from it". In other words, ownership is a very broad concept that includes moral and legal elements.

But let's start at the beginning. Can we legally own data? In other words, is it possible to own something that is (at least in part) immaterial—as digital data is (see [26])? The law answers this question affirmatively; intellectual property rights protection is an example. It gives people or organisations the right to control intellectual resources that are in part, or even entirely, immaterial.

Within the European Union, the EU General Data Protection Regulation (GDPR) grants special protections to so-called personal data, that is, data that refers to a specific identified or identifiable natural person. Names and addresses are clearly personal data; but IP addresses or genomes are too [27]. Personal data is seen as disclosing things about people and their lives that they may

want to be confidential or even private, and people may suffer harm if this data and information are known or used by others. For these reasons, not only GDPR, but most jurisdictions place restrictions on the collection and use of personal data. But there are crucial differences in how personal data is protected. To put it very generally, in Europe, the predominant view has been to see personal data and information as belonging to people in a moral sense, without being considered property in the legal sense. This means that personal data is not seen as something to be sold, or something that has a market value. The protection of personal data is ensured through privacy rights.

According to European Law, the question of whether data can be owned has multiple layers. One layer refers to the fact that any data has to be categorised as either personal or non-personal data. Personal data is protected by a number of fundamental individual rights, such as the right to be informed, the right of access, the right to rectification, the right to erasure, the right to restrict processing, the right to data portability, the right to object, and rights in relation to automated decision-making and profiling (see Chap. 3 GDPR). These individual rights continue to exist as long as the data has not been anonymised— this means that, taking into account all the means reasonably likely to be used, the data does no longer relate to an identified or identifiable person (i.e. all links to do so have been destroyed). In other words the conception of personal data within the GDPR cannot be aligned with a third party owning somebody else's personal data.[4] It also means that, in the European context, the question of ownership only arises regarding non-personal data. And this is where the next layer comes in: as data does not easily fit into either one of the traditional legal categories of material or immaterial, it cannot be subsumed under property that is moveable or intellectual property. The European Commission itself stressed that current

---

[4]The question of lawfulness of processing of special categories of personal data according to Article 9 GDPR has to be seen apart from any kind of possible ownership and is therefore not discussed here.

intellectual property laws are not a suitable tool for data governance [28].

In the United States, debates about whether personal information should or could be viewed as property have been complex. Some authors see property rights as the best way of protecting personal data [29]. Partially, this notion is rooted in the important role that property rights play in American self-conception. Property rights, understood—in William Blackstone's deliberately provocative description—as 'that sole and despotic dominion which one man claims and exercises over the external things of the world, in total exclusion of the right of any other individual in the universe' [30], are woven into the very foundations of American society and legal culture. Even for those scholars who say that this ideal has never been implemented in actual practice, property rights have nevertheless played a much more important role in the United States than in Europe.

In U.S. discourse, treating personal data as property has served the important purpose of overcoming the shortcomings of U.S. data protection systems [31, pp. 507–508]. In contrast to the European Union, who have a data protection law that applies to the processing of all personal data and expands its territorial scope even beyond European borders, American privacy laws are sector-specific; they are tailored to specific fields such as healthcare or financial services. This has led some scholars to argue that, because American privacy laws are relatively weak, property rights are the best, or even the only, way to ensure people's control over their data.

Other authors (e.g. [32, p. 1295]) disagree with this stance. They argue that "the raison d'etre of property is alienability" [32, p. 1295]. The meaning of this statement becomes clear only if we take a closer look at how property rights are organised: It is best conceived as a bundle of entitlements, rather than as one single right. It is the bundle of rights, rather than one specific characteristic, that sets property rights apart from other entitlements to things. Within that bundle, there are some "stand-out" rights that characterise the bundle.

To use an example from the physical world: When someone has borrowed a book from a library, the book is in her possession. She is enti-tled to do a lot of things: to read the book, to control who else gets to read it, and she can use it for other purposes such as place a laptop on top of it for a videoconference. She can exclude other people from even looking at it. But there are things that this person who has taken a book from the library is not entitled to do: She must not sell or destroy the book. These additional entitlements are reserved to the person or entity that holds property rights. In other words, the bundle of rights granted to a person due to mere possession (e.g. having the book in your house after having taken it from the library) is less "thick" than the bundle of property rights. Property rights include all rights that other forms of possessions include (the right to possession, income, etc., as listed below) plus the right of alienation (selling or destroying).

Another example of the difference between weaker forms of possession on the one hand, and property rights on the other, is renting a flat. As a lawful tenant I am entitled to determine who can enter the flat, how it is decorated, and what is done inside. But only the owner (here: the holder of property rights) holds the additional rights that are also in the bundle, such as selling the flat. (The fact that I am not normally allowed to destroy my flat, even if I hold property rights, illustrates that even property rights are not unlimited—even they can be restricted to protect important other rights and interests. In the interest of public safety and security I am not allowed to burn down my flat, or to neglect it to such an extent that it becomes a public nuisance).

Back to digital data. But how does this difference between property rights and "weaker" forms of possession that apply to tangible goods such as books or flats work with intangible things such as data? As noted, although data has a tangible, material element, including the technical infrastructures that enable its collection, storage, and use, at least a part of them is immaterial.

In order to answer this question it is helpful to unpack the bundle of rights and entitlements that make up property rights. Denise Johnson [33], drawing upon Honore's famous work in the 1960s [34], names the following entitlements as part of the bundle of property rights:

1. The right to **possess**. Just as the example of the library book, or the rented flat, below, the person who rightfully possesses has exclusive control of a thing. When the thing that is owned is intangible, then, as Honore put it, possession is the right to exclude others from using or benefitting from the thing. Moving to the digital realm, for data in the healthcare domain, such as imaging data and lab results, it is very difficult to conceive what such "exclusive" control would look like. When an imaging department that does a cardiac perfusion scan on a patient owns the imaging data (because the patient may have agreed to this when signing the consent form for the procedure) "exclusive control" means that they can share the data with third parties—they can even sell the data. But does it mean that they can exclude the patient from accessing their own perfusion scan?, Wherever GDPR is applicable, this stance would be difficult to argue—because as long as the perfusion scan is seen as personal data—i.e. as data that is linked to an identified or identifiable person (note that this includes pseudonymised data)—then the patient has a right to access—or even initiate the erasure—of her own data even though she does not hold property rights to it [35].

2. The right to **manage** gives people the right to decide who can use the thing that is possessed, and how. It includes the right of lending or contracting out (see also [36]). This right seems relatively unproblematic in connection with digital data, except that it may be difficult to exclude patients from using their own data as long as this data is considered personal data—as explained in point (1). Referring to our example of the perfusion scan explained above, this means that the entity that holds property rights to the perfusion scan data can decide who gets access to it, for what purpose it can be used, and who can commercialise it. They may not, however, be able to refuse patients access as long as the imaging data can be linked to an identified or identifiable person.

3. The right to **income** allows the property rights holder to allow others to use the thing and to pay her for this use. This right is closely related to the previous one, namely the right to manage; the difference between the two is that the right to income focuses on the money that one receives in return—for other people using the thing, for example (see also [36]). This seems no more difficult to enforce in the case of digital data than it is with owning a physical object.

4. The right to **capital**—which is the right that allows a person to alienate the thing, namely to give it away, to consume it, to change it, or to destroy it. The problem here is that it is not so easy to decide what "consuming" or "destroying" data means. Physical things are consumable and rivalrous: They can be 'used up', and the use of the good by one person affects the use of the good by others. Many authors argue that the same cannot be said for digital data, as they are considered to be neither consumable nor rivalrous: The perfusion scan data does not disappear, or deteriorate, if lots of people use it; and one research group using it does not detract from the utility of the data for another. Having said this, whereas the data itself is not consumable or rivalrous, their value can be: the value of a dataset can be highest for those who have exclusive use; and it can, of course, be affected by many people using it. Think of proprietary information such as search algorithms, or information on commercial mergers that are likely to affect stock prices, for example. For these reasons, digital data is best described as simultaneous [26]: It can be in more places than one at the same time, it can be copied and used by several people at the same time, independent of what the others are doing, and it leaves traces even when it is deleted. Because the value of data can be rivalrous, it is arguably this multiplicity of data that is the key difference between physical entities and digital data with regard to the right to capital. In situations where those holding property rights to data cannot

control all copy of the dataset (or do not even know where all the different copies are), the right to capital may be difficult to enforce.

5. The right to **security** protects the rights-holder from expropriation. In Quigley's words [36, p. 633], it is "the assurance that a person […] will not be forced to give it up without adequate recompense." It is not difficult to conceive of this right with respect to digital data.

6. The power of **transmissibility** means that the rights holder can give the thing that s/he owns to somebody else, either before or after his/her death. Also here, it is not difficult to imagine this right to be applied to digital data (for the instrument of post-mortem data donation specifically, see [26, 37]).

7. The **absence of term**: This means that the length of ownership is not time-limited.

8. Now we are moving into the provisions within the bundle of property rights that are duties and liabilities rather than entitlements: The first one is the **prohibition of harmful use**, meaning that even the person who owns a thing is not free to do with it whatever she pleases; the boundaries of her freedom are the rights of others. In the physical world this is best described with a knife: Even if I hold all entitlements of the bundle of property rights to the knife I am not allowed to use it to cut into another person. With regard to data, the prohibition of harmful use raises really interesting questions: Does this only mean that the data owner herself is not allowed to use the data in a harmful way? Or does it include a duty to actively prevent that others can use the data in a harmful way? Does this mean that restrictions of data sharing may be required as a preventive measure? These questions remain open.

9. Those who hold property rights are also **liable to execution**; which means that the thing that is owned can be taken away for the repayment of a debt, for example. It is conceivable that this would apply to digital data: if the data has commercial value, ownership

of a dataset could be taken away to pay for something that the rights holder owns.

10. Last but not least, property rights have a **residuary character**: This means that, even if the property rights holder has given away many entitlements within the bundle (e.g. she has leased her property to someone else), she still holds whatever is left of the bundle. To the extent that the bundle of property rights can be applied to digital data, the residuary character does not pose any additional complications.

In sum, many of the entitlements and duties within the bundle of rights that constitute property rights—which were originally developed for physical things—cannot be neatly transposed to digital data. Because of the multiple nature of digital data (the ability of digital data to be at several places at the same time), it is more useful to speak about the right to control data in the context of medical imaging than about data ownership. Because of the complexities laid out in this chapter, and because of the moral and legal connotations of the term, the notion of ownership tends to confuse more than it clarifies when applied to digital data.

14.5   Conclusion

This chapter started with the diagnosis that we are amidst an "AI ethics bubble", where especially corporate interest in ethics of AI and machine learning is extremely high. Technology corporations and other businesses provide funding for ethics institutes and endowed chairs on AI ethics at leading universities, and co-opt academics into the ethics governance of their own companies. The pitching of "ethics" against "regulation" has been part of this process.

Taking the stance that ethics and regulation, albeit having different emphases, complement and require each other, rather than being clearly separable, this chapter then opened up the "ethics bubble" of AI. Our diagnosis was that most of the ethical concerns identified and discussed in this context map against the so-called FAT paradigm. It orders concerns in several clusters, including fairness, accountability, and transparency. While this typology is extremely helpful, we proposed to take a step further and go beyond the FAT paradigm. In order to do so, we suggested to go beyond the toolbox of medical ethics and draw more strongly upon the instruments in the growing field of data ethics. This is necessary, we argued, because the reference point of medical ethics is the physical body, which has clear boundaries. The same does not apply to people's data bodies, which are far from clearly bounded: Data is multiple in the sense that it can be in several places at the same time.

What, then, does this mean for the question of data ownership? Who owns the data that medical imaging departments work with? The final section of this chapter seeks to answer this question by discussing how the "bundle of rights" that make property rights can be applied to digital data. We conclude that because of the multiple nature of digital data, some of the entitlements and duties within the bundle of property rights can be applied to digital data only with difficulty.

References

1. Moss E, Metcalf, J. The ethical dilemma at the heart of big tech companies. Harvard Business Rev. 2019. https://hbr.org/2019/11/the-ethical-dilemma-at-the-heart-of-big-tech-companies. Accessed 24 Apr 2020.
2. Ochigame R. 2019. The invention of "ethical AI". The Intercept. https://theintercept.com/2019/12/20/mit-ethical-ai-artificial-intelligence/?comments=1. Accessed 24 Apr 2020.
3. O'Neill C. Weapons of math destruction: how big data increases inequality and threatens democracy. Crown. 2016.
4. Ford M. Rise of the robots: technology and the threat of a jobless future. New York: Basic Books; 2015.
5. Frey CB, Osborne MA. The future of employment: how susceptible are jobs to computerisation? Technol Forecast Soc Chang. 2017;114:254–80.
6. Chockley K, Emanuel E. The end of radiology? Three threats to the future practice of radiology. J Am Coll Radiol. 2016;13(12):1415–20.
7. Grace K, Salvatier J, Dafoe A, Zhang B, Evans O. When will AI exceed human performance? Evidence from AI experts. J Artif Intell Res. 2018;62:729–54.
8. Obermeyer Z, Emanuel EJ. Predicting the future—big data, machine learning, and clinical medicine. N Engl J Med. 2016;375(13):1216.
9. Yeung K, Howes A, Pogrebna G. AI governance by human rights-centred design, deliberation and oversight: an end to ethics washing. The Oxford handbook of AI ethics. Oxford: Oxford University Press; 2019.
10. European Commission Ethics Guidelines for Trustworthy AI. 2019. https://ec.europa.eu/digital-single-market/en/news/ethics-guidelines-trustworthy-ai. Accessed 16 May 2020.
11. Haenlein M, Kaplan A. A brief history of artificial intelligence: on the past, present, and future of artificial intelligence. Calif Manag Rev. 2019;61(4):5–14.
12. Surden H. Structural rights in privacy. SMUL Rev. 2007;60:1605.
13. Prainsack B. Precision medicine needs a cure for inequality. Curr Hist. 2019;118(804):11–5.
14. Choi H. Deep learning in nuclear medicine and molecular imaging: current perspectives and future directions. Nucl Med Mol Imaging. 2018;52(2):109–18.
15. Choi H, Ha S, Im HJ, Paek SH, Lee DS. Refining diagnosis of Parkinson's disease with deep learning-based interpretation of dopamine transporter imaging. Neuroimage Clin. 2017;16:586–94. https://doi.org/10.1016/j.nicl.2017.09.010.
16. Schönberger D. Artificial intelligence in healthcare: a critical analysis of the legal and ethical implications. Int J Law Inform Technol. 2019;27(2):171–203.
17. Esteva A, Kuprel B, Novoa RA, Ko J, Swetter SM, Blau HM, Thrun S. Dermatologist-level classification of skin cancer with deep neural networks. Nature. 2017;542(7639):115–8.
18. Lakhani P, Sundaram B. Deep learning at chest radiography: automated classification of pulmonary tuberculosis by using convolutional neural networks. Radiology. 2017;284(2):574–82.
19. Pesapane F, Volonté C, Codari M, Sardanelli F. Artificial intelligence as a medical device in radiology: ethical and regulatory issues in Europe and the United States. Insights Imaging. 2018;9(5):745–53.
20. Finn E. What algorithms want: imagination in the age of computing. Cambridge, MA: MIT Press; 2017.
21. Vladeck DC. Machines without principals: liability rules and artificial intelligence. Washington Law Rev. 2014;89:117.
22. Jannes M, Friele M, Jannes C, Woopen C. Algorithms in digital healthcare. An interdisciplinary analysis. Gütersloh: Bertelsmann Stiftung; 2019.
23. Dwork C, Hardt M, Pitassi T, Reingold O, Zemel R. Fairness through awareness. In: Proceedings of the 3rd innovations in theoretical computer science conference; 2012. p. 214–26.
24. Taylor M. Genetic data and the law: a critical perspective on privacy protection. Cambridge: Cambridge University Press; 2012.
25. Metcalf J, Crawford K. Where are human subjects in big data research? The emerging ethics divide. Big Data Soc. 2016;3(1):1–14. https://doi.

org/10.1177/2053951716650211. Accessed 16 May 2020.

26. Prainsack B. Data donation: how to resist the iLeviathan. In: The ethics of medical data donation. Cham: Springer; 2019. p. 9–22.

27. Goddard M. The EU General Data Protection Regulation (GDPR): European regulation that has a global impact. Int J Mark Res. 2017;59(6):703–5.

28. European Commission Legal study on ownership and access to data. Final report. 2016. https://www.op.europa.eu/s/n2Qc. Accessed 16 May 2020.

29. Murphy RS. Property rights in personal information: an economic defence of privacy. Georgetown Law J. 1996;84:2381–217.

30. Blackstone W.. Of property in general. Commentaries on the laws of England. 1765–69; Book II: Chapter I. 1979. https://avalon.law.yale.edu/subject_menus/blackstone.asp. Accessed 12 May 2018.

31. Purtova N. Property rights in personal data: learning from the American discourse. Comput Law Secur Rev. 2009;25(6):507–21.

32. Litman J. Information privacy/information property. Stanford Law Rev. 2000;52:1283–313.

33. Johnson DR. Reflections on the bundle of rights. Vermont Law Rev. 2007;32:247. https://lawreview.vermontlaw.edu/wp-content/uploads/2012/02/johnson2.pdf

34. Honoré AM. Ownership. Making law bind: essays legal and philosophical. Oxford: Clarendon Press; 1961. p. 161–92 (Originally published in Guest AG, ed. Oxford essays in jurisprudence. Oxford: Oxford University Press; 1961. p. 107–47).

35. Thorogood A, Bobe J, Prainsack B, Middleton A, Scott E, Nelson S, Corpas M, Bonhomme N, Rodriguez LL, Murtagh M, Kleiderman E. APPLaUD: access for patients and participants to individual level uninterpreted genomic data. Hum Genomics. 2018;12(1):7.

36. Quigley M. Property and the body: applying Honoré. Med Law Rev. 2007;17:457.

37. Krutzinna J, Floridi L, editors. The ethics of medical data donation. Cham: Springer International Publishing; 2019.

Artificial Intelligence and the Nuclear Medicine Physician: Clever Is as Clever Does

15

Roland Hustinx

Contents

For several years now, the role and place of artificial intelligence (A.I.) in radiology have been discussed and debated in all strata of the radiological field. From university hospitals to private centers, from large companies to countless start-ups, from scientific societies to medical associations, all are very actively and vocally involved. The U.S. Centers for Medicare and Medicaid Services' (CMS) decision in September 2020 to provide its first-ever reimbursement of a radiology A.I. algorithm is expected to open the door to broader coverage of imaging A.I. software in the clinics. The feeling in radiology is that A.I. is no longer a prospect, it is a reality. The physician's attitude has shifted from the fear that "A.I. will replace radiologists" to the belief that "radiologists who use AI will replace those who don't." A.I. has been much less present in the field of nuclear medicine (NM), which is distinct from radiology as a medical specialty in most countries. However, they share similar technologies, in particular the cross-sectional techniques used in hybrid imaging, e.g. CT and MRI. There is no reason that the advances, solutions, and new problems highlighted by A.I. in the radiological field should not be observed sooner or later in the NM field. Some of our practical specificities, such as the complication of dealing with short-lived isotopes for scheduling the clinical activity, or the complexities of individual dosimetry in treatments with radiopharmaceuticals, should, on

R. Hustinx (✉)
Division of Nuclear Medicine and Oncological
Imaging, University Hospital of Liège, GIGA-CRC
In Vivo Imaging, University of Liège, Liege, Belgium
e-mail: rhustinx@chuliege.be

the contrary, constitute excellent fields where A.I. helps our practice. Nonetheless, it is indisputable that NM is lagging behind radiology in the clinical implementation of A.I. Whatever the reasons, increased susceptibility of the NM techniques to local methodological variables, difficulty to gather large curated datasets or perhaps smaller market less attractive for the industry, we do not seem close to seeing any reimbursement of an A.I. add-on in our field. It is only a matter of time, however, and it should give NM physicians the opportunity to better prepare and contribute more actively to shaping how A.I. will be integrated into our practice. The question is essentially twofold: what would be the role of NM physicians in a medical era where A.I. is more and more present, and what must we learn and do to shape this future.

In this chapter we shall consider successively the benefits of A.I., the threats and the obstacles that accompany its implementation, and finally the possible steps that need to be taken for a successful and mutually satisfactory embedment of A.I. in clinical nuclear medicine. These questions shall be considered looking at the three axes of involvement of A.I. in the field of NM: Physics, i.e. how A.I. will impact image acquisition and reconstruction; operational, i.e. how A.I. will optimize health care delivery through improved scheduling and overall organization; clinical which encompasses all applications aiming at improving the interpretation of the studies (not limited to the images) in terms of diagnostic accuracy, prognostic and predictive value or individual pre-treatment dosimetry.

15.1   I Am Looking Forward to More A.I. in My Practice Because…

15.1.1   The Images Will Look Prettier

In theory, we nuclear medicine physicians should benefit from the introduction of A.I. in all three fields, and the physics applications are probably the most obviously welcome. Indeed, we will be looking at images obtained with lower injected activity, i.e. lower patient's exposure [1]. Studies will be shorter to acquire, leading to improved patient's comfort and experience, fewer movement artifacts, and also increased throughput. X-ray exposure may also be reduced by using deep learning (DL) for attenuation correction, hence removing the need for low-dose, attenuation correction only, CTs [2]. A.I. has the potential to further enhance the image quality through improvements in the co-registration of the CT and SPECT/PET parts of hybrid studies. This may have major implications in particular in studies where misregistrations may have significant clinical implications. This is the case for instance when using the diagnostic CT study along with the [^{99m}Tc]MAA SPECT/CT study for determining the activity of [^{90}Y]-labeled microspheres to inject during selective intra-arterial radiation therapy. In summary, considering the images and their content as a product, we will be working with better-quality material, and nobody would argue against that.

Furthermore, improved, faster, and more robust automated AI-based segmentation algorithms will streamline the data analysis. For instance, [^{18}F]FDG PET/CT is key in the management of diffuse large B cell lymphomas (DLBCL), and the metabolic tumor volume (MTV) appears to be a metrics that further improves its prognostic value. The current consensus tends towards using a fixed maximum standardized uptake value (SUV$_{max}$) threshold of 4, but even when semi-automated, the process is tedious, time-consuming, and imperfectly reproducible [3, 4]. Automated algorithms based on DL have been proposed for this task [5], and in all likelihood most of us should see those as a welcome addition to our daily routine.

15.1.2   My Life Will Be Easier

The introduction of A.I. into the operation of the NM department should also benefit to the physicians, through optimization of the resources. This has been demonstrated in radiology departments [6], and it should prove even more relevant in NM, which is dealing with isotopes, including short-lived ones. Patients scheduling, radiopharmaceutical preparation, and report generation are operational activities all susceptible to benefit from A.I., provided that the physicians, radiopharmacists, and administrative staffs strongly contribute to framing the A.I. intervention and fully stay on top of the processes. The worst-case scenario would be an A.I.-supported take-over by non-medical, bureaucratic supervisors who would consider that A.I. provides them with all the insight needed to optimally manage an NM Department, without a significant contribution from the physicians. A basic task, often overlooked, but which is responsible for a significant waste of time for the NM physician is to recover and organize previous studies, not only in NM but also in other modalities. It is often difficult to streamline a process that involves different providers, for the PACS and the different viewers that may coexist in a department. Operational A.I. would be of great value in this setting.

15.1.3 My Patients Will Be Better Off

More generally, NM physicians are used to looking at images but also at data. Radiomics and A.I. will provide more data, more reliable data, and new ways at interpreting these data. NM should therefore be a fertile ground for these developments in diagnostic and prognostic applications in general. However, we must first study the terrain before attempting to consider the practical impacts that can be expected in clinical NM. Activity profiles are very different in academic centers and public and private services. They also vary from country to country, in Europe and across the world. Some services work primarily with single-photon NM, i.e. bone scan, myocardial perfusion scintigraphy, and a range of studies performed less frequently such as kidney, thyroid, or parathyroid scans. These studies, when added together, constitute a significant contribution to the production of these services. The relative contribution of hybrid imaging (SPECT/CT) also varies considerably from center to center. In yet other departments, most of the activity relates to PET/CT, and some

regularly perform a large number of non-FDG studies, such as radiolabeled PSMA ligands. In addition, theranostic approaches, with the accompanying treatment procedures, also occupy very different places in NM centers. Therefore, it is clear that considering the potential impact of A.I. in the field of NM involves first trying to understand the major trends in the future development of the specialty itself. A systematic review published in 2019 showed a strong imbalance in A.I. applications towards oncology, which accounted for 86% of all publications in A.I. and radiomics fields [7]. Hence, one may infer that those centers where oncology, and more specifically high-end, tertiary or quaternary-care oncology, is more prevalent, will experience the most immediate impact of A.I. on their clinical practice. Neurology and cardiology are probably the next in line in terms of clinical implementation. From the physician's perspective, the initial steps in this clinical implementation process should be quite exciting. We can expect to benefit from a growing number of A.I. toolkits designed to perform dedicated and highly focused tasks, such as characterizing lung nodules using [^{18}F]FDG PET and CT, or recognizing normal patterns, e.g. non-pathological studies in whole-body bone scans with [^{99m}Tc]-labeled diphosphonates. Such tasks should prove to be of great benefit to the specialty, and our patients, by improving the quality and reliability of the diagnostic information contained in our reports. We would always maintain a holistic, human-centered approach to the NM imaging field, as we would use these A.I. tools to merely complement an otherwise unchanged process of interpreting images and quantitative data that supports them. Personalized dosimetry may also be helped by A.I. and thus gain further acceptance in the clinical field. For instance, similar to diagnostic studies, A.I. may lead to shorter acquisition times for the [^{177}Lu] SPECT studies or better model and predict voxel-wise dosimetry measurements. Again, the final decision, i.e. should we treat the patient and if yes, the activity to be administered, would remain in the physician's hands, albeit better armed for making those decisions.

With all of these largely positive elements, the transition to AI-augmented nuclear medicine should be smooth and easy. All we have to do is learn how to use the new tools first and then how extensively to trust them. Just as we use quantitative algorithms that compare individual studies to population-based normality, like the Cedar-Sinai program in MPI or Parametric Statistical Mapping (SPM) in FDG brain PET studies, and many more. These are useful tools, fully integrated into the clinics, but the conclusions of which do not replace those of the NM physician. Obviously, however, this is not the full story. Indeed A.I. undoubtedly contains threats to the practice of nuclear medicine as we know it, and as some us might want to keep it. And other obstacles exist in the way of a smooth implementation of A.I. in clinical NM.

15.2   I Am Wary of More A.I. Because…

15.2.1 I Don't Understand It

This represents perhaps the greatest obstacle on A.I.'s path towards clinical nuclear medicine. As stated previously, we as NM physicians are used to dealing with data, numbers, values, quantitative measurements in addition to looking at images. We understand the relationship between these numbers and results, and the physiological, biological, or biochemical processes that underlie them. We easily translate time/activity curves into glomerular filtration rate. We understand how to translate counts/pixel into the SUV, as a semi-quantitative measurement of the glucose metabolism. We also understand and know very well all the factors that affect the variability of the SUV. We also know that we could, if we wanted to, obtain absolute measurements such as the glucose metabolic rate in mmol/min/g. tissue. Every nuclear medicine physician knows the difference between filtered back-projection and iterative reconstruction. We have been trained to master the basics of physics and instrumentation,

and we are able to speak or at least listen to our fellow physicists and engineers. However, our training in computational science and our understanding of probabilistic learning is quite limited. For many of us, the leap to radiomics is reasonably doable, because they are quantitative features that answer formulas, and for which we can assess confounders. Basically, the good old SUV is nothing more than a basic radiomic function. The more advanced features remain very similar whether they represent a measure of signal heterogeneity, shape or intensity, e.g. the biological phenomenon responsible for the accumulation or distribution of the tracer. The leap to A.I. is much more difficult, because our scientific background has not prepared us for it. We do not have the mental tools to fully understand the basics of a U-Net architecture. Without even considering DL, the more basic learning machine algorithms, such as the random forests and support vector machine, are not entirely part of our natural domain of competence. Furthermore, the relationship between the images, the quantitative features abstracted from the images and the biology, is lost after going through the DL process. Moreover, with A.I. in medicine, high performance is often associated with high opacity. Hence the call for explainable and interpretable A.I. Some authors have gone further in distinguishing explainability and causability [8]. The former "highlights decision-relevant parts of the used representations of the algorithms and active parts in the algorithmic model, that either contribute to the model accuracy on the training set, or to a specific prediction for one particular observation." The later refers to "the extent to which an explanation of a statement to a human expert achieves a specified level of *causal understanding* with effectiveness, efficiency and satisfaction in a specified context of use." In other words, an algorithm is explainable if we understand the effect of variables on all the moving parts that constitute the algorithm, and it fits the causability criterion if the end result, i.e. the conclusion at the end of the computation, is efficiently and transparently actionable.

15.2.2 I Don't Trust It

Obviously, it is difficult to trust processes that are poorly understood, which is why explainability and causability are prerequisites for trust. Beyond that, A.I. is not free of risk, in particular it can generate errors. For example, image reconstruction with DL can lead to artifacts and alterations that could have clinical impact [9]. Machine learning algorithms, even the smartest, can be fooled by minute alterations to the input data and completely mishandle the data, in a way that humans are not subject to [10]. This is the so-called "adversarial machine learning" well known in the A.I. community, and the concept has been extended to the field of radiomics [11]. This raises the specter of an initially effective and fully validated A.I. algorithm turning into a mill generating mislead interpretations and erroneous decisions. The validation process itself needs to be validated. The medical literature is not devoid of papers that, although peer-reviewed in a seemingly appropriate fashion, are methodologically impaired in a severe way. Many questions arise concerning the statistical methods for assessing the performance of an algorithm. Most articles in NM use the area under the receiver operating characteristic curve (AUC ROC) as the main metric for assessing the performance of the model when the outcome is binary, i.e., recurrence/no recurrence, malignant/not malignant, etc. Yet in presence of unbalanced data, the AUC artificially inflates the performance of the model [12]. There is a need for at the very least using the most appropriate test, e.g. AUC and F-score, depending on the sample distribution and hypothesis, and also probably to develop more specific tests [13].

Further improving and perfecting the A.I. should be accompanied by further safeguards. Current typical A.I. models are essentially static, in that they have been trained using samples corresponding to a population that was fully validated at the time the model was built. They are efficient in test sets that correspond to their training sets. Those static algorithms may be subject to concept drift, which means that even though a task was at first efficiently and reliably fulfilled, it is no longer the case when the patient population evolves or when the technique changes. So ideally, the algorithms should not stop learning, i.e. they should adapt along with modifications introduced in the sets of data to analyze. This is the continuous learning or continual A.I. [14]. The algorithm learns to learn, incrementally adapts to new characteristics found in the input data, constantly updating its feature selection to better fit its changing environment. Intuitively we may realize the advantages of such process, but we also realize that it should be associated with a constant "revalidation process." Indeed, the catastrophic inference or forgetting may occur when extreme outliers wreak havoc into an autonomously relearning algorithm. To put it simply, even fully validated and trustworthy A.I. algorithms at the time of marketing and clinical implementation need to continuously go through extremely stringent quality controls.

15.2.3 I Don't Want It

The ultimate, and most compelling, question is "where does the physician fit in this puzzle?" Say we end up with a multitude of A.I. algorithms dedicated to a multitude of specific tasks, possibly running in parallel and selected depending on the patient's medical profile and issue at hand. Say those algorithms are constantly learning, and one way or another, the process is safeguarded by multiple checkpoints. Once we get there, the role of the physician could go either way: The physicians remain in charge of the patient's care, responsible before the law, they keep receiving the medical fees, and thus decide when and how to use the A.I. tools. Or the physicians do not have the knowledge and expertise to correct the A.I. tools when they are wrong; they do not even know when an A.I. tool is wrong, and they are surrounded by so many effective A.I. tools that the gestalt, which was the heart of the medical profession, is no more than the vestige of a bygone era, in so much so that the physicians no longer enjoy the confidence of the public and health care providers. The debate remains very vivid in the radiology community. The prophecy

G. Hinton playfully made in 2016 ("People should stop training radiologists now. It's just completely obvious within five years that DL is going to do better than radiologists") has not been verified yet, but the question remains circulated in the decision circles. The Dutch Finance Minister Wopke Hoekstra very recently commented that "The work of the radiologist to a significant extent has become redundant, because … a machine can read the images better than humans who studied 10 years for it" [15]. The answers coming from medical and scientific organizations are only half-convincing. They argue that as the medical demand is increasing, A.I. will take care of the automated, time-consuming tasks, always in support of the physicians, whose number will remain stable, hence improving the cost/effectiveness ratio of the radiological profession. They add that "AI will still make mistakes, which can be easily corrected by a human, by a radiologist. But will not be possible for AI to correct itself" [15], which as we have seen represents more wishful thinking than hard truth. Furthermore, considering the balance "who corrects who," past experience with computer-assisted diagnosis is not uniformly encouraging as, in some instances, radiologists tend to ignore or overturn the computer prompts, even when they are correct [16]. Needless to say, implementation of A.I. in the clinics has massive implications in terms of legal responsibilities, but this topic would deserve a full chapter.

15.3   How to Proceed? Let's Be Practical!

Radiology is ahead of nuclear medicine, and seems caught in a circular argument: A.I. is there to stay, it's going to be faster, more powerful, and more reliable for organizing the departments and providing the clinicians with the most relevant information, yet radiologists need to remain totally in charge and in full control.

The key issues are probably the validation of the A.I. algorithm and its endpoint. A typical approach is to compare the A.I. with the human truth. A good example is provided by Sibille et al.

who identified, located, and segmented over 12,000 regions in 629 FDG PET/CT studies performed in lymphoma and NSCLC patients [5]. A DL algorithm using both the PET and the CT data performed very well for these tasks, with 87.1% sensitivity and 99% specificity in classifying the lung cancer patients, and 88.6% localization accuracy in the same population. Similar results were obtained in the lymphoma patients. In this case, the network is trained to do as well as the physician. It does not reach this level of performance, but close enough, and is thus proposed as an adjunct to the physician's interpretation. In this case, we do not know the ground truth, we do not know who is right in the discrepant cases (human "gold standard" or DL?), but it does not matter, as the product is designed to help the physician accomplishing his task, including the potential flaws. This is a very marketable product, because it does not change the paradigm, the physician remains in charge, and the product being a tool that automates and accelerates a process. It has been trained to replicate the human's process, and it is designed to be checked by humans.

Following this approach does not fully take advantage of the capacities of A.I. Zhao et al. recently went further with their report on DL for diagnosing metastatic involvement on bone scintigraphy [17]. They studied over 12.000 cases, and the endpoint was clear-cut, i.e. the presence or absence of bone metastases in the scintigraphy. They showed an overall accuracy of 93.4%, with 92.6% sensitivity and 93.9% specificity and an AUC of 0.964, consistent across cancer types. This compared favorably with the performances of experimented NM physicians, as in 13/200 cases read in parallel, A.I. was correct and all three physicians were wrong, compared to only 6 cases where it was the reverse. And this was obtained at lightning speed, as only 11 seconds were needed for interpreting 400 cases, which is…fast! As a comparison, it took an average of 136 minutes for the NM physicians to read those 400 studies, e.g. almost 3 studies per minute, which for a human being, is also quite fast. This paper is a good case study. Published in a prestigious journal, the conclusion is unequivocal: A.I.

is faster, better, and cheaper than the physicians. Case closed. In this model, there is no need for a physician in control, no A.I. at the service of the physician, and no A.I. as a complement or support to the physician. A.I. wins, period. Yet in order to go further and implement such algorithm in the clinic, one must first answer a few questions. The study deals with planar scintigraphy, although SPECT is recommended and routinely performed. That is relevant because the benefit of A.I. was primarily in terms of sensitivity. Also, adding the CT further improves the diagnostic accuracy. The ground truth is also debatable, as explained in the methods. And finally, the algorithm is the perfect example of a black box. Hence, this tremendous amount of work (over 12.000 studies!) published in a high-level journal, provides very little chance of effective clinical translation, if NM physicians are asked to give their opinion. The imaging technique is not up to date, the gold standard is weak, the method is questionable, and the algorithm is opaque. Similarly to some extent, major critiques were addressed after the publication of a paper reporting on a DL algorithm outperforming radiologists for interpreting mammographies, even though this study was methodologically very solid [18, 19]. One may wonder whether A.I., to be accepted, must be clamped and its power limited.

In order to get out of this labyrinth and come to the situation where not only nuclear medicine physicians coexist with A.I. but patients also truly benefit from this development, a multistep approach is required. First, physicians must identify unmet clinical needs, taking into account the bigger picture. This means identifying the weak points of our techniques, in terms of accuracy or reproducibility, in diseases and clinical situations where it makes a difference for patients. [^{18}F] FDG-PET/CT is quite effective in identifying residual disease at the end of treatment for diffuse large B-cell lymphoma. The advantage of developing A.I. for this task would be marginal at best, and difficult to establish. The impact would be quite different were it to predicting or assessing early response to immunotherapies, which can be very effective but in a limited number of patients and with significant costs, both monetary and in terms of morbidity. Theranostics is a major field for the development of A.I. in nuclear medicine, to help the physicians in identifying those who would benefit from the treatment based upon the diagnostic companion study, tailor the treatment through fast personalized dosimetry, and finally reliably and rapidly assess treatment success, or failure. Second, we need to acquire the minimal knowledge necessary to get on speaking terms with those who will actually develop and build A.I. This goes through changing how the research teams are organized, developing strong collaborations outside the faculty of medicine, and probably partnering with the industry. This also implies revamping the education and training of residents to account for this evolution. We have to get better in statistics and computational sciences. Third, we need to build multicenter networks. It is very unlikely that single-center protocols will manage to gather the amount and diversity of data necessary to develop A.I. algorithms directly applicable to the routine clinical practice. We need to account for the diversity in the hardware performances, acquisition and reconstruction algorithms, and population types. And finally, we need to set the highest standards for validation, not only regarding the methodology surrounding the development and testing of the A.I. model but also the clinical relevance of the question being solved and the clinical appropriateness of the population sample being investigated.

If we can fulfill these criteria, i.e. if we identify the need, comprehend the methods, and put ourselves in a situation such as to produce reliable and reproducible results, then and only then will we be fully prepared for the next phase, i.e. enthusiastically promoting and advocating the A.I.-augmented nuclear medicine to the clinical world.

Acknowledgements The author wishes to thank Nadia Withofs, MD, PhD for fruitful discussions.

References

1. Schwyzer M, Ferraro DA, Muehlematter UJ, Curioni-Fontecedro A, Huellner MW, von Schulthess GK, et al. Automated detection of lung cancer at ultralow dose PET/CT by deep neural networks—initial results. Lung Cancer. 2018;126:170–3. https://doi.org/10.1016/j.lungcan.2018.11.001.

2. Shiri I, Ghafarian P, Geramifar P, Leung KH, Ghelichoghli M, Oveisi M, et al. Direct attenuation correction of brain PET images using only emission data via a deep convolutional encoder-decoder (Deep-DAC). Eur Radiol. 2019;29:6867–79. https://doi.org/10.1007/s00330-019-06229-1.

3. Burggraaff CN, Rahman F, Kassner I, Pieplenbosch S, Barrington SF, Jauw YWS, et al. Optimizing workflows for fast and reliable metabolic tumor volume measurements in diffuse large B cell lymphoma. Mol Imaging Biol. 2020;22:1102–10. https://doi.org/10.1007/s11307-020-01474-z.

4. Barrington SF, Zwezerijnen BG, de Vet HC, Heymans MW, Mikhaeel NG, Burggraaff CN, et al. Automated segmentation of baseline metabolic total tumor burden in diffuse large B-cell lymphoma: which method is most successful? J Nucl Med. 2021;62(3):332–7. https://doi.org/10.2967/jnumed.119.238923.

5. Sibille L, Seifert R, Avramovic N, Vehren T, Spottiswoode B, Zuehlsdorff S, et al. (18)F-FDG PET/CT uptake classification in lymphoma and lung cancer by using deep convolutional neural networks. Radiology. 2020;294:445–52. https://doi.org/10.1148/radiol.2019191114.

6. Curtis C, Liu C, Bollerman TJ, Pianykh OS. Machine learning for predicting patient wait times and appointment delays. J Am Coll Radiol. 2018;15:1310–6. https://doi.org/10.1016/j.jacr.2017.08.021.

7. Sollini M, Antunovic L, Chiti A, Kirienko M. Towards clinical application of image mining: a systematic review on artificial intelligence and radiomics. Eur J Nucl Med Mol Imaging. 2019;46:2656–72. https://doi.org/10.1007/s00259-019-04372-x.

8. Holzinger A, Langs G, Denk H, Zatloukal K, Muller H. Causability and explainability of artificial intelligence in medicine. Wiley Interdiscip Rev Data Min Knowl Discov. 2019;9:e1312. https://doi.org/10.1002/widm.1312.

9. Antun V, Renna F, Poon C, Adcock B, Hansen AC. On instabilities of deep learning in image reconstruction and the potential costs of AI. Proc Natl Acad Sci U S A. 2020;117(48):30088–95. https://doi.org/10.1073/pnas.1907377117.

10. Zhou Z, Firestone C. Humans can decipher adversarial images. Nat Commun. 2019;10:1334. https://doi.org/10.1038/s41467-019-08931-6.

11. Barucci A, Neri E. Adversarial radiomics: the rising of potential risks in medical imaging from adversarial learning. Eur J Nucl Med Mol Imaging. 2020;13:2941–43. https://doi.org/10.1007/s00259-020-04879-8.

12. Cook J, Ramadas V. When to consult precision-recall curves. The Stata Journal. 2020;20:131–48. https://doi.org/10.1177/1536867x20909693.

13. Flach P. Performance evaluation in machine learning: the good, the bad, the ugly, and the way forward. In: The thirty-third AAAI conference on artificial intelligence (AAAI-19). 2019.

14. Pianykh OS, Langs G, Dewey M, Enzmann DR, Herold CJ, Schoenberg SO, et al. Continuous learning AI in radiology: implementation principles and early applications. Radiology. 2020;297:6–14. https://doi.org/10.1148/radiol.2020200038.

15. Turner J, Ward P. Dutch debate intensifies over future shape of AI. 2020. https://www.auntminnieeurope-com/indexaspx?sec=sup&sub=aic&pag=dis&ItemID=619384.

16. Nishikawa RM, Schmidt RA, Linver MN, Edwards AV, Papaioannou J, Stull MA. Clinically missed cancer: how effectively can radiologists use computer-aided detection? AJR Am J Roentgenol. 2012;198:708–16. https://doi.org/10.2214/AJR.11.6423.

17. Zhao Z, Pi Y, Jiang L, Xiang Y, Wei J, Yang P, et al. Deep neural network based artificial intelligence assisted diagnosis of bone scintigraphy for cancer bone metastasis. Sci Rep. 2020;10:17046. https://doi.org/10.1038/s41598-020-74135-4.

18. McKinney SM, Sieniek M, Godbole V, Godwin J, Antropova N, Ashrafian H, et al. International evaluation of an AI system for breast cancer screening. Nature. 2020;577:89–94. https://doi.org/10.1038/s41586-019-1799-6.

19. Haibe-Kains B, Adam GA, Hosny A, Khodakarami F, Shraddha T, Kusko R, et al. Transparency and reproducibility in artificial intelligence. Nature. 2020;586:E14–6. https://doi.org/10.1038/s41586-020-2766-y.

Correction to: Radiomics in Nuclear Medicine, Robustness, Reproducibility, and Standardization

Reza Reiazi

Correction to:
Chapter 3 in: P. Veit-Haibach, K. Herrmann (eds.), *Artificial Intelligence/*
Machine Learning in Nuclear Medicine and Hybrid Imaging,
https://doi.org/10.1007/978-3-031-00119-2_3

The corresponding author of Chapter 3: Radiomics in Nuclear Medicine, Robustness, Reproducibility, and Standardization, "Reza Rezai", was incorrectly spelled, which has been corrected to "Reza Reiazi".

The updated version of the book can be found at https://doi.org/10.1007/978-3-031-00119-2_3

akin to sonic logs recorded in the wells. This is also known as 'pseudo interval velocity transform' *(PIVT)*. However, an improved version known as 'Seislog' with relatively better resolution was developed by Lindseth (Lindseth 1979), which was used for 2Dsesismic data with more reliable results. Seislog provides better information about lateral change in lithology and porosity, helpful for stratigraphic correlation and interpretation of layer properties (Fig. 8). It is a simple and convenient method suited for 2D seismic data. Each trace may be a considered a 'pseudo sonic log' which makes correlations easy as would be in a profile of actual sonic logs recorded. However, with recent development of sophisticated impedance inversion techniques, it is seldom used, its utility being limited to 2D seismic data.

Acoustic Impedance Inversion (AI)

Acoustic impedance inversion operates on post-stack normal seismic data and yields P-impedances. Essentially the process depends on statistical extraction of wavelet from seismic data with or without logs. If well data is available, *a priori* model for acoustic impedance inversion is usually built from logs. The reflection coefficient series derived from sonic and density logs are used to extract statistically the wavelet from seismic data. The derived wavelet is used to compute the response of the model reflectivity series at the well for comparison with the seismic data as a check. The starting model may be iteratively updated in a way till a reasonable match with seismic is met and the estimated wavelet is considered appropriate. Inversion of seismic volume data is then carried out with the wavelet to create an impedance sequence somewhat similar to deconvolution. The inversion process involves broadening of the limited seismic bandwidth by adding low frequencies and high frequencies to deliver impedance sections of superior resolution. Low frequencies are obtained from the low-frequency trend, which forms the basis of impedance or velocity structure, derived from sonic logs by filtering out high frequencies (Fig. 9). The trend added to the inverted impedance traces provides scope for making quantitative interpretation. In the absence of well data, the low-frequency trend can be

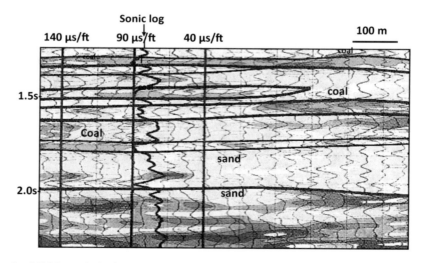

Fig. 8 Example of Seislog velocity inversion carried on seismic traces in which the amplitudes *(Rc)* are converted to interval velocities *(CVL)*. Each trace is like a sonic log which makes interpretation and correlation of lithologic layers easier and more accurate. Note the excellent match of inverted velocity with sonic (solid black trace) at the well. High impedances represent sands and the low impedance as coals, colored green (After Mummery 1988)

derived from seismic NMO stack velocity, and used as *a priori* information during the inversion process. Inversion of data lacking in high frequency components in seismic may end up in outputs wanting in resolution for defining thin layers. High-frequency enhancement to achieve larger bandwidth is done by tweaking the high-frequency signals in data above the noise level. This is performed by advanced processing techniques of deconvolution.

Acoustic impedance sections make it simpler to identify lithological and stratigraphic details which help estimate reliably the reservoir properties such as porosity, fluid content, pay thickness and areal extent. An example of a stack seismic and the acoustic impedance section, derived by inversion is shown (Fig. 10). The impedance log derived from well logs is overlaid

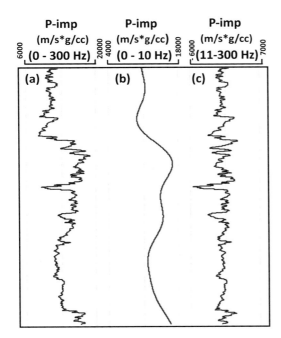

Fig. 9 An example showing the filtering of a broadband impedance curve derived from well sonic and density data. (**a**) Initial broad band (0-300Hz), (**b**) filtered with low pass(0–10 Hz) and (**c**) filtered with high pass (11-300Hz)frequencies. The low pass curve (0–10Hz) yields the crucial low velocity trend used in impedance inversion to obtain absolute impedance values. The high pass curve (**c**) shows finer velocity variations but is straight without any trend. (Image courtesy of Arcis Seismic Solutions, TGS, Calgary)

on the impedance section for quality check (Fig. 10b). The improved resolution of the inverted impedance section showing excellent correlation with the log measured impedance curve lends confidence in generation and interpretation of impedance data. Consequently, inverted impedance volume has the advantage as it can be used straight away to interpret three-dimensional geobodies from a 3D seismic volume.

Elastic Impedance Inversion (EI)

Elastic impedance is more involved and is an angle-dependent inversion performed on prestack gathers. The technique exploits geological information from near angle traces as well as far angle traces, manifested by the P-amplitude variability with incident angle across a prestack gather. The CMP gather at the well position is picked up and different angle ranges are selected to generate angle stacks. Given the V_P, V_S and density log curves, the elastic impedance, which is the angle dependent P-impedance, is calculated and for each input partial angle stack of the gather, a unique wavelet is estimated for preparing the synthetic trace. The inverted elastic impedances derived from the angle stack traces are compared for quality check. However, there can be some practical problems in the approach. Amplitudes of the near-offset traces are related to the changes in acoustic impedance, and can be calibrated with well log curves or synthetic seismograms. By contrast, if a far-offset or a far-angle stack has to be calibrated with the log data or synthetic seismograms, there are no corresponding set of log curves that could be used for the purpose.

Elastic inversion outputs are angle dependent near-angle and far-angle P-impedances (referred as elastic impedance) from prestack gathers, in contrast to normal incidence P-impedance (acoustic inversion) extracted from post stack data. The advantage over acoustic inversion is that it adds more information to rock-fluid properties. While the near-trace normal P-impedance provides structural/stratigraphic

areas. Modelling has become an integral part of interpretation work-flow to aid and validate interpretation, as in cases of direct hydrocarbon indicators (DHI) where AVO modelling is widely practiced (Chapter "Shear Wave Seismic, AVO and Vp/Vs Analysis"). The input geologic models can be structural or stratigraphic, for which seismic responses can be computed in 1D, 2D or 3D mode depending on the objective. Once the input model parameters are given, the seismic response is computed and then compared with recorded seismic for an acceptable match. Generally it may involve repetitive computations and comparisons. Each time a discrepancy between computed response and real seismic is observed, the model parameters are suitably modified, response recomputed and compared until a desired match with actual is achieved to infer the geology. However, it may be underscored that modelling results are not unique as several variability in the input parameters to the model can have the similar causal response.

Seismic Forward Modelling

1D Modelling, Synthetic Seismogram

One dimensional (1D) seismic model is by far the simplest to create response of the earth in the form of a trace and is known as synthetic seismogram which is elaborated in detail in Chapter "Seismic Interpretation Methods". It is the most elementary and common example of forward modelling to represent seismic response of the earth. The synthetic seismogram is essentially a trace output by convolving a seismic wavelet simulating the acquisition source with the reflectivity series, an array of points aligned vertically in depth as earth's subsurface reflectors. The reflectivity series is generated from log curves which measure the density and velocity of rocks at the well. The synthetic seismogram is then matched with field seismic trace for well tie (Fig. 2). The purpose and process of generating synthetic seismogram, the challenges involved in

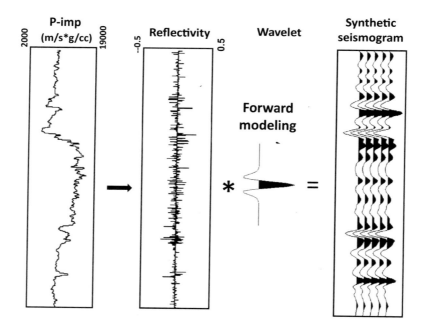

Fig. 2 Figure illustrating forward modeling work flow. It computes the one dimensional seismic response (synthetic seismogram) of a given geologic model, a reflectivity series by convolving it with a chosen seismic wavelet usually a zero-phase Ricker wavelet. The reflectivity series is derived from the impedance curve calculated from the sonic and density measurements in the well logs. The star denotes the mathematical process of convolution. (Image courtesy of Arcis Seismic Solutions, TGS, Calgary)

seismic match at the well and the possible reasons for mismatch are also described in Chapter "Seismic Interpretation Methods". Proper matching of synthetic seismogram with real seismic not only provides insight to typical seismic response of subsurface rocks at the well, but also indicates the quality of resolution in the acquired data. In cases where the synthetic—seismic match is poor, it is important that the causes for the mismatch analysed, instead of ignoring the exercise by putting it away. Analysis can help get insight to the mistie problem to sort out certain other related aspects like ensuring the ground location of the well, well velocity and sonic measurements and the seismic data processing efficacy.

Choice of Wavelet

In seismic modelling, choosing a wavelet and its polarity is extremely important as it decides the seismic response. A Ricker, zero-phase wavelet of a chosen dominant frequency with SEG normal polarity (+ve Rc, peak) is commonly used for computing the model response. When the polarity of the seismic reflections are unclear, as is in many cases, wavelets in both SEG normal and reverse polarity are used to compute synthetic and decide on the appropriate wavelet that best fits the seismic. A zero phase symmetrical Ricker wavelet with even side lobes shows maximum amplitude at zero time, that is, the arrival time of the wave(reflection) is without delay with respect to actual interface depth (Fig. 3a). Ricker wavelet is simple to realize, useful for resolving power and convenient for picking reflection events (peak/trough) and for these reasons are most widely used. However, seismic acquisition systems commonly use dynamite on land and air-gun sources for offshore, which generate minimum phase wavelets, a front-loaded wavelet with asymmetrical concentration of energy and side lobes (Fig. 3b)., where the reflection arrival time is delayed. As can be seen the wavelet has longer duration than its zero-phase equivalent and offers relatively less resolving power. For minimum phase recorded data and not processed for zero-phase it

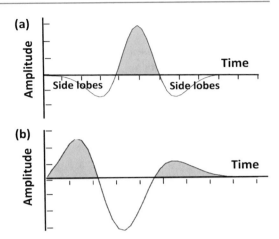

Fig. 3 Schematic showing wavelet characteristics. (a) Zero phase Ricker wavelet, symmetrical with even side lobes and maximum amplitude at the centre. It is used commonly for computing synthetic seismograms as amplitude maxima denotes the reflection arrival time without delay. (b) Minimum phase wavelet is asymmetrical with uneven side lobes and energy concentrated n the early part (front loaded). This produces maximum amplitude of reflection delayed in time with reference to the reflector depth.

may require a minimum phase wavelet for computing synthetic seismogram. Often both the types of wavelet with normal and reverse polarity are used for computing synthetic to find the best fit with seismic.

Seismic interpreters prefer to work with data offering better resolution, and the seismic minimum-phase data is processed close to zero-phase data. Vibroseis source, however, has no such problems as it produces the embedded zero-phase wavelet, the 'Klauder' wavelet (Chapter "Seismic Reflection Principles: Basics"). Some prefer to use the source wavelet that is measured during generation, often a practice in marine offshore surveys. Nonetheless, a more common option these days is to extract the wavelet from the stacked data being interpreted. This is done either by using a statistical method for estimation of the wavelet, or from comparing the seismic trace at the location of the well with the impedance reflectivity derived from the well log data to find the best-fit wavelet.

2D/3D Modelling, Structural and Stratigraphic

Structural Modelling

Tectonically complex areas are known to impact seismic wave propagation in a relatively intricate way and generates poor images which can be confusing and challenging to interpret. The subsurface with various kinds of deformed and dipping layers cause several problems including (a) focusing and defocusing effects; (b) absorption and transmission losses; (c) inter-bed multiples; (d) severe lateral and vertical near-surface velocity variations, (e) generation of mode converted waves, (f) scattering and (g) noises. Many of these impediments in 3D acquisition are, however, mitigated during data processing such as by efficient prestack migration. In highly tectonized zones such as in fold and thrust belts, the steep structural dips and complicated geometry of deformed fold, thrusts, overthrusts with associated fault splays, commonly show frequent lateral and vertical velocity variations. This adds to complications in wave transmission and reflection, resulting in creating obscure images despite prestack depth migration (PSDM), that do not depict the subsurface correctly. Another area where wave propagation can be intricately affected is in zones of high-pressured shale and salt diapirs with associated near-vertical structures and characterized by significant velocity

contrast with surrounding sediments. Reflection P- seismic also produces poor and unreliable images below gas chimneys and especially below salt overhangs, failing in accurate delineation of salt geometry and associated flank traps for exploration. Other geologic examples of poor or no seismic imaging include those of formations underlying thick section of high-velocity basalts and salt intrusive rocks and fault zones below the foot wall of reverse faults, often referred as 'fault shadow' area.

How does one interpret this kind of data unless has some kind of basis to start with? In such cases the use of 2D/3D forward modelling tool offers clues to understand the complex deformations and help map subsurface stratal geometry from seismic. Modelled response may be used to test diverse options of structural geometry to find out which configuration gives the best match to the recorded seismic data to help reduce uncertainties in interpretation. It also gives an assessment of what best can be achievable in seismic and accordingly reprocess the data to look for the solution. Such an example of computed response of a depth model of a salt dome with beds abutting against flanks which are often interesting for hydrocarbon exploration is shown in Fig. 4. The synthetic behaves as a guide to interpret actual seismic as the synthetic response shows the salt dome geometry, reflection arrival times and amplitudes and more

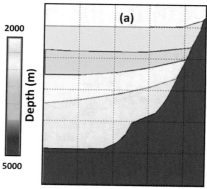
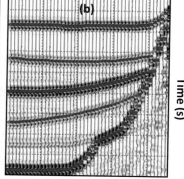

Fig. 4 An example illustrating utility of a 2D forward modeling. (**a**) Geologic model of a salt dome in depth showing beds abutting against its flank and (**b**) synthetic seismic response computed for the model. Synthetic models help realize seismic image in terms of arrival time, amplitudes and the geometry of beds with salt dome flank which guides interpretation of field seismic. (Images courtesy of Arcis Seismic Solutions, TGS, Calgary)

importantly the beds abutting against the salt flank which may be potential strati-structural traps. Structural modelling in fold and over-thrusts belts is most useful and often indispensable to guide interpretation of structural folds and over thrust planes in the subsurface.

Stratigraphic Modelling

Stratigraphic modelling may be more elaborate due to the involvement of larger number of variables as model input. In addition to geometry of the geologic structure, variations in rock-fluid properties, i.e. density, porosity, fluids and contacts, bed thickness and most importantly lateral changes in velocities, are also to be taken into consideration. A relatively simpler strati-structural trap, gas sand reservoir with water contact on one flank and facies changed to silt at the crestal part of the anticline is modelled to interpret the observed high amplitude seen on the flank of the structure (Fig. 5). This was necessary to confirm interpretation because of misgivings about the unusual disposition high amplitude anomaly limited to the flank instead of the crest of the structure. The modelled amplitude

response confirmed the interpreted geologic model as gas sand and clearly demonstrates the gas and water saturated sands limits thus delineating the reservoir areal extent with the fluid contact. It, however, did not pick the fault perhaps due to its small throw. Another interesting modelling application is exemplified where it is used for validation of a high amplitude anomaly suspected to be gas sand. Responses of three likely geologic models with different lithology and fluid content were computed and compared with observed seismic (Fig. 6). The one with best fit offers the obvious answer and that showed the anomaly was caused by calcareous shale (Fig. 6c). Many times the interpreter may be handicapped by data without access to prestack gathers and modelling in such cases may come in handy for authentication of DHI anomalies. Subtle variations in amplitude and waveform observed in seismic often may necessitate modelling to guide or corroborate interpretation in making reliable prediction of reservoir parameters.

2D/3D forward modelling requires the input of a geologic section in depth with density and

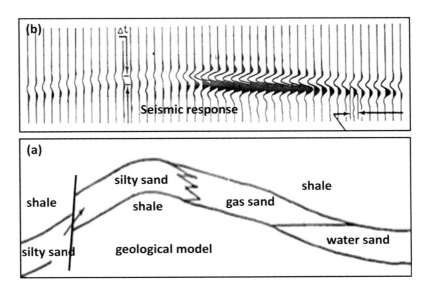

Fig. 5 Showing example of stratigraphic modeling of a strati-structural trap used for validating interpretation of a high amplitude seismic anomaly. (**a**) geologic model of gas sand with water contact on one flank of an anticline and changing to silt facies at the crestal part (**b**) The computed seismic response. The modelling confirmed the interpretation of gas sand. Note the decrease in amplitude with approach of the water contact. Stratigraphic modelling needs increased number of variable inputs. (After Schramm et al. 1977)

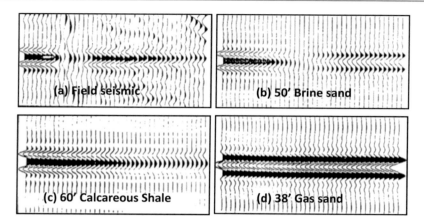

Fig. 6 Another example illustrating utility of seismic model for interpreting a high amplitude seismic anomaly at (**a**). Three lithologic layers with varying thickness and fluid content at (**b**), (**c**) and (**d**) are modeled to match field seismic (**a**), suspected as a gas sand. The response at (**c**) matches the best and helps to interpret correctly the high amplitude anomaly, caused by the calcareous shale (After Neidell 1986)

velocity assigned to each of the individual layers and a wavelet to generate the seismic response. The input also includes an assigned overburden velocity function to transform the depth to time in the modelled version to indicate arrival times of different events. The 2D synthetic is commonly generated by simple convolution process using ray-tracing procedures, a fast and usually an adequate representation of the earth model. The 3D modelling, on the other hand, involves a more detailed wave equation approach to get improved responses needed in structurally complex areas. 3D modelling also has applications in fundamental research projects for creating, checking and/or calibrating processing algorithms. Wave equation solution takes into consideration the propagation effects such as refraction, diffraction and attenuation and requires migration and other necessary processing steps to provide accurate model response. Typically, the wave equation modelling is seldom a part of common interpretation work flow.

Ideally, forward modelling may be used before undertaking expensive and intricate acquisitions (Chopra and Marfurt 2012) such as multi-component 3C/3D, time lapse 3D and wide angle surveys aimed at solving specific engineering and geologic problems. This may include surveys planned to get more information on fractured reservoirs, reservoir monitoring and fluid-flow surveillance and for mapping of sub-salt and sub-basalt Mesozoics particularly at large depths. Responses are simulated for a wide range of layouts of source and receiver line geometry and other crucial recording parameters such as spread length, bin size, fold and range of azimuth etc., for designing a survey for performance evaluation of different sets of configurations. This not only decides the feasibility of such a survey but helps decide the most favourable cost-effective option to choose for conducting the survey. Sophisticated data acquisition techniques may fail at times in providing desirable geological information if the survey is not object-specific or lack suitable parameterization of survey elements or in the extreme unachievable.

Limitations of Forward Modelling

One of the critical issues for achieving a good 'model-actual' match is the selection of the wavelet for computing model response. Response calculated commonly with a Ricker wavelet, for subtle as well as complicated stratigraphic models may not have satisfactory match with actual seismic, necessitating more

appropriate wavelet for computation. This would require, ideally, the knowledge of exact seismic wavelet at the depth where the feature is to be imaged. The source wavelet, though known at the surface, changes shape due to propagation effects and is hard to determine it precisely at the particular depth. For this reason, the wavelet is often estimated statistically from the seismic constrained by log data and used for computing model response. But again, the estimated wavelet can greatly differ from the real wavelet away from the well due to variations in attenuation, facies change, multiples, or acquisition parameters on the ground. Another problem, faced in stratigraphic modelling for hydrocarbon reservoir characterization is the appropriate choice of geologic parameters from the large number of viable variables and their numerical values as input to the model. Often the lack of adequate knowledge about the laterally varying velocity field can be a great impediment. It may be also mentioned that solutions offered by modelling including 3D, as stated earlier, are not unique as

the computed seismic response can match more than one geologic version of the model.

Inverse Modelling Types

Referring to Fig. 2, in the forward modelling process the model input of log curves are displayed on the left and the computed seismic output response on the right. Turning around the display with seismic as input on the left and the impedance curve as output on the right, would represent the reverse process of forward modelling, called the inverse modelling (Fig. 7). As mentioned earlier, inverse modelling is a process where the subsurface geologic model is synthesized from the seismic data. Seismic interpretation in the context can be considered a good example of inverse process.

Inversion of seismic data to obtain the geologic information is a great innovation in seismic technology, immensely useful in hydrocarbon exploration and production. Seismic inversions

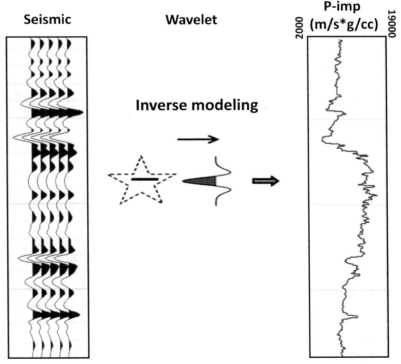

Fig. 7 A schematic illustrating the general workflow of inverse modeling, which is the reverse process of generating a synthetic seismogram. Forward modeling generates seismic from a geologic model where as inverse modeling generates a geologic model from the seismic data. The star with a dash inside denotes the mathematical process of deconvolution (Image courtesy: Arcis Seismic Solutions, TGS, Calgary)

enhance resolution and deliver details of layer properties that are not feasible to get from normal stacks or amplitude slices. Inversions can be of several kinds such as: (1) operator based; (2) recursive; (3) model based; or (4) geostatistical (stochastic).

Operator-Based Inversion

The seismic wave changes amplitude and frequency during propagation in the subsurface by physical processes such as absorption, scattering and refraction etc. To obtain the true amplitude and frequency response that can be causally related to interfacial and layer properties, it will need appropriate corrections for the losses caused by wave propagation. Reversing these effects is achieved to certain extent mathematically during data processing. Compensating for attenuation losses, deconvolution and migration are a few examples of such processes in which operator-based inversions work mathematically in the reverse way, to compensate for the propagation effects. Operator-based inversion is essential and is indispensable in data processing workflow to provide reliable data for interpretation. Nonetheless, the operator based compensation cannot fully compensate and negate the effects to restore the real responses, as that would entail the actual retrograde process of propagation occurred in the earth to be physically reversed, by all means an impossibility.

Recursive Inversion

Recursive inversion is of an earliest and elementary type. It essentially assumes that seismic amplitudes are proportional to reflection coefficients (reflectivity) and transforms the amplitudes in the input seismic traces to acoustic impedance traces. If reflectivity is known at one level by tagging to impedance values measured in a well by the logs, it can be computed at the next level and is a recursive process of inversion. This, however, does not fully satisfy the basic assumption, proportionality of amplitude to

reflection coefficient as the wavelet effect is not removed. Consequently, the wavelet side lobes (wavelet length) which are present, impede resolution. Also, the results are produced within the initial existing seismic bandwidth and the method does not offer a significant advantage relative to interpreting conventional seismic data. On the other hand, a broadband reflectivity series, representing the subsurface reflection interfaces, can be obtained by removing the embedded wavelet from the seismic traces, a process somewhat similar to deconvolution. However, the removal of the wavelet from the trace to arrive at a suitable reflection coefficient series is not unique, and there can be more than one geologic solution. To overcome this mathematical limitation, some inversion methods adopt ways to get constrained with *a priori* model for the possible solution within the seismic bandwidth leading to model based inversion techniques

Model-based Inversion

An important aspect of seismic interpretation is to carry out detailed investigation of seismic properties to extract information pertaining to reservoir lithology and rock properties including hydrocarbon fluids. One way to approach this goal is to convert the observed seismic through an inversion process into impedance and velocity which are principal physical properties of a rock. Model based inversions are deterministic in nature and are achieved by performing inversion on a seismic trace constrained with *a priori* model (well data), attempting essentially to improve resolution. With advances and innovations made in inversion techniques, the elastic moduli, the bulk modulus (k), shear modulus or rigidity (Mu), Poisson's ratio (σ), Young's modulus (E) and density of rocks can be estimated to provide more and better information on rock-fluid properties for reservoir evaluation. Because of its efficiency and quality, most companies now use model based seismic inversion to increase the resolution and reliability of the data to improve estimates of porosity, pay thickness and fluid saturation.

Geostatistical (Stochastic) Inversion

Geostatistical inversion is performed on post or pre stack seismic data and is a probabilistic approach to estimating reservoir properties away from the well on prospect scale. The technique uses integration of multidisciplinary data from many sources and allows obtaining multiple earth-model realizations, each of which honours the seismic as well as well data. Interestingly, this also helps bring out the degree of uncertainty in the results that can be quantified. The earth-model estimation is constrained with the seismic, regional geostatistical data as well as the measured high resolution acoustic impedance data from the well logs to match the known geological patterns in the area. Essentially many different input models are generated using distributions of earth property models from well data to compute synthetics for comparing it to the input seismic data. The error between the synthetic and the seismic being inverted is minimized in an iterative way leading to the final output inversion model. Oddly, the large number of realizations generated are sometimes averaged to represent a single best fit property model (Cooke and Cant 2010), as it is considered close to the deterministic inversion (model-based inversion).

Seismic Inversion, Types of Attributes

Reflectivities are caused due to contrast in impedances across the interfaces in the subsurface. The resultant amplitudes observed, however, are controlled by variations in properties of rocks either above or below or both, across the interface. The amplitude attribute information is thus limited to information of the interface and on relative variation in rock properties across it. By contrast, the impedance, the product of density and velocity, is a distinctive property of a layer, entities that are measured directly in a well by sonic and density logs and can be calibrated with seismic. Thus, while impedance is a layer property, the seismic amplitude is representative of the layer property. If quantitative interpretation of seismic data for thin reservoirs is to be attempted, it is to be based on analysis of layer property, the impedance attribute instead of the interfacial reflection amplitude attribute. Seismic inversion achieves this by transforming seismic reflectivity to inverted reflectivity or the impedance.

Seismic inversion can be done with post stack or prestack data and most techniques employ *a priori* model which is typically built from well log data. Constrained with a model, not only helps increase resolution but also reliability in the inverted results that improves confidence in estimation of reservoir properties. Seismic inversion techniques that enable to quantitatively estimate the important rock properties are listed.

- Interval Velocity *(Vp)* inversion
- Acoustic impedance *(AI)* inversion, thin bed reflectivity
- Elastic Impedance *(EI)* inversion
- Simultaneous inversion*(SI)*-
- Density inversion
- AVO inversion

Interval Velocity Inversion (Vp)

One of the simplest forms of inversion is the decades-old velocity inversion, an example of recursive inversion. Reflectivity at an interface can be expressed simply as

$$Rc = (V_2 - V_1)/(V_2 + V_1),$$

ignoring the densities. It assumes the post stack seismic trace amplitude as a log of measure of normal-incident reflection coefficients, Rc with time. If velocity V_1 of the first layer is known, from the above simple equation, velocity of the second layer V_2 can be estimated. Similarly, velocity of the following layers can be estimated successively to produce a plot of interval velocity with time. Velocity inversion technique essentially transforms the seismic reflectivity trace to a continuous velocity log *(CVL)* in depth domain (Chapter "Seismic Reflection Principles: Basics"),

Printed in the United States
by Baker & Taylor Publisher Services

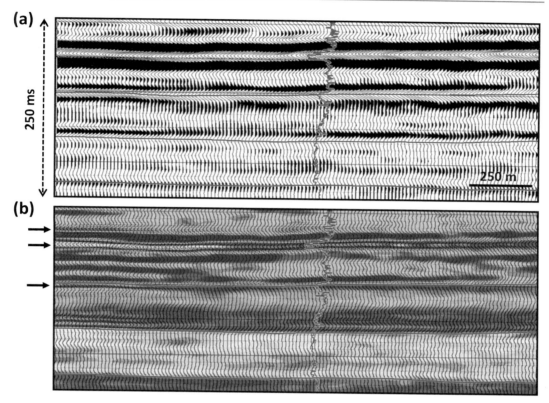

(a)

250 ms

250 m

(b)

Fig. 10 Example of acoustic impedance inversion from seismic. (**a**) seismic stack section and (**b**) the derived inverted impedance section. The log measured impedance curve is overlain on both the sections for comparison to demonstrate the improved resolution and better match of details contained in amplitude and arrival time, the angle-dependent P-impedance in elastic inversion provides details on lithology and fluid information contained in the far traces. Analysed together, much more useful information can be retrieved than the acoustic inversion alone can achieve. the inverted section with the measured log impedance. Thin layers are clearly seen and correlated accurately with lateral impedance changes indicating variance in the layer properties that can be predicted with confidence. (Images courtesy of Arcis Seismic Solutions, TGS, Calgary)

details contained in amplitude and arrival time, the angle-dependent P-impedance in elastic inversion provides details on lithology and fluid information contained in the far traces. Analysed together, much more useful information can be retrieved than the acoustic inversion alone can achieve.

Simultaneous Inversion (SI)

Elastic inversion delivers angle-dependent P-impedances that can characterize lithology, porosity and fluid content of reservoirs. However, inclusion of S-impedance in analysis can help estimate the properties more accurately with better reliability. *Simultaneous inversion (SI)*, a technique that employs angle or offset-limited sub-stacks similar to elastic inversion but more rigorous in using full Zoeppritz's equations to deliver P-impedance, S-impedance, Poisson's ratio ($\sim Vp/Vs$) and density. One of the major advantage of simultaneous inversion *(SI)* over elastic impedance *(EI)* is that many geologic layers exhibiting similar *P*-impedances can be segregated by S-impedance delivered by *SI*. Conjoined studies of *P*- and *S*- impedances, *Vp/Vs* ratio and density essentially minimise prediction risks of reservoir parameters for characterization (see Chapter "Shear Wave Seismic, AVO and Vp/Vs AnalysisShear Wave Seismic, AVO and Vp/Vs Analysis"). Simultaneous inversion deliverables lend more credibility to estimation of reservoir rock-fluid properties and are commonly used as inputs to reservoir modelling. Particularly, the *Vp/Vs* (Poisson's ratio) information helps provide solutions to several important reservoir parameters such as, fluid content, quality of reservoir, clay content etc., for which the simultaneous inversion is considered an essential tool for reservoir characterization. Besides being useful in distinguishing hydrocarbon bearing sands from brine saturated sands and shale, which cannot be discriminated based on only P- attribute, it has also other useful applications in reservoir and drilling engineering fields mentioned later under AVO inversion. Shear impedance section, derived from simultaneous inversion, by itself can also be useful in detecting subtle seismic onlaps, toplaps and stratal interfaces, not perceptible in inverted P-impedance section because of feeble contrasts.

Density Inversion

Of the three vital parameters, P-, S- impedance and density, the density is the most difficult one to quantify from seismic. Bulk density can be related to important reservoir parameters such as porosity, fluid type and saturation and its estimation is useful for improved reservoir characterization. Often in marine set-ups, P-impedance of young reservoir sand is similar to that of shale and with Vp/Vs values showing wide scatters, it is difficult to distinguish sand from shale. In such cases, density helps as a dependable discriminator of reservoir sand as the density of reservoir sands usually exhibits considerably lower values than shales.

Density can impact significant changes in amplitude with varying offsets (Quijada and Stewart 2007). Shear wave (P-SV) reflections are known to be more sensitive to density contrasts at large incident angles (about 40^0) than the P-reflections, characterized by amplitude increase with increasing angles. It is thus possible to estimate density by inversion using very large offsets on prestack data. However, such large angle incident data are not commonly used because of operational constraints and wherever recorded, shows high amount of noise deteriorating the reflection quality unfit for meaningful study. A small amount of noise greatly impacts

reliability of density estimation and remains an arduous task. Nevertheless density determination from seismic continues to remain an important issue under study.

AVO Inversion

Analysis on AVO attributes like amplitudes, intercepts and gradients were discussed earlier in Chapter "Shear Wave Seismic, AVO and Vp/Vs AnalysisShear Wave Seismic, AVO and Vp/Vs Analysis". AVO response for a reservoir is modelled using Zoeppritz's equations, where the contrasts in P- and S-impedance, density and Poisson's ratio are known at a well. Conversely, from pre-stack seismic data, constrained with the log data and using angle-dependent seismic reflectivity, P-and S-reflectivies are determined which are subsequently converted to P-and S-impedance attributes. This is known as AVO inversion and a process through which the AVO attributes, the intercept and gradient intercept information is also obtained.

This is also achieved by simultaneous inversion. Essentially both AVO and simultaneous inversion deliver the same goods, the latter being a more evolved and robust technique that directly transforms prestack amplitudes into impedances without the intercept and gradient attribute information. Once P-impedance, S-impedance and density are obtained, a number of elastic modulii other than bulk and shear such as Young's modulus (E), V_p/V_S ratio, Lambda-Rho, Mu-Rho and Poisson's ratio can be determined. These are important parameters having applications in several fields in petroleum exploration industry. Lambda-Rho and Mu-Rho, products of elastic modulii and density and are used as fluid and matrix indicators. Young's modulus and Poisson's ratio denote stiffness and strength of rock respectively and are geomechanical rock properties needed to build mechanical earth models (MEM). MEM helps planning and designing parameters for reservoir stimulation such as fracking tight reservoirs and in drilling to avoid borehole related problems (see Chapter "Seismic Wave and Rock-Fluid Properties").

AVO inversion is extensive and needs integration of all types of data—seismic, geological, borehole, rock physics, and petrophysics.

Though several inversion techniques are available, the approach to adoption of a particular inversion will depend on the geologic objective and the type of data at hand. Notwithstanding, the type of inversion adopted, the recursive, model-based, or geostatistical, the impedance volumes generated have generally inherent significant advantages. These include increased frequency bandwidth, enhanced resolution and thereby providing more reliable estimate of layer property that helps in integrated approach to geological interpretation. However, since the inversion process transforms seismic amplitude directly into impedance values, special attention needs to be paid to true amplitude preservation to ensure that the amplitudes represent the actual geological effects. The seismic data therefore essentially needs rigorous reconditioning of data to be free of multiples, acquisition imprints, coherence noise, and improved signal-to-noise ratio and resolution.

The inverted impedance sections may be displayed in wiggle-variable area mode for clarity to judge the quality of the all-important seismic tie with well before proceeding to quantify rock properties. Display in variable density mode may be avoided as it does not show small mismatches in seismic well calibration that can be important. One of the simplest quality check for inversion is a comparison between the initial seismic and the inverted impedance section, if the two sections look similar the exercise is meaningless.

Thin-bed Reflectivity Inversion

Reflections from thin beds below 10-15m (λ/4) are usually unresolvable due to seismic bandwidth and side lobes of the source wavelet impeding resolution. Special processing techniques are used to improve resolution by removing the wavelet from the seismic data to achieve the subsurface reflection coefficient series. This is known as thin-bed reflectivity processing, a post stack technique which uses time varying wavelets for deconvolution. This is somewhat likened to spiking deconvolution, but uses spectral decomposition techniques, to eliminate the wavelet to improve resolution for defining thin beds. However, as the reflectivity series constitutes of spikes, it becomes difficult to correlate horizons and needs to be filtered with high band pass. The filtered output is a high resolution seismic section, where beds much below the tuning thickness can be tracked and correlated (Fig. 11). Thin-bed reflectivity inversion is a post stack operation which transforms the reflectivity to acoustic impedance. The inverted section can be extremely useful in providing thin layer properties for reservoir delineation and characterization. While the low frequency component obtained from seismic can introduce some amount of uncertainties, as without its addition, the inverted traces would not provide absolute values of impedances. Nevertheless, it should not be a great impairment because the inverted impedance sections can still be useful as their lateral changes, constrained with geologic data can be interpreted to predict variability in layer properties qualitatively for providing inputs to reservoir modelling.

Phase Rotation to Harmonize Seismic Data

The 3D seismic volume data processed for zero-phase, often are not exactly zero-phase with some amount of residual phase delay still remaining in the data. This may be checked and necessary time corrections made by appropriate phase rotation of data volume. Synthetic seismograms, computed with zero phase wavelets, or wavelets extracted from seismic data using statistical process are correlated with seismic trace at all the wells for calibration. The correlation may show varying order of phase shifts at the wells due to residual phase delays and the least common multiple of these phase shifts may be determined and applied to seismic data to harmonize the phase in the 3D volume. Though strictly the data is not zero-phased, the rotated wavelet can be considered close to it and with

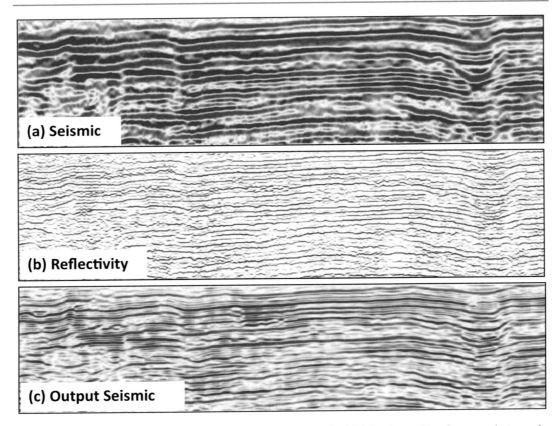

Fig. 11 Example illustrating thin bed reflectivity inversion (**a**) the band limited seismic segment, (**b**) the deconvolved data with seismic wavelet removed showing the reflectivity series and (**c**) the high resolution seismic output after high band pass filter for convenient correlation of reflections by character in interpretation. (Image Courtesy: Satinder Chopra, Calgary)

minimal time delay for arrival times of reflections. This is illustrated in a real example where the 3D seismic zero-phase data required a phase rotation of 63°, for harmonizing data which shows better match with synthetics (Fig. 12). The synthetic traces computed with zero-phase (Fig. 12a) and the rotated zero-phase wavelet (Fig. 12b), show perceptible difference between the two traces with the phase rotated trace showing better match with the seismic trace at the well (Fig. 12b). The phase rotation of 63° in the example entails time correction of about 7ms. An extended form of Fig. 12, composited with well logs, computed synthetic traces and seismic segments spliced with synthetic trace is displayed in Fig. 13.

Phase mismatches can be as high as 90 degrees, entailing time delay of the order of 10ms. The time delay correction of 10 ms (always negative) applied to arrival time for a pay at a depth of 4 km could impact its depth considerably by change of 12-15 m. For uncorrected phase data, the time delay would result in higher reservoir depth predicted from seismic based on uncorrected phase data. Nonetheless, as far as the prediction of the oil pay top is concerned, it may not impact because drilling would encounter the reservoir top earlier than predicted. But seismic data uncorrected for phase could create problems with tying the actual pay tops at the wells and lead to erroneous correlations of the target horizon. Such mistie problems could also hamper

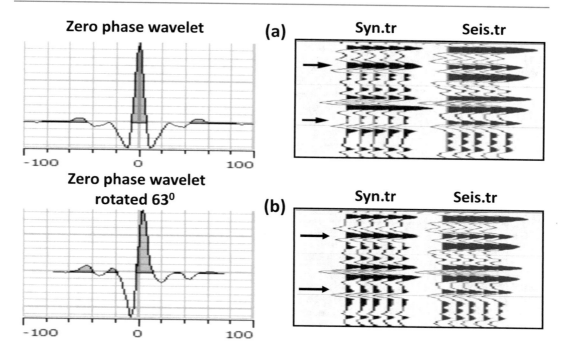

Fig. 12 Example demonstrating need for phase correction of zero-phase seismic data. (**a**) the zero phase wavelet and the computed synthetic seismograms and (**b**) phase rotated wavelet and computed synthetic at a well (velocity and density logs shown in Fig. 13). The real seismic trace at the well is juxtaposed to both the synthetics (**a**) and (**b**). Note the change in the synthetic trace computed with phase corrected wavelet (**b**) and its improved match with seismic (marked). This shows need for phase correction of seismic data prior tinversion. (Image courtesy: Satinder Chopra, Calgary)

accuracy with the extracted attribute slices used for reservoir characterization, particularly for thin reservoirs. It is therefore essential to correct the residual phases to improve prediction precision.

Seismic Inversion in Reservoir Modelling and Management

Inversion provides elastic modulii of rocks that leads to determination of physical and mechanical properties of rocks. Information on these critical parameters helps better reservoir management aimed at optimum production with minimum cost. Inversion outputs assist in solving problems ranging from reservoir delineation and characterization, identification of flow barriers, by-pass oil, reservoir modelling and monitoring to cite a few amongst several others.

Reservoir modelling and simulation requires the vital parameters such as reservoir thickness, porosity, permeability and hydrocarbon saturation at all places over the prospect. These parameters, which vary laterally and vertically, however, are measured and known only at limited locales at the wells. Herein, comes the utility and significance of seismic inversion. Inversion of 3D volume data provides the rock parameters in the areas in-between and away from the wells and provides inputs to help build geocellular modelling, the three dimensional reservoir modelling prepared in depth domain. Extracted layer properties from inversions performed in depth volumes can be conveniently and seamlessly imported to reservoir geologic and engineering data platform which are also in depth domain. Simultaneous inversion of better imaged and more accurate PSDM data, is a powerful tool for

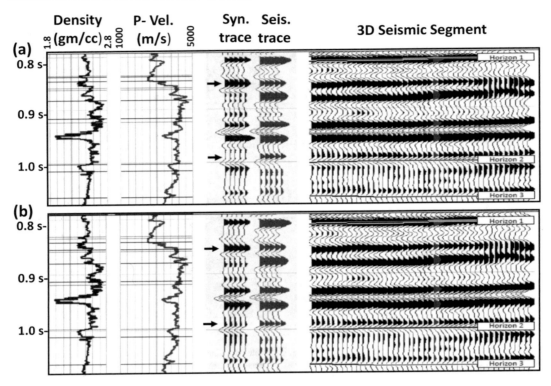

Fig. 13 Shows extension of Fig. 12 with composite panels of velocity and density curves and computed synthetics zero phase Ricker wavelet (**a**) and phase corrected wavelet (**b**). The real seismic trace at the well is also plotted alongside for comparison. The perceptible improvement in synthetic trace computed with corrected phase and the good match with the seismic (arrow marked) in (**b**) demonstrates presence of residual phase in the 3D zero-phase data which needs correction. Note the improvement in the reflection characters and match with synthetic that helps pick the correct phase of the target horizon to derive the attributes with more precision. (Image courtesy: Satinder Chopra, Calgary)

exploration and production and forms an integral part of work flow in the industry (Kessler et al. 2017).

However, choice of the inversion technique may be made judiciously depending on the geologic need, the quality of seismic data and more importantly the nature of the rock-fluid properties in the particular area considered. This requires detailed study of rock and fluid properties measured by the well-logs and arduous rock-physics-modelling (*RPM*) for calibration with seismic. Seismic may also need reconditioning of data and preferably corrected for zero-phase for robust well-tie prior to attempting seismic inversion for using the inversion outputs as inputs to geocellular modelling for reservoir characterization and flow simulation.

Limitations of Inversion

All model-based inversion techniques essentially consist of three components, (a) computation of an initial impedance model, (b) extraction of a wavelet and (c) broadband seismic data. Seismic rock physics modelling may also have to be made to have insight to problems related to production engineering for feasibility study before attempting inversion, especially stochastic inversion. Building an initial appropriate earth model, though usually constructed from the log data comprises of some of the rock-fluid properties measured and the others interpreted. The vital parameters, such as effective porosity, permeability and hydrocarbon saturation are log interpreted with imposed interpreter's bias and can impact building a seismic rock-physics model to analyse and establish the links between seismic and rock properties.

Accurate wavelet estimation for computing synthetic is the most critical factor for the success of any seismic inversion and in turn depends on an accurate seismic-well tie. The selected seismic wavelet strongly influences the seismic inversion results and, consequently assessment of the reservoir properties. Lack of an appropriate low frequency trend would prevent the transformed impedance traces from having the absolute values of impedance and the trend derived from sonic log or seismic could impact quantitative interpretation of reservoir parameters. The well to seismic calibration must be meticulous in matching phase and polarity. Often the data to be inverted is not actually a zero-phase and may end up showing shifts with log impedance curve as already discussed under phase rotation. This may require several repeated calibration exercises to determine the phase corrections to be effected by rotating the phase of processed seismic data. Density determination may be another issue as it may not be feasible to achieve by inversion for reasons stated earlier. The inversion process is very sensitive to the quality of seismic data which needs reconditioning and if noise and phase corrections are not properly taken care, it may offer unacceptable solutions in the framework of a multi-disciplinary integrated workflow.

One of the major inherent problem may be in transforming the dimensions of measurement, from microscopic log data to macroscopic seismic data. Because model computed response can be same with differently varying model parameters, inversion results may not offer an exclusively unique solution as mentioned in comprehensive and powerful stochastic inversion. Many times, the subtle changes in reservoir rock and fluid properties, though detectable, may have ambiguity in quantification of parameters from inverted data, even at moderate depth where the data quality is considered good. This only underscores the rigours of taking care of initial small steps involved which eventually matter for the success of application of seismic inversion in reservoir management.

References

Chopra S, Marfurt KJ (2012) Evolution of seismic interpretation during the last three decades. The Leading Edge 31:654–676

Cooke D, Cant J (2010) Model-based seismic inversion: comparing deterministic and probabilistic approaches, CSEG RECORDER, 34

Kessler D, Kosloff, D, Codd J, Bartana A (2017) Depth imaging—more than PSDM, Fifteenth International Congress of the Brazilian Geophysical Society, 1–3

Lindseth RO (1979) Synthetic sonic logs—a process for stratigraphic interpretation. Geophysics 44:3–26

Mummery RC (1988) Discrimination between porous zones and shale intervals using seismic logs. The Leading Edge 6:10–12

Neidell NS (1986) Amplitude variation with offset. The Leading Edge 4:47–51

Quijada MF, Stewart RR (2007) Density estimations using density-velocity relations and seismic inversion. CREWES Res Rep 19:1–20

Schramm MW Jr, Dedman EV, Lindsey JP (1977) Practical stratigraphic modelling and interpretation. AAPG Memoir 26:477–501

Seismic Pitfalls

Abstract

All seismic anomalies are not related to geology. Spurious anomalies and misinterpretation of seismic images often lead to drilling results, substantially different from that predicted, leading to exploration setbacks. This is commonly referred as 'seismic pitfalls'. Seismic pitfalls can originate due to inadequacies in data acquisition, processing, and interpretation of subsurface geology. Pitfalls can also be caused due to natural fetters such as technological system limitations such as of seismic wave propagation, time-domain recording and complex geological subsurface in nature. Awkwardly, pitfalls are also at times caused by misinterpretation of data due to deficient workflow, personal bias and eagerness for quick-fix solutions given by the work-station.

While seismic successes are widely publicized, failures for some reason, are scarcely reported. This chapter elaborates the various sources of seismic pitfalls and highlights some of the failures with case examples. Pitfalls, however, will continue to be an upshot of seismic prediction, though can be mitigated to a large extent by synergistic interpretation of multi-set data by experienced and skilled interpreter.

In simple geological settings such as layer-cake deposits, the seismic images generally replicate the subsurface stratal geometry and are easy and straight forward to interpret (Fig. 1). But in complex structural and intricate stratigraphic settings, such as in highly tectonic belts of overthrusts and recumbent folds, salt/shale tectonic areas and complicated depositional systems on shelf margins and slopes, seismic images may not replicate and represent the subsurface stratal geometry. Structural complexities in tectonized zones, rapid variations in sedimentary thickness and lithology, growth faults and roll-over structures, shale and salt structures often cause rapid lateral velocity variations. This together with structural geometry related problems create complications in seismic elastic wave propagation and impede generation of reliable seismic reflections. Aberrations and obscure images create spurious anomalies which can make interpretation difficult and ambiguous. All anomalies observed in seismic are not related to geology and misinterpretation of such spurious anomalies often lead to drilling results substantially different from that expected. This can land an interpreter in a 'spot' and allegorically speaking, in a 'pit'. Such seismic anomalies that cause setbacks in exploration and predicament for the interpreter are commonly referred as 'seismic pitfalls'.

Seismic pitfalls can befall due to any or all of the limitations of seismic technology, the data acquisition, processing, interpretation (API) of subsurface geology. Pushing data interpretation beyond the confines, too, can at times generate flawed predictions leading to pitfalls. Clearly, this needs to be avoided through understanding

Fig. 1 Seismic segment displaying an image replicating the subsurface stratal geometry in a simple geologic setting. Interpretation of such images are easy and straight forward (image: courtesy ONGC, India)

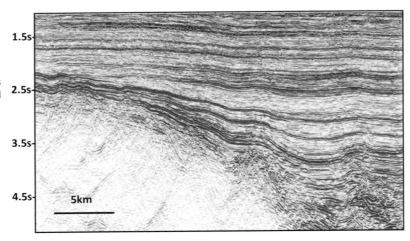

of the whole gamut of seismic technology and its limitations - the seismic data acquisition, processing and interpretation and the subsurface geological aspects. Pitfalls are described succinctly in a monograph by Tucker and Yorston (1973) who classified the pitfalls under three main types: (1) stratal geometry (2) seismic velocity and (3) seismic recording and processing. The first two categories of pitfalls are nature's creation (described at the end of this chapter) and some of these, of more complex type, may even be beyond the realm of current seismic technology for a solution. The pitfalls originating from data acquisition, processing and interpretation happens to be under human control and can be avoided to a large extent.

Pitfalls, discussed by Tucker and Yorston (1973), were mostly from old 2D seismic vintage where pitfalls could be aplenty due to reasons traced to the then prevalent inadequacies, in data acquisition and processing. Tremendous improvements in modern day seismic technology and techniques in acquisition and processing have made it possible to obtain much better subsurface images and avoid to a great extent many of the earlier geometry and velocity related artefacts that can cause pitfalls. Acquisition of 3D and 3D-3C seismic data with improved equipment and techniques followed by sophisticated volume processing techniques have made a tremendous change in acquiring quality images

having high signal-to noise ratio and improved resolution. Surface-consistent deconvolution and statics, azimuthal velocity analysis, one-pass prestack time and depth migration and demultiple and noise suppression techniques, have in recent times made seismic offer reasonably dependable and representative subsurface images and have reduced chances of pitfalls to considerable extent. However, pitfalls continue to exist and the causatives can be categorized under the heads as discussed below.

Seismic Technology (API) Related Pitfalls

Acquisition Related Artefacts

Spurious anomalies or artefacts may originate due to limitations, intrinsic to the data acquisition technique or in their faulty planning and execution. Seismic recorded amplitude and derived velocity are the principal attributes, and their lateral and spatial variations are extensively used for interpreting subsurface geology. But how accurate and reliable are these attributes in a recorded reflection signal to truly represent the rock and fluid properties? The common and most important seismic property, the reflection amplitude recorded at the surface is dependent on the source generated energy, the wave propagation mechanism in the subsurface, the receivers on the ground and the subsurface geometry and type of reflector. Consider for instance land data acquired with dynamite source. The shot-hole depth and charge size are generally decided below the weathering zone and in a medium where the charge would be exploded, for effective energy transmission. However, changes in shot hole depths and in type of medium, variations in lateral velocity and thickness of the near-surface shallow weathering zone, planting of geophones vertically upright and with firm contacts with ground, are some of the important factors which hinder to a large extent the recording of true amplitude response of the rocks. Each of these elements in the scheme of acquisition has the potential to contaminate amplitudes and randomly. Additionally, the survey geometry, shooting direction and recording parameters may not be optimally parameterized for the specific geologic objective and can suffer in image quality required for interpretation. Often the 3D data contains noise including acquisition foot-prints due to acquisition design or unavoidable ground conditions which distort the amplitudes. Although the processing techniques are well advanced and designed to remove the acquisition deficiencies, it may still be inadequate to eliminate the aberrations fully. After all, how effective the processing can be if the data is acquired with geophones lying horizontally on ground or with poor ground contact due to improper planting? These on-land problems fortunately are fewer in marine data, which is generally far superior in quality to land data. Nevertheless, the true reflection amplitude is hardly ever precisely retrieved, despite corrections attempted in processing. Consequently, all seismic attributes extracted from amplitude have an element of uncertainty in exactness that can breed pitfalls.

Processing Linked Snags

Often when the data is considered unsatisfactory for meaningful interpretation, it is requisitioned for reprocessing or special processing. Reprocessed data, however, may not improve the entire seismic section from top to bottom with improvements restricted to a part of the data and that too may be at the cost of the rest. For instance reprocessing may improve the shallower events but cause deterioration in the deeper events or the other way round. In either case it can be problematic, particularly in virgin or less explored areas where the interpreter seeks information from the entire vertical section to understand basin evolution in entirety to help evaluate the plays and prospects. Processing in its dispensation can also introduce artefacts and cause faulty interpretation of geologic anomalies and especially so in complex tectonic fold and thrust belt zones.

Velocity, besides amplitude is the other vital attribute that builds the foundation of exploration seismic technology and can be another major source for breeding pitfalls. Seismic velocity is an apparent velocity derived from optimal stacking of traces (stack velocity) in common depth point gather (CDP) and is used albeit with a correction, in several applications in processing and interpretation methods. Picking velocities based on reflection semblances precisely during velocity analysis on NMO gathers, is important and needs to be done judiciously. Since reflection quality commonly deteriorates with depth, velocity picking can be often subjective in these greater depth ranges. Stack velocity is influenced, among other things by the quality of reflections, the stratal dips and the recording spread length and over all, the way it is picked from velocity analysis. Interval velocities used for inferring rock properties are deduced from stacking velocity can be highly sensitive to subjectivity and ambiguity, especially when computed for small intervals (Chapter "Seismic Reflection Principles—Basics"). Some may think the depth migration as the panacea to provide true velocity and depths which is not true as discussed in Chapter "Evaluation of High-Resolution 3D and 4D Seismic Data". Essentially if the kernel, the primary reflection is poor or not recorded, neither a good fold stack nor a migration stack attempt to improve data quality can be successful. Consequently, seismic velocity being susceptible to factors external to geology can provide much scope for misguiding interpretation.

While remarkable improvements in 3D seismic data acquisition and processing can vastly improve the data quality, it has also become extremely sensitive to the processing work-flow, the parameters and the algorithms used. Processing work-flows comprise a number of modules and each with options of choosing the type of software and needs suitable parametrization. Depending on these factors, processing output can deliver different images for the same data set leading to different interpretations. Sophisticated migration processes do improve images but at times different algorithms can lead to overreach processing marvels and can strongly impact image outputs to baffle the interpreter (Fig. 2). One version of depth migration (Kirchoff) is interpreted as a salt diapir whereas, the other migration version (Beam) suggests vertically folded beds. The two versions are significantly diverse and add to interpreter's problem, though in this case the regional geologic syndrome can decide accordingly whether the data is from the salt or highly tectonized basin.

Interpretation Linked Pitfalls

Seismic data acquisition and processing though deliver excellent high resolution seismic images, it can sometimes be worryingly susceptible to faulty or inadequate data interpretation due to lack of geologic understanding (Fig. 3). Often pitfalls originate from interpreter's flawed geologic perception or the way the interpretation workflow is managed to achieve the task. Different people view the same data differently and can end up with diverse interpretations. Image visualisation by the intuitive human mind can be deceptive and often an interpreter starts 'seeing' features in seismic data that one's brain urges to see. Guided by instinct or intuition, the interpretation may ensue in fallacy. For instance a channel feature may be confidently mapped out of image perception that is non-existent in the subsurface. It is important to have instinct and imagination for an interpreter but it is also necessary to be aware of one's proneness to bias. Seismic interpretation can be likened to an inversion process that does not provide unique solutions. Reflecting on viewing and visualizing the data in different ways, discussing the inferences for possible ambiguities that can arise with

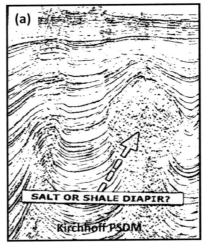 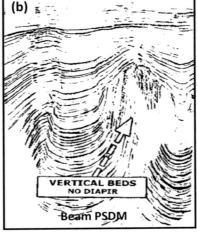

Fig. 2 Example showing impact of different migration processing algorithms in resulting seismic images that can be baffling for interpretation to breed pitfalls. The seismic data was processed with prestack depth migration algorithms (**a**) Kirchhoff and (**b**) beam migration and show contrasting results that have significant geological consequences as annotated

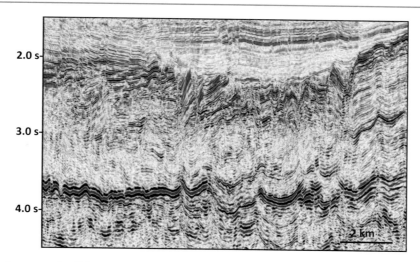

Fig. 3 Seismic segment in offshore showing high quality image in a tectonically disturbed geologic setting which can be difficult to interpret. Though advanced acquisition and processing techniques can create excellent images, lack of proper understanding of geology may impede proper interpretation which requires skill, experience and knowledge of depositional systems and tectonic styles (image: courtesy ONGC, India)

peers, seeking opinions and welcoming criticisms can help reduce the source of potent pitfalls.

Many of the pitfalls, in the author's opinion, may be arising out of quick-fix solutions by work-station based interpretations, employing fast and powerful softwares. Work-stations and softwares are extremely useful and indispensable but these are only tools. Their capabilities and limitations must be well understood for their judicious application. The usefulness of the software depends on the type and quality of data and often the software design can be geology-specific. Software algorithms too, may have innate assumptions of certain physical factors that may not be in tune with the specific geology of the area. Workstations provide accurate results but may not offer the solutions and over-reliance on softwares without human supervision may lead to risks of interpretation pitfalls. Often interpretation is carried out without adequate integration of geological, geophysical, petro-physical and engineering data. Integration is an unrelenting and an involved process which needs critical evaluation by the human brain. Notwithstanding the above discussions, often to confirm or corroborate interpretation results one may require re-acquisition or reprocessing of data, which, unfortunately, may not be always feasible because constraints of accessibility of data or time due to other pre-commitments.

Some of the common interpretation pitfalls often can be traced to interpreter's lack of skill and experience. Seismic tie with wells is the most important stepping stone to reservoir delineation and characterization which is identification of the target reflection horizon from the well and its lateral correlation. Precise well calibration and correlation defines the geometry of the reservoir and the rock properties. Correlations are based on reflection character which comprises of amplitude, phase (peak/trough), frequency, waveform and the dip attitude. Commonly, horizon correlations are done in auto-track mode because it is fast and supposedly accurate. However, auto-tracking cannot recognize splits in reflection waveform or lateral polarity changes caused by variations in rock and fluid properties and may not yield desired accuracy in areas of poor and/or patchy reflections (Chapter "Seismic Interpretation Methods"). Auto-tracking and contouring may lead to flawed maps resulting in erroneous reservoir geometry and hydrocarbon volume estimates. Faults and their delineation is another area where impromptu alignment and lack of fault attribute

Fig. 4 Seismic segment in offshore showing an example of amplitude related pitfall. The inferred high amplitude DHI anomaly is due to a basalt flow sill and underscores the importance of polarity information (image: courtesy ONGC, India)

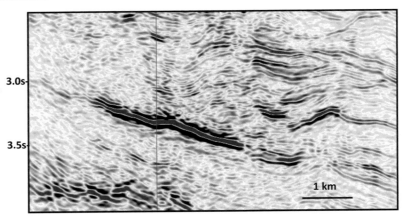

analysis can generate pitfalls by mapping pseudo fault closures as structural traps. Powerful softwares such as 3D volume interpretation for horizon correlations and auto mapping of faults are welcome but not without manual supervision.

Amplitude-Related Pitfalls

Many pitfalls unfortunately accrue from casual interpretation of seismic amplitudes in data without analysing the polarity and adequate understanding of the geology involving the rock properties. Since the advent of 'bright spots' as hydrocarbon indicators, high amplitude anomalies are often considered by many as related to hydrocarbon sands irrespective of the geological setting and recommended for drilling without adequate analysis for validation. As a rule of thumb, high amplitudes associated with rocks of old age and at greater depths are unlikely to be hydrocarbon indicators and in fact may be considered a discouraging criterion for hydrocarbon. High impedance hydrocarbon rocks are more likely to show 'dim spots' and such strong amplitude anomalies may be due to water saturated calcareous sandstones or limestones or intrusive sills which need thorough investigation before drilling. The key in these cases is the reflection polarity which may be unknown to the interpreter and with no access to prestack gathers or AVO analysis software, it can result in pitfall. In an offshore example, the strong amplitude interpreted as hydrocarbon sand turned out to be Upper Cretaceous intrusive sill

(Fig. 4). In another case, a genuine-looking, high amplitude offshore channel cut–and-fill sand prospect in super deep waters, drilled for gas, encountered thick section of mudstones without trace of reservoir rock and hydrocarbon (Fig. 5). The bright amplitudes, investigated later by AVO modelling showed the strong amplitude caused by high Poisson's contrast between the facies within the mudrock section, without significant impedance contrast (Nanda 2018).

Pitfalls can also occur due to overreliance on attribute slices interpreted in isolation without considering the vertical sections. An inconsistent amplitude pattern on time slices may appear as a hydrocarbon bearing geologic feature (e.g. channel crevasse'/fan complex) and interpreted without seeking corroborative evidences or appropriate depositional model. The interpreter with sound knowledge of geology and seismic techniques would be in most cases able to differentiate genuine amplitude anomalies from artefacts related to data acquisition and processing issues. The artefacts may be caused due to wave propagation effects, reflector geometry and tuning thickness which can greatly influence amplitudes. Problem of identifying the correct reflection phase and polarity, as often is the case with composite reflections, to ascertain the nature of reflectivity (Rc) for inferring correct lithology, correlation of horizon and its precise depth can be yet another reason for ambiguous interpretation. Polarity, crucial for validation of high

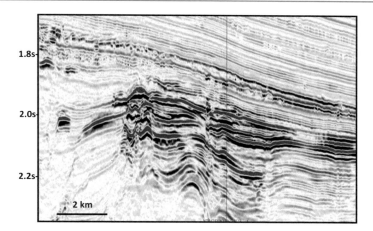

Fig. 5 Example of an offshore deep water seismic DHI anomaly showing amplitude related pitfall. The high amplitude anomaly drilled for a prospective channel-fill gas sand in super deep offshore proved to be massive mudstone formation. The high amplitudes are caused mainly due to high contrasts in Poisson's ratio within the massive mudstone section and not due to impedance (image: courtesy ONGC, India)

amplitude anomalies and thin hydrocarbon-charged sand layers, may sometimes be incorrectly interpreted. However, there are several instances where high amplitude anomalies authenticated by positive AVO analysis has also led to dry wells. This could be because of shortcomings in the presumptions made in AVO technique, discussed in Chapter "Shear Wave Seismic, AVO and Vp/Vs Analysis".

In yet another interesting example, two similar looking Pliocene 'bright spots' in offshore, stacked vertically, one above the other and expected to be gas bearing, on drilling turned out to be normal grade oil bearing sands (Fig. 6).

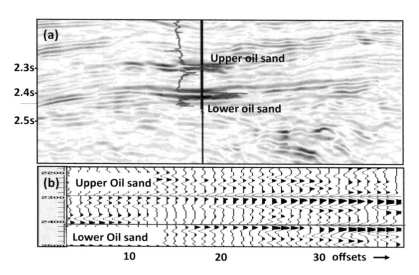

Fig. 6 The figure displays two similar seismic strong DHI anomalies drilled for gas but proved oil bearing. (**a**) Seismic high amplitudes (red, negative Rc) caused by the oil sands and (**b**) validated by AVO class 2(n) anomalies. Log evaluated reservoir properties for the two sands are similar except for considerable difference in oil saturation and permeability. Note with similar amplitude and AVO anomalies, the highly dissimilar productivities of the sands could not be predicted (images: courtesy ONGC, India)

The seismic angle gather later showed both the sands as Class 2(negative) AVO anomalies with weak amplitudes in the near traces and increasing with offsets (Nanda and Wason 2013). The sands have similar density and porosity values but with considerable difference in permeability and saturation on logs (Nanda and Wason 2013).With similar seismic amplitude and AVO anomalies, the significantly different production potential of the sands could not be predicted. Presence of oil, though unexpected, was a heartening welcome and so would not be included under pitfalls. The examples are cited to underscore the uncertainties in interpretation of data (see Chapter "Shear Wave Seismic, AVO and Vp/Vs Analysis"). There may be similar surprises in many cases, the pitfalls cropping up due to lack of proper understanding of the intricate relationship between rock-physics and seismic response which, ironically can be made only after the well is drilled.

Velocity-Related Pitfalls

Seismic velocity, as has been earlier mentioned, is by far the most essential element of seismic technology applied in petroleum exploration. NMO stack and migration in processing, quantifying reservoir rock-fluid properties and monitoring EOR processes, all are dependent on apt velocity information for dependable results. Estimation of accurate average velocity is vital as errors in depth prediction to reservoir (pay) top and its thickness can lead to disappointing drilling results. An appraisal well encountering the pay top deeper than predicted can end in water and, upset the exploration plan. Determining variability in lateral velocity has always been a difficult and challenging task despite employing techniques such as tomography in prestack depth migration (see Chapter "Evaluation of High-Resolution 3D and 4D Seismic Data"). Most interpretations suffer from various degrees of depth prediction errors depending on the degree of lateral velocity variation and an error of 10–15 m is generally considered acceptable. Figure 7 is an example which illustrates how the actual structural geometry of the reservoir proved substantially different from that mapped in time domain because of severe lateral variation in the overburden velocity in the area. Proper

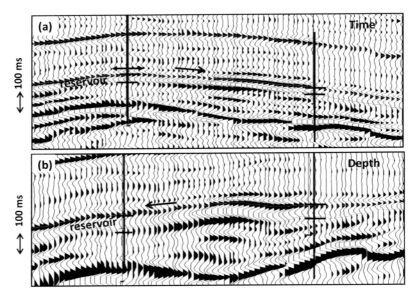

Fig. 7 Displays the seismic segment in (**a**) time and (**b**) depth, illustrating velocity related pitfall. The time section (**a**) shows the reservoir with a crestal reversal (arrow) and higher time values at the well to right. However, the depth migrated section (**b**) does not bear out the reversal and in contrast shows continuing up dip to become shallower at the well at the right. Note the change of low-frequency look of reflection sin (**b**) due to stretch in depth section (images: courtesy Hardy Energy, India)

understanding of the geological reasons accounting for such velocity variance in the overburden is desirable which helps predict depths with more confidence and reliability.

Case Example

Velocity related pitfalls can be due to presence of localised high or low velocity zones above the reservoir, such as an extra patch of carbonate mound having high velocity or a channel filled with low-velocity clay that can cause serious discrepancies in depth predictions. These are known as "time anomalies", 'pull up'/ 'pull down' or 'sag' effects which the interpreter must be careful to notice. A case example of 'sag', an artefact, caused by low-velocity is shown (Fig. 8). The channel morphology and the continuous and parallel internal reflections configuration within the channel, indicates low-velocity clay-fill. Typically the artefacts occur vertically below the structures and usually give them away. The 'sag' seen at the reservoir level being vertically below and the causative being confirmed by drilling as channel-fill clay confirms the sag as 'time anomaly', also known as 'velocity anomaly'. The channel-fill feature was mapped and appropriate corrections for the low-velocity

artefact led to predicting depths with confidence. Drilling results confirmed the pay top at shallower level than that expected from the time map showing a structural low and adding to reserves (Nanda et al. 2008). However, unnoticed, such artefacts in 2D data can be potent breeders of pitfall.

Interpretation is a scientific art which provides solution to inverse problems and suffers from usual innate shortcomings of uncertainties because solutions are not unique. Lack of adequate expertise, and more significantly, impromptu application of information without due verification may cause an interpreter to stumble, despite having excellent seismic images to work with. The risks, however, can be mitigated to a great extent by the skill and experience, though cannot be completely eliminated. A careful and mindful interpreter is open to inferences from all kinds of validations possible to lessen uncertainties and cut down exploration and development risk. Seismic 'pitfall' is a normal and professional hazard for an interpreter to occasionally get ditched. Nevertheless, the challenge lies in bouncing back out of the pit, getting wiser each time from experience so as to avoid repeats of such stumbles in the future.

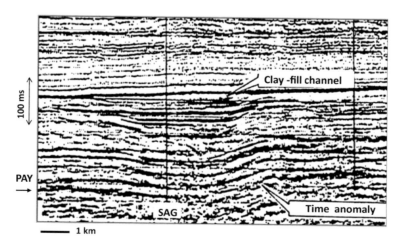

Fig. 8 Another example of seismic segment showing velocity related pitfall ('time anomaly'). Though drilled on a time-low, the pay top was actually encountered much shallower because of lower over burden velocity due to the channel-cut filled with low velocity clay. Note the channel cut morphology and the parallel and flat reflections with init typifying clay fill which resulted in 'sag' (pull down), vertically below at all levels below including the reservoir. The sag is a 'velocity anomaly' artefact (after Nanda et al. 2008)

Natural System-Related Pitfalls

Wave Propagation Complications

The over-simplified assumptions of homogeneous and isotropic elastic media of earth are not valid, as in nature the seismic wave propagates in anelastic, heterogeneous and anisotropic media of varying degrees. The propagation mechanism gets further complicated with complex structural and stratigraphic strata with strong lateral velocity change that radically distorts subsurface image quality. Imprecise and blurred images are formed due to irregularity and rougosity of reflectors which cause heavy scattering of energy. Add-ons problems such as generation and recording of mode converted waves (P-SV), intrabed (peg-leg) multiples, and attenuation losses, and ambient ground noises further help deteriorate the seismic images.

Seismically the most challenging areas are the highly contorted fold and overthrusts belts, the subsalt and the sub basalt formations where it is generally difficult to image the objects properly.

The major issues are mostly the strong velocity and density contrasts, for instance between salt and the surrounding beds, where generation of converted P-SV-P waves and scattering due to heterogeneities within the salt/basalts are likely to be high. Consequently imaging of the beds abutting against salt-flank are also poor due to wave transmission (refraction) through the salt core. Particularly complex salt structures with near vertical dips and overhangs are big challenges for precise imaging. Davidson et al. (2013) in their article have succinctly described the various issues concerning imaging of salt including lateral velocity variation and anisotropy within the salt mass and the ensuing uncertainties in interpretation leading to pitfalls.

An example of uncertainty in imaging geometry of relatively simple salt diapirs indicating related exploration risks is illustrated in Fig. 9. Reservoirs abutting against the salt flanks constitute potential stratigraphic traps for hydrocarbon exploration with salt acting as an excellent updip lateral seal. The trap geometry, however, depends on defining exactly the salt core

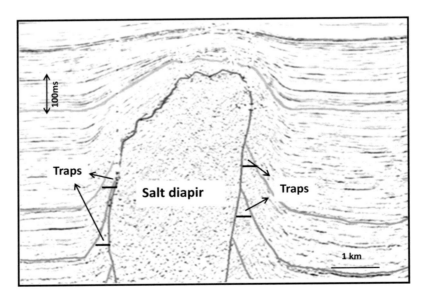

Fig. 9 Illustrating an example of a poorly imaged salt diapir due to wave propagation related issues, and can potentially lead to pitfalls. The uncertainty in delineation of the salt boundary and the linked traps formed at its flank scan lead to pitfalls in exploring salt associated traps. Note the small lateral extent of the traps and the steep dip of beds that allow very little margin of error for drilling at proper location to find hydrocarbon. Drilling structurally too high up may miss the reservoir while lower, down dip may end in water

boundary as well as the lateral termination of the beds with their dips. The interpreted geometries of the salt core and the dipping beds as shown in the Fig. 9 is dubious and can vary differently depending on individuals. The uncertainties in clear definition of the up-dip flank traps consequently poses problems as to decide precisely the drilling locations to drill for hydrocarbons. As it can be made out, the margin of error in defining the space for drilling location is too small, varying between the reservoir being altogether missed if drilled much up-dip and encounter water, drilled much down-dip. This would lead to pitfalls severe enough to upset exploration endeavours for such prospective traps. Sophisticated migration processes do improve images but as has been earlier mentioned migration cannot improve quality of a reflection which could not be recorded properly because of wave propagation problems.

Sub-basalt imaging also suffers from reasons similar to salt due to strong impedance contrasts between the basalt and the surrounding strata and scattering caused due to heterogeneity and rugosity of the eroded basaltic surfaces (Zhou et al 2010). Often thick basalt sections, as the Decan traps in Indian peninsular, consist of multiple flows with thin layers of sediment lying in between the flows, known as intratrappeans. The alternating low impedance Intratrappean beds cause severe transmission loss, one of the possible reasons for poor imaging of sub-basalts. An example of a pitfall during a frontier exploration venture for sub-basalt is shown in Fig. 10, where Mesozoic sequence beneath the basalt (Deccan trap) is known to exist. The Mesozoic angular unconformity with basalt, forming a potent up-dip trap is clearly seen on seismic and the mapped prospect drilled. Drilling was terminated thousands of meters deep into the basalt without any evidence of sedimentary reservoir section. The strong stratal dips seen in seismic turned out to be within the massive basalt section interlaced with thin intra-trappean beds deposited between the episodic lava flows. Though, seismic forward modelling to a large extent could mitigate risk but the number of unknowns such as the basalt thickness, number of thin intratrappean layers and their properties and disposition within the basalt make it a difficult exercise.

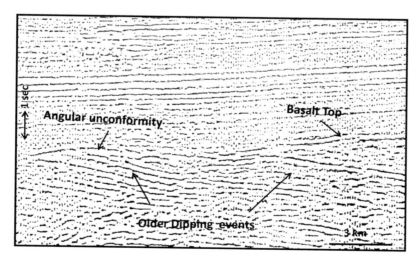

Fig. 10 Illustrating another example of a pitfall related to ambiguous imaging of sub-basalt Mesozoics, the exploration target. The dipping beds in the seismic segment were interpreted as an angular unconformity Mesozoic prospect against the over-lying basalt. Drilling proved the seismic dipping events to be from with in the basalt, linked to intratrappean layers deposited during breaks of episodic basalt flows (image: courtesy ONGC, India)

Anisotropy

Anisotropic formations such as with fractures and thick layered shales have strong azimuth dependent velocities and their presence in the overburden can create significant complications in wave propagation and contaminate recording of *P*-and S-reflections (Chapters "Seismic Wave and Rock-Fluid Properties" and "Shear Wave Seismic, AVO and Vp/Vs Analysis"). Recent advances in seismic processing and imaging techniques can handle anisotropy in improving images including those of steep structures but are yet to become an integral part of regular processing workflow in practice. Nevertheless, the complicated anisotropic behaviour of velocity field requires anisotropy coefficients which are often not realizable and continues to remain a practical issue. Regardless of advanced and sophisticated acquisition, processing and interpretation (seismic API) techniques, there are natural limitations, innate in seismic technology and subsurface geological complexities. These cannot be completely remedied leading eventually to some unavoidable pitfalls. Strangely, as technology has advanced, so has the complexity of geologic targets to be explored and the issue continues.

Time Domain Data Recording

The single most important and fundamental shortcoming in the seismic technology is the recording of seismic data in the time domain. Though the time values are ultimately converted to depth by velocity, the spatially varying velocity field over the area remains unknown for accurate seismic depth predictions. Seismic measurements of arrival time of reflection signals, their amplitudes and attributes are controlled by velocity, and lack of its precise information can be a great impediment in the interpretation of data. Prestack depth migration (PSDM) mitigates the problem to a great extent. But it cannot offer a perfect solution without a priori knowledge of velocity which has to follow

from the data itself, 'a chicken first or egg first' paradox! Seismic velocity, constrained by the velocity measured at the well is used for accurate time-depth conversion at the well but elsewhere, away from the well, it remains worrisome due to its uncertain velocity field. A well-defined accurate overburden velocity field is essential for time to depth conversion and efficient depth migration. Ironically, this most crucial attribute happens to be the most common source of pitfall.

Geological Impediments, Vagaries of Nature

Seismic properties and attributes are deployed to exploit geological information on rocks and fluid properties and their vertical and lateral variation. What if the two different rocks have similar seismic property or marginal difference that is insensitive to seismic response? Even with the best quality of seismic data acquired, processed and interpreted with sophisticated techniques, prediction uncertainties at times can still remain due to inexplicable reasons for the vagaries of the nature. For instance, explanation for 'bright spot' seismic anomalies caused by light oil due to its large amount of dissolved gas remains contentious (Chapter "Seismic Wave and Rock-Fluid Properties"). Likewise, the exact nature of seismic response of 'fizz gases', referred to small amount of free gas/ dissolved gas in water, is another such baffling issue.

Impairments can also happen due to unforeseen seismic response of the ultimate sum impact of the individual properties within the rock. In favorable geological and petrophysical setup, response of individual parameters may add-up to produce a clear discernible seismic response, whereas in another situation they negate one another to be hardly perceptible. Under these circumstances, accurate and unambiguous prediction can be hampered due to difficulty in discriminating the effects of individual parameters from the combined seismic response of the rock (Chapter "Seismic Wave and Rock-Fluid Properties").

Case Examples, Vagaries of Nature

In general, Plio-Plistocene offshore hydrocarbon sands show excellent images, best suited for rigorous AVO and Vp/Vs attribute analysis. Despite excellent data quality and stringent authentication of the anomalies, for some inexplicable reasons, a few tested dry, in the proven hydrocarbon block. One major reason for prediction uncertainty can be due to fact that myriad rock types with varying facies and properties in diverse geologic environment demonstrate similar seismic attributes. Figure 11 is such an example from offshore, east coast, India where a stack of high amplitude anomalies are seen in near and far-stacks and drilled for gas. The log measured low Vp/Vs ($\sim$ 1.8) also suggested hydrocarbon but on testing it was found to be a good quality water-saturated sand. This is contrary to the fact that similar seismic anomalies and Vp/Vs ($\sim$ 1.8) values have typically proved good oil sands in the area (Nanda 2017). The higher value Vs of the water-sand resulted in the low Vp/Vs, but the falsity is inexplicable and could not have been foreseen. Yet, in another inexplicable case of seismic pitfall in the same area, a 'bright spot' validated by clear class-3 AVO was drilled and notwithstanding the log indication of a low Vp/Vs (1.8) value, the sand on testing produced water (Fig. 12). Such unforeseen and unpredictable vagaries of geology can lead to pitfalls beyond interpreter's reach.

Other common pitfalls may include cases where a mapped high amplitude and low impedance layer, thought to be gas reservoir, may be an organic-rich shale and carbonate mounds on shelf edges mapped from seismic do not turn out to be porous reef. On the other hand, during drilling for a deeper target, poor or transparent reflection event associated with an old and deeper feature was discovered as oil sand by serendipity. This though shows the uncertainty in interpretation, thankfully is not considered a pit fall because of positively encouraging results. Strong amplitude anomalies, easily noticeable in seismic are usually the preferred natural picks as prospects for exploration. In contrast, how many of no or poor amplitude anomalies, that could be potentially hydrocarbon bearing are detected and singled out as exploratory objects?

Serendipity brings unexpected good results in contrast to pitfalls that fetch setbacks and are always welcome though the causes for the serendipity are rarely analysed unlike pitfalls. One of the most important event of serendipity in the

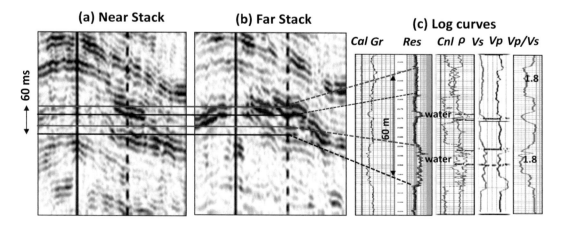

Fig. 11 Example of a pitfall related to unpredictable geologic nature. Amplitude anomalies seen in the near and far angle-stacks (**a**) and (**b**) were drilled for gas but were found to be water saturated sands on testing. This is despite the logs (**c**), among other positive indications, showing the low Vp/Vs (1.8), typically a proven indicator of good oil-sand in the area. Note the unusual increase in Vs despite slight decrease in Vp, resulting in low Vp/Vs. The unforeseen character of the unique sand was a big geologic surprise (Image courtesy: ONGC, India)

(a) Near Stack   **(b) Far Stack**   **(c) Prestack gather**   **(d) Log curves**
Cal Gr Res Cnl ρ Vs Vp P_i Vp/Vs

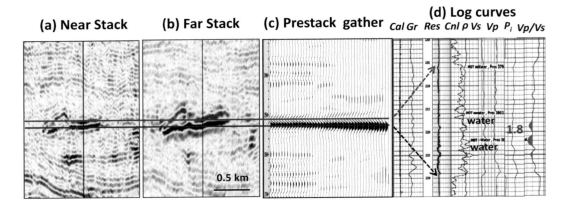

Fig. 12 Another example of a pitfall related to vagaries of geology. The 'bright spot' anomaly with class-3 AVO and low *Vp/Vs* value of 1.8 on log, proven hydrocarbon indices in the area on testing found water-bearing for inexplicable reasons. The slightly higher *Vs* and lower *Vp* explains the resulting low *Vp/Vs* but the issue of water saturation is incomprehensible (after Nanda 2017)

industry is the finding of hydrocarbon in fractured basement, almost all the giant and large hydrocarbon fields of fractured basement are serendipitous finds (Chapter "Fractured-Basement Reservoirs"). The serendipity thus being always welcome as a windfall do not qualify to be included in pitfalls, but it is mentioned here to underscore the point that uncertainties remain in seismic data evaluation, which at times result in pitfalls and at other times in serendipity.

Seismic Limitations

Seismic reflection is essentially based on impedance contrasts and cannot detect stratigraphic boundary between two rock types if they have little impedance contrast. Yet in an example cited earlier (Fig. 5), strong contrast in Poisson's ratio caused high amplitude anomalies without significant impedance contrast. Seismic imaging is reasonably sensitive to changes in rock-fluid property at shallow depths but with sensitivity deteriorating with increase in depth, it suffers in quality. This may lead to imprecise definition of reservoir geometry, particularly of the thin reservoirs at greater depths. Despite best-quality data, acquired and processed, prediction of rock properties from seismic in many such circumstances may be ambiguous and end as interpretation pitfalls. Further, as was earlier demonstrated seismic responds to all the elements of a rocks, the framework, matrix and pore fluid, and the seismic attribute variability may be difficult to attribute to a specific rock property and may not be unique (Chapter "Shear Wave Seismic, AVO and Vp/Vs Analysis").

Synergistic interpretation of multi-set data by an experienced and skilled interpreter in many cases can mitigate pitfalls to a large extent. The interpreter needs to be aware of acquisition and processing artefacts and try to work on several variants of data sets. Seismic attribute evaluations can be checked for conformity with geologic and well data for a convergent solution to mitigate occasional pitfall befalling the interpreter. Pitfalls and serendipity are chance factors and are inevitable components of hydrocarbon exploration. The unexpected and undesirable results are unfortunately termed pit falls whereas the desirable ones are welcome as serendipity. Nonetheless, pitfalls and its converse complement 'serendipity' will continue to play their roles in exploration, of course with the difference; pitfalls bring unhappiness while 'serendipity' brings happiness to all.

References

Davidson I, Jones IF, Waltham D (2013) Seismic imaging of salt diapirs: problems and pitfalls. In: Thirteenth international congress of the Brazilian Geophysical Society, pp 1–6

Nanda NC (2017) Quantitative analysis of seismic amplitudes for characterization of Pliocene hydrocarbon sands, eastern Offshore, India. First Break 35:39–45

Nanda NC (2018) Analysing a seismic pitfall-pliocene superdeep high amplitude anomaly. CSEG Recorder 30–33

Nanda NC, Wason A (2013) Seismic rock physics of bright amplitude oil sands—a case study. CSEG Recorder 38:26–32

Nanda N, Singh R, Chopra S (2008) Seismic artifacts—a case study. CSEG Recorder 33 (view issue)

Tucker PM, Yorston HJ (1973) Pitfalls in seismic interpretation. SEG Monogr Ser 2:1–50

Zhou B, Hatherly P, Peters T, Sun W (2010) Experience with the issue of seismic surveying over basalts. ASEG Ext Abs 1–5. 10.1081/22020586.2010.12041919

Unconventional Reservoirs Exploration and Production-Seismic Role

Oil Sands, Heavy Oil, Tight Oil/Gas, BCGAs and CBM

Abstract

Unconventional reservoirs differ from conventional hydrocarbon reservoirs because of their poor matrix porosity and permeability and are characteristically difficult to produce hydrocarbon. Unconventional reservoirs occurring worldwide are of various types some of which namely the oil sands, heavy oil, tight oil and gas, high pressured basin centred gas accumulations (BCGA) and coal bed methane (CBM) are discussed in this chapter and the rest in subsequent chapters.

Unconventional reservoirs invariably need external stimulus in the form of secondary and enhanced oil recovery processes for hydrocarbon production and are briefly dealt. The role of seismic to help explore and exploit these unconventional reservoirs by way of locating the plays and monitoring reservoir stimulation processes are included. Application of AVO and fracture detection to locate 'sweet spots' in CBM reservoirs and BCGAs are outlined.

Reservoirs are historically defined as sedimentary rocks having porosity and permeability. Such sedimentary rocks capable of hosting and producing hydrocarbons are considered conventional reservoirs. Rocks with low matrix porosity and permeability sometimes also host hydrocarbon which do not flow on its own and need external stimulus for commercial production. These are known as unconventional reservoirs.

Other major differences from conventional reservoirs may include process of migration and accumulation. Conventional reservoirs host hydrocarbons migrated from non-porous source rock such as shale or limestone, whereas, unconventional reservoirs may store hydrocarbons that were formed within it. Unconventional reservoirs are of varied types and a graphic of some of these along with conventional reservoirs, on land with geologic disposition is shown (Fig. 1).Unconventional reservoirs are also comparatively more difficult to explore and exploit commercially. Primary recoveries from these reservoirs are mostly low and often uneconomical. Primary recovery refers to the process of oil rising to well head at the surface by self-flow or pumped out by artificial lift devices. Commercial production from unconventional reservoirs, excepting naturally fractured basements reservoirs, invariably require some kind of external stimulus to improve oil mobility and promote permeability for commercial production. These processes are referred to secondary oil recovery and enhanced oil recovery which are expensive. Secondary recovery involves methods such as gas or water injection to displace the oil making it flow. Enhanced oil recovery (EOR), also known as tertiary recovery, on the other hand is a process in which the oil property is changed to make it more amenable to flow to surface such as the thermal and chemical methods.

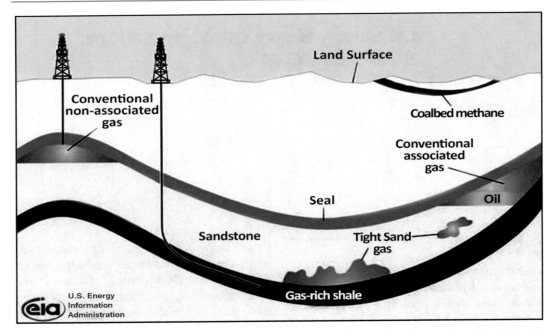

Fig. 1 Schematic geology showing gas resources of unconventional and conventional reservoirs on land with their representative locale of occurrences in the subsurface

Conventional reservoirs in structural and stratigraphic traps are relatively easier to be identified in seismic for exploration and exploitation. But with passage of time conventional oil and gas prospects becoming lesser and rarer, explorationists are pressed to look for other unconventional habitats to tap hydrocarbon so as to replenish the gradually depleting reserves. Shale and fractured basement oil and gas reserves are two such unconventional hydrocarbon resources that are being exploited economically in many places in the world. Technological advances and changes in economic scenario in the world have since made unconventional reservoirs as economically alternate viable resources. Shale oil and gas production in massive scale in the last decade in USA and to some extent in China has turned out to be a feasible unconventional source, notwithstanding the high costs and ecological problems.

Unconventional reservoirs may be classified as:
1. Oil sands, Heavy/extra heavy oil and Tight oil/gas
2. Basin-centred Gas Accumulations

3. Coal-bed methane
4. Shale Oil/Gas and Oil shale
5. Gas Hydrates
6. Fractured Basement reservoirs

The three unconventional reservoirs at the top are discussed in this chapter, the rest, the Shale oil/gas and Hydrates and the Fractured - Basement reservoirs are dealt in following Chapters ("Shale Oil and Gas, Oil Shale and Gas Hydrates and Fractured-Basement Reservoirs").

Oil Sands, Heavy/Extra Heavy Oil

Oil Sands

Oil sands also known as 'tar sands' and 'bituminous sands' are mixture of highly porous under- consolidated sands, clay, water and bitumen. Bitumen and tar though are synonymous, are actually quite different. Bitumen is a thick, sticky, highly viscous form of crude oil, formed by decomposition of vegetal matters, while tar is a residual matter from the process of coal distillation. Bitumen is composed of a mixture of hydrocarbons and exits naturally in a solid or semisolid state due to escape of lighter factions, unlike the conventional petroleum that occurs in natural liquid form. Oil cannot be produced from bituminous sands by conventional methods unless bitumen is separated and treated. Canada's Athabasca oil sands are the best example of this kind of reserve.

Extraction of Oil

Oil sands soaked with high viscous bitumen cannot produce commercial oil directly like the conventional reservoirs without secondary or enhanced recovery techniques. Primary production after treatment is low, about 5–6% from the biodegraded and highly viscous Athabasca oil sands. Extraction of oil from the oil sand depends upon how deep is the oil sand; if it is near the surface, bitumen is mined and the oil extracted by treating bitumen. For deep deposits, wells are drilled and oil made to flow or pumped out by deploying thermal methods of enhanced oil recovery, a process of heating the reservoir to reduce viscosity of the oil to make it flow. The different thermal methods used for treating such reservoirs are described below. Surface mining is less expensive but are more damaging to environment, while the in situ recovery methods are more expensive but much less damaging to the environment. Most productions from the oil sands in Canada are reported to be by surface mining.

Heavy/Extra Heavy Oil

Heavy and extra-heavy oil, deposits are similar to unconsolidated oil sands but they are saturated with oil instead of bitumen. The most widely used definition for heavy oils is based on the API gravity and generally oil grades of 10–20° API are considered heavy and grade less than 10° API considered extra or very heavy oil. Heavy oils are formed mostly due to biodegradation of normal oil by microbial activity aided by oxidation and tend to have low reservoir pressure and low gas-oil ratio (Santos et al. 2014). The heavy oil reservoirs mostly occur in shallow formations and close to unconformities and are exploited by drilling wells.

The highly porous unconsolidated sands of Orinoco Belt in Venezuela, is the largest deposit of its kind. These are sometimes described as oil sands which can be misleading. Orinoco sands are different from Athabasca oil sands. Orinoco sands are non-bituminous and are of relatively lower viscosity and may be subsumed under heavy or extra-heavy oil category.

Production of Oil

Heavy/extra heavy oils being highly viscous and immobile, similar to oil sands require stimulation to make oil flow to the well head for production. The primary production and recovery rate reported is typically low, 8–12 % as in Orinoco sands, Venezuala, but slightly better than the Athabasca oil sands (5–6%) because of lack of viscous bitumen. Without secondary or enhanced oil recovery (EOR), process, the productivity from such formation is uneconomical. Reservoir stimulation methods are of many types and depend on the type of the reservoir rocks, their physical and mechanical properties and depth of occurrence. Of all the secondary and EOR processes, the thermal methods are most commonly and widely used for producing heavy oil, and are discussed.

Thermal Methods

Heating lowers viscosity of heavy oil in a reservoir and facilitates mobility (Fig. 2). Viscosity decreases rapidly with increase in temperature and adding a small amount of heat can change mobility especially in reservoirs at lower range of temperatures (Zaydullin 2013).Thermal methods widely used include Cyclic Steam Stimulation (CSS), Steam Assisted Gravity Drainage (SAGD), Steam flooding and In-situ combustion (ISC).

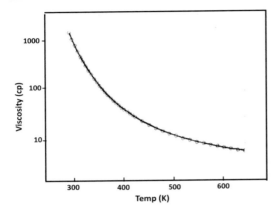

Fig. 2 Graph plot of viscosity of heavy oil versus temperature showing lowering of viscosity with increase in temperature. Note the initial rapid rate of decrease in viscosity, which becomes relatively lower with further rise in temperature, signifying that small amount of heat initially can appreciably change the mobility of oil in lower temperature range (after Zaydullin 2013)

Cyclic Steam Stimulation (CSS)

Heat in the form of steam is injected into the reservoir under high pressure and temperature and the well is shut for long enough to allow the heat to settle in to reduce viscosity of the oil around the well bore. After a period of time the well is opened to produce oil. The change in oil property, the viscosity, promotes mobility of oil to flow but gets dissipated after a period of time. This necessitates, the process to be repeated in cycles to increase recovery and hence the name cyclic steam stimulation (CSS). The number and duration of cycles, however, vary depending on the type of reservoir rock and oil properties. The EOR method involves a single well used as an injector and then as producer and is more suited for thick reservoirs and at moderate depth. The CSS is also known as 'huff-n-puff' or cycle steam injection (CSI) method.

Steam Assisted Gravity Drainage (SAGD)

It **is** an advanced method of steam simulation which requires a pair of horizontal wells, one a few meters structurally above the other. High pressure steam is continuously injected into the

upper wellbore to heat the heavy oil for reducing viscosity and mobilize it to the lower wellbore by gravity, for production. The method is better suited for horizontal wells where greater length of reservoir is accessible for the purpose of displacing more oil to recover.

Steam Flooding

Steam flooding method uses two sets of wells, one set to inject steam (injectors) that drives the oil to the other set meant for production. It differs from the cyclic steam simulation (CSS) in the functioning of the process. It is a combination of enhanced oil recovery (EOR) and secondary recovery method where after lowering the viscosity of oil, the high temperature steam is displaced by steam and hot water which drive the oil to the production well (Zaydullin 2013). Cyclic steam injection, steam flooding and Steam-Assisted Gravity Drainage (SAGD) methods are widely used recovery methods of heavy and extra-heavy oil production in sandstone reservoirs depending the reservoir geometry- type of rocks, thickness and depth of occurrence.

In-Situ Combustion (ISC)

Also known as fire flooding, in- situ combustion (ISC) is yet another thermal EOR process which involves burning part of the oil in-situ in the formation to recover rest of the oil. The in-situ fire is kept burning by continuously injecting oxygen enriched air through a well to lower the viscosity of the unburned oil in the vicinity, promoting mobility to flow (Zhang et al. 2019). The process is similar to that in the steam-flooding process except for the steam, instead of being injected from outside is produced within the reservoir by the burning fire. Steam is generated by vaporization of formation water during in-situ combustion and oil is driven towards the production well by the steam of combusted gases and the water. ISC mechanisms are largely a function of oil composition and rock mineralogy, the geological parameters playing a major role in the combustion process (Zhang et al. 2019).The

ISC process is usually complex and it is difficult to monitor and control the combustion front that makes the oil flow into the well.

Tight Oil/ Gas

Tight oil/gas is normal crude oil or gas trapped in tight reservoirs which are essentially very low permeable, low porous formations, mostly found on land. The reservoirs may include sandstones, siltstones, mudstones, carbonates and shales. Tight gas reservoirs producing mainly dry natural gas and are more common though significant quantities of gas also are produced from low-permeability carbonates, shales, and coal seams (Holditch 2006).Oil and gas in tight shale reservoirs, however, may be better termed 'shale oil/gas' to differentiate it from 'tight oil/gas'. Shale oil and gas has become an economical source of hydrocarbon and is separately described in Chapter ("Shale Oil and Gas, Oil Shale and Gas Hydrates"). 'Tight gas sands' are also sometimes referred as 'basin-centered gas accumulations' (BCGA), though BCGAs are uniquely different and are discussed under the head below. Gas in coal seams is known as coal-bed methane (CBM) and is deliberated in the chapter at the end.

Oil/Gas Production

While heavy oils are difficult to produce due to the low mobility of the fluid, tight oils and gas are hard to flow because of the low permeability of the rock. Consequently tight oil/gas reservoirs require unique stimulation processes and unlike in heavy oil, the secondary recovery technique involves increasing the permeability of the reservoir matrix rock instead of promoting the mobility of the fluid to flow. This is usually achieved by hydraulic fracturing and acidizing the tight formation to improve permeability. Fracturing, also known as "fracking" is described under shale oil and gas dealt in Chapter ("Shale Oil and Gas, Oil Shale and Gas Hydrates"). Acidizing involves pumping acids in to the well to dissolve calcite cement in carbonate rocks such as the limestones and dolomites. During process

of diagenesis grains in the rocks get cemented resulting in poor porosity and permeability of rocks. Acid besides dissolving cements can also create vugs in the carbonates, resulting in increased pore space and connectivity allowing more passage for hydrocarbon to flow. However, acidizing in carbonate rocks can be tricky and may also result in other unanticipated effects such as producing hydrogen sulfide gas (H_2S), which would damage the pipelines flowing oil and gas. Detailed knowledge of the rock minerology and rock physics, particularly the geomechanical rock properties are essential before venturing acidization.

Seismic Role

Most unconventional reservoirs are discovered only after drilling which is usually targeted for conventional prospects. Post drilling, the formation evaluation from well logs and the testing results showing no fluid influx confirm heavy oil and the tight reservoirs having low matrix porosity, permeability and hydrocarbon saturation. While the conventional prospects are easy to identify from seismic, it may be difficult to foretell unconventional reservoirs and differentiate them on the basis of porosity, permeability and viscosity from the seismic in the early stage of exploration. However, heavy oil and tight sand reservoirs are likely to show high velocity and density though gas saturation can offset the response in the latter case. With known and calibrated geology from a drilled well in the area, seismic can help identify and delineate heavy oil and tight oil prospects based on strong amplitudes and high impedance.

While tight reservoirs are artificially fractured and acidized, the heavy/extra heavy oil reservoirs are treated with thermal methods to produce. Seismic can help monitor secondary and enhanced recovery processes of fracturing (see Chapter "Shale Oil and Gas, Oil Shale and Gas Hydrates") and thermal heating. Success of thermal methods depends on the efficiency of the thermal front that sweeps through the volume of oil reservoir, in heating the oil sufficiently to mobilize flow. It is therefore necessary to ensure the heat front generated at the injector well sweeps the oil to the desired production well to allow flow. Sometimes faults, fissures, and permeable layers present in the heterogeneous formation surrounding the reservoir may divert or dissipate the heat resulting in poor production despite incurring huge expenditure. Seismic cross- well tomography can assist in monitoring the heat front in in such circumstances.

Cross-Well Tomography

Cross-well tomography (see Chapter "Borehole Seismic Techniques") provides a geological cross section of the formation between the two wells and in the event of the sweep not being effective, the tomography enables to identify the possible factors that obstruct heat transmission such as faults, permeable paths and heterogeneity in the subsurface rocks between the injector and the producer well. Heavy oil in formations behaves as semisolid ad exhibits higher seismic amplitude and velocity but after heat is applied the oil becomes less viscous, resulting in lowering the seismic properties. The low velocity track in the travel-time tomogram would thus monitor the path of the heat front. But monitoring heat front would need two surveys one before and the other after, similar to time lapse 3D. The seismic can thus help in making decisions to change or redesign the plan to achieve the goal.

Basin-Centered Gas Accumulations (BCGAs)

Basin-centered gas accumulations (BCGAs) are essentially low permeable, gas saturated tight reservoirs with abnormal pressures and other unique characteristics. The BCGAs are reported mostly in USA and are well researched. Though BCGAs are categorized as unconventional reservoirs, they have all the components of a petroleum system similar to that of conventional reservoirs, but with some noteworthy differences

in the type of accumulations. Law (2002), who has extensively studied the accumulations, in his seminal paper characterizes the BCGAs as regionally pervasive gas saturated accumulations in abnormally pressured low permeability reservoirs and commonly without presence of down-dip water. BCGAs are also referred as 'tight gas sands', 'deep basin gases' and 'continuous accumulations'. However, the nomenclatures do not encompass and satisfy all the characteristics of BCGAs (Law 2002). The terminologies were used by criteria based on typical features of the discovered accumulations. For instance, BCGAs are known to occur at moderate depths, ~ 2450–3500 m in Greater Green River Basin and ~ 1980–3660 m in Appalachian Basin (Law 2002), which are not deep enough in the basin (Law 2002). Similarly BCGAs occurrences are not always continuous as they are known to occur as discrete layers in Mesaverde Cretaceous sands in San Juan basin (Hart 2006). Some BCGAs also show departures such as having free water below the gas (Law 2002).However, the most common unique characters of all BCGAs are that these are low permeability reservoirs, abnormally (either over or under) pressured and occurring down-dip from regionally known water-saturated rocks. With such widely varying characteristics of the BCGAs discovered, the exact mechanism of their occurrence seems complex and yet to be fully understood.

Types of BCGAs

BCGAs are of two types, *direct* and *indirect*, based on their source rock characteristics. *Direct* BCGAs, result from gas-prone (kerogen III) sources such as humic coal beds and carbonaceous shales while the *indirect* BCGAs are formed from liquid prone source such as lacustrine and marine shales with kerogen I and II type (Law 2002). Source rock is the critical factor causing the different characteristics of the two types of BCGAs. This is because the type of source behaves differently in the pressure-temperature mechanism during burial and thermal maturity stages for generating gas. While gas in *direct* BCGAs is generated from the source with kerogen type III, gas in *indirect* BCGAs is caused from thermal cracking of oil generated from the kerogen type I and II source. Consequently, the BCGAs, controlled by the type of source, differ in their basinal disposition for accumulation contingent to migration distance and type of seal. Most of the known accumulations in USA belong to the *direct* type though there may be hybrid systems in which gas-prone and liquid-prone sources both contributed to BCGAs (Law 2002).

'Direct' BCGAs

Direct BCGAs with gas prone kerogen as source are likely to occur in the basinal lows, proximal to the generating source situated at basin centres and entailing short distance migration. With increasing burial depth, the generated gas is expelled and migrates to nearby low permeable sandstone reservoirs for accumulation. The accumulation process involves displacing free water in the reservoir and developing overpressures, the mechanism described below. This also explains why most BCGA reservoirs are found without water contact. Another unique aspect of *direct* BCGAs is the trapping mechanism, the overpressures at the top of gas accumulation behave as the seal and consequently they do not require structural or stratigraphic traps with lithological seals. The high pressured seal is transitional and typically cuts across the strata (Fig. 3).

'Indirect' BCGAs

Indirect BCGAs, on the other hand, controlled by oil prone source, may have short or long migration of gas which has generated from thermal cracking of oil in a later metagenesis stage due to increasing depth of burial. These accumulations, unlike *direct* BCGAs are buoyancy driven similar to process of normal oil accumulation. These accumulations need lithology related trapping mechanism, as structural or stratigraphic traps and may occur without or with down-dip water contacts similar to conventional reservoirs.

Abnormal Pressure and BCGAs Reservoirs

Abnormal Pressure (High Pressured)

High pressured formations are commonly compaction related and are caused by confined pore water under specific geologic conditions (Chapter "Seismic Wave and Rock-Fluid Properties"). However, generation of hydrocarbon in the source rock during thermal cracking of kerogen during metagenesis also causes high pressures, a process believed to be the main enabler for expulsion (Chapter "Seismic Stratigraphy and Seismo-Tectonics in Petroleum Exploration"). With increasing burial depth, as more and more gas is generated and expelled, it migrates to nearby low permeable sandstone reservoirs. At some stage when the gas generated and expelled are high, at a rate exceeding the rate at which gas from the reservoir is moved updip by migration, it ensues high pressure. As the updip migration is relatively a slower process due to low permeability of the reservoir, the expelled gas pressure exceeds the capillary pressure of pore water and forces the free water out resulting in gas-saturated overpressured accumulations (Law 2002; Bartberger et al. 2002). As regards to low abnormal pressure accumulations, both direct and indirect BCGAs, post accumulation may undergo uplifts and erosions causing loss of good amount of gas and result in under- pressures.

BCGAs Reservoirs

BCGAs are in tight reservoirs of low matrix porosity and permeability and usually comprise of sandstones and siltstones deposited under environment ranging from fluvial to marine. The reservoirs may be thin, lenticular and isolated layers or may be of considerable thickness consisting of vertically stacked multiple reservoirs embedded in thick highly rich organic shales. The reservoir properties would vary accordingly, depending the on depositional environment and style. Thick blanket sands such as delta front and beach sands are expected to have better lateral continuity compared to lenticular fluvial channel sands. In thick vertically stacked multiple reservoirs of *direct* BCGAs, presence of interbedded

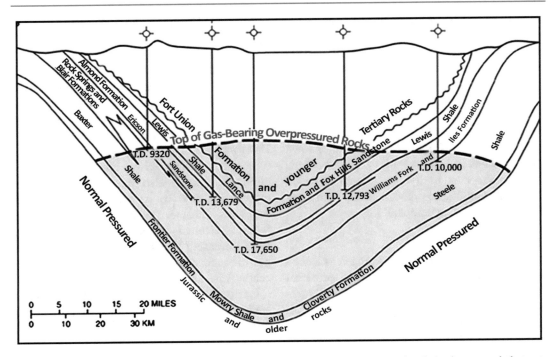

Fig. 3 Geologic profile Illustrating occurrence of '*direct*' BCGAs in overpressured formation at the basin centre. Note the unique, characteristic of BCGAs with the top of water-bearing layers, however, are not uncommon (Law 2002).

overpressured gas formation behaving as seal that cuts across formations. The 'direct' BCGAs do not need a trap with lithographic cap (after Law 2002)

The tight sandstone reservoirs need hydraulic fracturing (Chapter "Shale Oil and Gas, Oil Shale and Gas Hydrates") for gas production. Stacked thick sandstones may also develop natural fractures under tectonics which promotes permeability. Fractures can also develop in the reservoirs where high rate of gas generation is sufficient to achieve critical pore pressure and create fractures (Cumella and Jay 2020). The locales of natural fractures that enhance productivity by promoting permeability are termed 'sweet spots'. Such 'sweet spots' may warrant horizontal or slant wells to encounter maximum swarms of fracture for better productivity.

Role of Seismic

Traditionally, deeper synclinal part of many basins are overlooked for exploration, for reasons which may include lack of structural highs, paucity of good reservoirs, expensive drilling for large target depths, likely overpressured formations and down-dip disposition to proven water bearing formations up-dip on the flanks. Nevertheless, the basin-centered gas accumulations, in particular the *direct* BCGA, can be interesting because the explorer is not required to evaluate elements of conventional hydrocarbon accumulation such as reservoir quality (porosity and permeability) and areal extent, fluid type and saturation and trap seals as these factors are immaterial. On the upside, the advantage is, BCGAs are laterally extensive with massive resource potential and can be an alluring gas play. However, the prime requisites for identification of BCGAs plays are the presence of rich source rocks, proximally located sandstone/ siltstones and requisite thermal maturity for gas generation and overpressured conditions that can be assessed from seismic.

Source and Reservoir Detection

Conjoined analysis of seismic facies analysis and seismo-tectonics (Chapter "Seismic Stratigraphy and Seismo-Tectonics in Petroleum Exploration") can evaluate the regional geologic setup of depositional environment and assess the source and its type, reservoirs and the overpressured regimes to identify prospective BCGA plays. Organic rich shales, the humic coal beds and carbonaceous shales, the prime requisites for BCGAs are normally soft formations of low seismic impedance whereas, the tight sandstone and siltstone reservoirs are of higher impedance. Ideally, the high impedance reservoirs embedded in thick low impedance source rocks would generate strong contrasts and would be well noticed in seismic as alternating reflections of strong amplitudes.

Overpressure Detection

Overpressured formations have low seismic properties and are usually identified from sonic velocity and density logs (Chapter "Seismic Wave and Rock-Fluid Properties") The change in trend showing lowering of velocity and density indicates undercompacted rocks and velocity reversal and constant density with increasing depth are typical of overpressured rock sections (Fig. 4a). Overpressured sections can also be detected from seismic stacking velocities (Fig. 4b) which does not show the expected increase in stack velocity with depth. Velocity volumes from high resolution 3D seismic data can be extracted and analyzed for pore pressures to predict overpressure (Chapter "Evaluation of High-resolution 3D and 4D Seismic Data"). Integrated analysis of regional geology, seismic stratigraphy and seismo-tectonics analysis for depositional and tectonic styles, depth of burial and regional thermal gradient for thermal maturity can help assess potential plays of these unconventional accumulations.

Fracture Detection, 'Sweet Spots'

Although BCGA have large areal extents, it may not be economically productive everywhere, particularly if the reservoirs are isolated and discrete. Tectonics related natural fractures in the reservoir, as mentioned earlier, can improve recovery and such locales called 'sweet spot's, are important to be delineated. Seismic attributes such as coherence and curvatures are widely used to map small faults and fractures (Chapter "Analysing Seismic Attributes") from 3D seismic data which can be useful in delineating the 'Sweet spots'. Swarms of natural fractures were found associated with subtle structural features in San Juan Basin, Wyoming, USA and the 'sweet spots' were delineated by mapping such subtle structural features from seismic by curvature attributes (Hart 2006). Relatively lowered seismic properties may also provide clues to 'sweet spots' in the tight sand reservoirs and may be validated by Class 1 AVO for gas saturation.

Coal-Bed Methane

Coal-bed methane (CBM), is also referred as coal seam gas (CSG) is a form of natural gas extracted from coal beds and has become an important source of energy in many countries. Coal beds have poor matrix porosity and permeability and acting as both source and reservoir rocks for methane, are classified under unconventional reservoirs. Coal is product due to transformation of vegetal organic matters of kerogen type III undergoing depth of burial subjected to increased heat and pressure over a long period of geologic time. During coalification process, the transformation generates large quantities of methane which may be thermogenic or biogenic depending on generation mechanism. Methane, generated as a result of thermal maturation of organic matter in catagenesis phase is called thermogenic (Chapter "Seismic stratigraphy and Seismo-tectonics in Petroleum Exploration"). Biogenic methane, on the other hand is generated by bacterial action on the coal beds occurring at shallow depth in the early stages of diagenesis.

The transformation process undergoes four stages of coalification subjected to increasing vertical pressure and temperature under continuing depth of burial. These are known as peat, lignite, bituminous and anthracite. Thermogenic

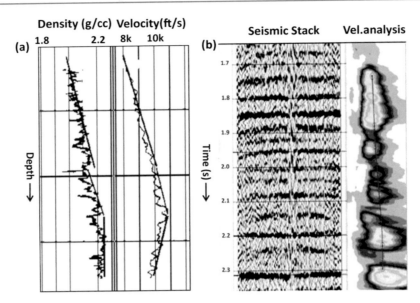

Fig. 4 Figure showing (**a**) the trends in sonic velocity and density logs and (**b**) seismic stacked segment with NMO velocity analysis. (**a**) The top line marks trend of normal pressured rocks, the middle for undercompacted and the last line for overpressured rocks. Note in the last leg, the density shows no change with increase in depth while velocity reverses, typical of overpressured sections. (**b**) NMO velocity analysis (right panel) used for picking velocity for seismic stack (left panel). The velocity panel shows no increase in velocity with depth, typical of overpressured sections (after Chopra and Huffman 2006)

methane generation begins around the sub-bituminous stage and increases significantly during the course of formation of high volatile bituminous coals to anthracite (Nikols et al. 1990). Beyond this further increase of burial temperature leads to a reduction of the amount of thermally generated methane.

The Coal Reservoir

Due to poor matrix porosity of coal, the methane generated is mostly adsorbed within the micro-pores of the coal matrix and in the lining of fractures present in the coal. This is unlike the conventional gas reservoirs where it is stored in intergranular pore spaces. Adsorption is the process of adhesion of liquid or gas molecules that are attached to the surface of a solid particle. Methane is also trapped within the fractures, called the cleat system that usually exists in the coal, as free gas or as gas dissolved in water.

Coal Cleats, the Fracture System

Cleats in the coal are the natural fractures caused by stress at the time of coalification. The cleats typically comprise of two main sets of natural fractures, known as 'face cleat' and 'butt cleat'. The coal cleat system is schematically presented in three dimensions as well as in planview showing the sets of fractures (Fig. 5). Face cleats are created parallel to maximum horizontal stress and are usually dominant, almost planar, persistent and laterally extensive. The subordinate fractures, the 'Butt cleats' are orthogonal to the 'face cleats'. The 'face cleats' are continuous throughout the coal seam while the 'butt cleats' are discontinuous, non-planar and commonly end at the intersection with face cleats (Rodrigues et al. 2014). Together they comprise the network of fracture/joint system within the coal sheets. Tertiary cleats of fractures/joints, with orientation different from that of the main cleat fractures may also be present in some coal beds. Termination of these fractures against the 'face' and 'butt' cleats

(a)

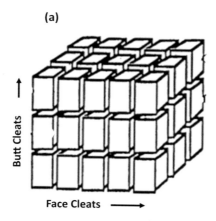

Butt Cleats

Face Cleats ⟶

(b) Butt Cleats

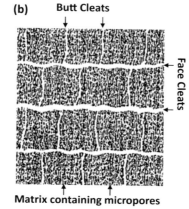

Face Cleats

Matrix containing micropores

Fig. 5 Schematics showing typical cleat system in coal (a) 3D view and (b) 2D plan view. Coal cleats consist two sets of fractures, the 'face cleats' and the 'butt cleats', caused by stress during coalification. The main fracture, the 'face cleat', parallel to maximum horizontal stress is along the bedding plane and the subordinate 'butt cleat', orthogonal to it. The cleat fracture network (a) and coal micropores (b) control storage and permeability for production of methane (Nikols et al. 1990)

suggest that they were formed later in time (Mandal et al. 2004). Large scale faults cutting across the coal beds and other strata with attendant fractures/joints may also be present due to tectonic activities and/or unloading of overburden during uplift and erosion, post coalification. The tertiary cleats and faults when present, augment density of the cleat fracture network and promote permeability. In Jharia coal field, India, of Gondwana age, four types of natural fractures consisting of face, butt, tertiary cleats and other fractures are reported based on C.T scan studies of cores (Mandal et al. 2004).

Cleat Porosity and Permeability

Coal matrix consists of micropores and has little primary inter granular porosity (Fig. 5b). The cleats present, however, provide secondary (fracture) porosity, usually of the order of 1–3%, and together with the micropores provide mostly the storage space for methane for adsorption in the molecular structure of the coal or in the lining of cleat fractures present in coal. Coal is thus usually modeled as dual porosity reservoir. The cleat system, besides storage capacity, provides permeability in the reservoir and plays the major role in methane production by providing the flow pathways in the poor permeable coal matrix.

The CBM reservoir permeability may vary from a few to tens of millidarcies depending on the intensity of the cleat system. The Jharia field shows the cleat porosity is determined as 3.01 to 5.93% and permeability in the range of 0.03 to 2.88 millidarcies (Mandal et al. 2004). This is despite the reported presence of four sets of natural fractures, which indicates that cleat systems can be complicated with the fractures sets not so well networked. The cleat permeability is also influenced by anisotropy, the horizontal permeability along the 'face cleats', parallel to bedding plane being more than the permeability in the orthogonal direction of the 'butt cleats'.

The potential of a coal reservoir depends on the amount of gas that can be recovered contingent to the intrinsic properties of the coal such as rank and quality of coal, its adsorption capacity, fracture density, interconnectivity in the cleat system and the seam thickness. The coal rank and composition is also important as its geomechanical properties can impact stimulation which most coal beds need for commercial production. The ranking of coal is classified by its degree of maturity, i.e., the extent to which metamorphic transformations have taken place. Coals ranked in terms of increasing carbon content, hardness, heat content and decreasing moisture are lignite, sub-bituminous, bituminous and anthracite, anthracite taking the highest rank. Cleat networks are more likely to be well developed in low volatile bituminous coals and the least in the lowest and the highest rank, the lignite and anthracite. Depth of occurrence also plays role as coal beds with deeper burial depths are susceptible to risk of closure of cleat fractures because of increased overburden pressure and cause permeability loss.

Methane Production

Coal reservoirs require stimulation like most unconventional reservoirs to produce methane. The methane adsorbed in the micropores and cleat system is held by pressure and when a coal reservoir is drilled, the pressure declines resulting in release of methane. The desorbed gas flows to larger pores of cleat system by diffusion and then to the well head driven by normal pressure gradient (Nikols et al. 1990). Diffusion is a process of fluid flow from a region of higher to lower concentration driven by gradient of concentration. Most coal reservoirs are water saturated and the

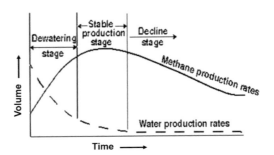

Fig. 6 Graph showing typical production curves for a US coal-bed methane well showing fluid flow volumes in different stages of production. In the initial stage of dewatering methane production is low with high volumes of water produced. After dewatering, methane production starts with little water and continues so till the decline stage is reached (*downloaded from Wikipedia*)

water needs to be pumped out to disturb the equilibrium that exits between the adsorbed methane in matrix and cleat system to initiate the diffusion process for gas to flow. Typically, the process produces water initially with little gas. After a period of time the gas production increases with commensurate decrease in water (Fig. 6).

As production continues, the pressure drop results in changing the geomechanical properties of

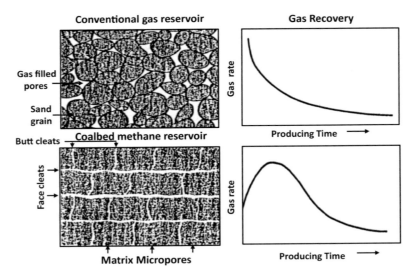

Fig. 7 Figure illustrating the contrasting methane production patterns in conventional and unconventional coal-methane reservoir. (**a**) Plan view of conventional reservoir showing intergranular porosity and linked methane production profile and (**b**) the planview of coal matrix with micropores and fracture system and production profile. Note the contrast in gas rates for the reservoirs (after Nikols et al. 1990)

the coal, affecting mainly the permeability. Permeability of coalbed methane reservoirs tends to increase with depletion of gas and strikingly in contrast to productions from conventional reservoirs where gas recovery decreases as shown in Fig. 7 (Nikols et al. 1990). This unique behavior is because of shrinkage of coal. As gas is liberated from the coal, the matrix shrinks resulting in widening the cleat fractures and ensuing increased permeability. Production from coal reservoirs depend on the efficiency of the cleat system to produce methane and more intense the interconnecting fracture network, better is the permeability for more gas production. Eventually, the productivity potential would depend on the amount of methane generated, the cleat fracture system present for storage capacity and flow (permeability) and the ability of controlling depressurization, the lowering of reservoir pressure.

However, many CBM reservoirs may not have effective cleat systems offering required permeability due to reasons ranging from lack of fracture density and interconnectivity, fractures cemented or constricted due to increased depth or other geologic reasons. In such cases, the

reservoir may require horizontal wells and expensive stimulation processes such as hydraulic fracturing (Chapter "Shale Oil and Gas, Oil Shale and Gas Hydrates"), to create cracks and fractures in the coal for facilitating better connectivity in the cleat system for improved permeability.

Seismic Role

Coal is typically a low-density and low velocity rock occurring between denser and higher velocity formations, such as sandstone and shale (Fig. 8). Coals exhibit density varying from about 1.0 to 1.4 gm/cc, whereas, the P- and S-velocities vary from around 1600–2400 m/s and 700–1400 m/s depending on the coal rank (hardness) and depth of occurrence. The coal velocities are usually lower by as much as a factor of two from the overlying and underlying rocks (Dombrowski et al. 1994). Consequently, the embedded extremely low impedance coal with large negative contrast at the top and positive at the bottom would be well imaged in seismic as a discrete reflector (Chapter "Seismic Reflection Principles—Basics") with strong amplitude response. In the initial exploration phase, coal bed methane plays can be easily detected and delineated by seismic mapping. Variations in amplitude may indicate possible change in coal thickness and character, presuming the overlying rocks continue to have similar properties laterally. The characteristic of extremely low impedance of coal is another way to map coal beds. The coal reflection offers an advantage in that it has high signal to noise ratio with strong amplitudes and low formation velocity and help extract several attributes from high resolution 3D seismic with confidence for evaluation. From known geology in the area and the depth of occurrence evinced in seismic, reasonable prediction can be done about the coal rank.

At later stage, with wells drilled, the seismic properties can be bench marked after calibration with well and petrophysical data. The high seismic amplitude and the low interval velocity may

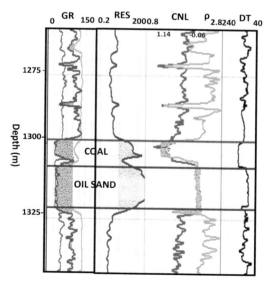

Fig. 8 Figure showing typical log response of an Eocene coal bed, India. Note the coal characteristic properties, extremely low density and velocity of coal overlain by high density and high velocity shale and underlain by sand (courtesy, ONGC, India)

be used to predict with more confidence the quality of coal seams in an area. For instance, significantly low velocity and high amplitudes attributes would imply soft coal such as lignite whereas, relatively higher velocity and lower amplitude would indicate hard coal anthracite. Both the coal ranks, however, are generally considered unsuitable for commercial methane production. A more accurate way of mapping coal ranks can be by impedance computed from seismic inversion. Further, the seismic coherence and curvature attributes can detect cleats and fracture network and help identify the favorable CBM reservoirs. Especially in cases of multiple coal beds embedded in thick formations causing as many strong reflection events, the attributes can distinguish the more potential CBM reservoirs for methane production. The sweetness attribute, based on strong impedance contrasts in rocks, can be another useful tool to map potential CBM reservoirs. The composite attribute 'sweetness 'primarily driven by stronger instantaneous amplitudes and lower instantaneous frequency (Chapter "Analysing Seismic Attributes ") can lead to thicker coal seams as potentially better CBM reservoirs and can be confirmed by AVO analysis, described below.

Seismic can also help during CBM field development stage by identifying the coal beds more suitable for fracturing and in monitoring the fracture process. Elastic parameters such as Young's modulus (E) and modulus of rigidity (μ) which denote the strength and brittleness of rocks can be estimated by seismic attributes from high resolution 3D data to delineate the favorable coal seams for fracking (Chapter "Shale Oil and Gas, Oil Shale and Gas Hydrates").

AVO Analysis for Coal

Use of AVO to authenticate 'bright spot' anomalies for gas sands is well known. Gas in low-impedance sands and with negative Poisson's ratio (Vp/Vs) contrast with respect to shale cap are characterized by Class-3 AVO anomaly, that is negative amplitudes in near trace becoming more negative with increasing offset and with negative gradient. Coal top reflections with strong negative contrast also show very high

amplitude anomalies similar to gas-sand associated 'bright spots' in normal stack sections. However, there is a major difference in the type of AVO for the two similar looking anomalies. While the Poisson's ratio contrast, which controls the AVO attributes, is negative due to gas in the sand reservoirs, in coal seam it is opposite, the contrast being positive. This is because of presence of cleats and fractures which raise the Poisson's ratio of coal (Gregory 1976). The Poisson's ratio mostly used as an index for identifying pore fluid in conventional reservoirs, can be used as indicator of fractures in rock matrix, the indispensable property in unconventional CBM reservoirs.

Laboratory measurements of dry coal samples indicate increase in compressional and shear wave velocities with increase in coal ranks while Poisson's ration decreases with increasing coal ranks (Dirgantara et al. 2011). Presence of cleat fractures, that are more likely to occur in higher rank coals, would lower both Vp and Vs but with more lowering of Vs due to reduced rigidity that leads to increased Poisson's ratio. Ramos and Davis (1997), from laboratory measurements have found higher Poisson's ratio for fractured coal than that of sand and shale and it increases with increase in fracture density (Fig. 9). Higher Poisson's ratio for the fractured coal thus ensues a positive Poisson's ratio contrast against overlying shale or sand and behaves as class - 4 AVO anomaly (Chapter "Shear Wave Seismic, AVO and Vp/Vs Analysis"). The AVO attributes for a CBM reservoir would show strong negative amplitude at near trace which decreases with increasing offset and with positive gradient (Fig. 10).

Coal depositions are typically wide spread over swampy back-bay lands in fluvio-deltaic environment and often the coal seams are vertically stacked with intervening sands or shales. The individual coal seams may be discontinuous and diachronous and in varying quality and quantity of organic matter depending on local structural reliefs and the influx of source and amount of vegetal matters. Coal, for this reason is often not regarded as a geologic marker. The different coal beds, thus, can be varying in their

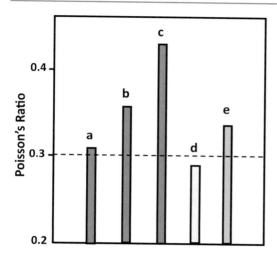

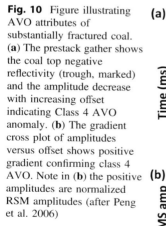

Fig. 9 Histogram displaying Poisson's ratio of coal with varying fracture densities and compared to sandstone and shale. (**a**) Coal with little fractures, (**b**) with moderate and (**c**) with substantial fractures, (**d**) sandstone reservoir and (**e**) shale. The lab-measured values show increase in Poisson's ratio with increasing fracture density. The Poisson's ratio for densely fractured coal is substantially higher than shale and water saturated sand stone (modified after Peng et al. 2006)

characteristics and mechanical properties and all of them may not have the requisite cleat-fracture network qualified to be CBM reservoir.

Constrained with well data the seismic attributes from 3D data can be useful in identifying the fractured coal beds and the 'sweet spots 'in the area validated by the simple and convenient method of AVO attribute cross-plots. Faults, cleats and fractures are the most important aspect og CBM reservoirs have dual favorable effect on CBM reservoirs as they promote storage and permeability, though in some cases the faults may lead to leakage of gas (Peng et al. 2006).

Limitations

Rock-fluid properties reported are mostly empirical, area-specific and/or based on lab-measured samples which may be different from the in-situ rock characteristics. Consequently, the modelled seismic responses may not always be exact and mismatch with real seismic data. Furthermore, the laboratory measurements pertain to the static elastic modulii of rock samples, and can be different from the dynamic moduli of the in-situ rock. It may also be mentioned that mechanical properties are more important than physical, particularly in monitoring secondary and enhanced recovery processes.

Fig. 10 Figure illustrating AVO attributes of substantially fractured coal. (**a**) The prestack gather shows the coal top negative reflectivity (trough, marked) and the amplitude decrease with increasing offset indicating Class 4 AVO anomaly. (**b**) The gradient cross plot of amplitudes versus offset shows positive gradient confirming class 4 AVO. Note in (**b**) the positive amplitudes are normalized RSM amplitudes (after Peng et al. 2006)

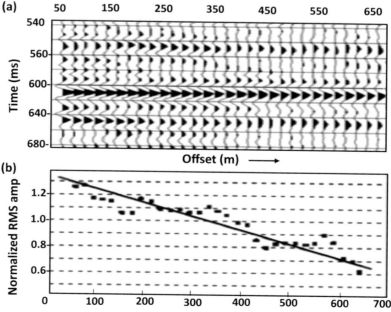

Relation between Poisson's ratio and fracture density in CBM reservoir may not be simple as coal is a complex rock. The fracture parameters such as, the size, orientation, type of fracture (open, closed, mineralized), and fluid content though influence the seismic response, factoring these elements in seismic modelling for fractures in coal under varying overburden and pore pressure can be difficult. Properties of coal and the overlying rocks can also vary depending on depositional environment, depth of burial and geologic age. For instance Permo-carboniferous Gondwana coals at deeper depth can exhibit vastly differ properties than of relatively younger Eocene coals at shallower depths. Poisson's ratio contrasts of coal can also vary with different cap rocks (Peng et al. 2006), such as shale and sand that rapidly show lateral facies change, typical of the fluvio-deltaic environment in which coals are deposited. This could impede reliability in predicting cleat fractures laterally away from the well.

References

Bartberger CE, Dyman TS, Condon SM (2002) Is there a basin-centered gas accumulation in cotton valley group sandstones, Gulf Coast Basin, U.S.A.

Chopra S, Alan H (2006) Velocity determination for pore pressure prediction. CSEG Rec 31, p

Cumella S, Jay S (2020) Geology and mechanics of the basin-centered gas accumulation. Piceance Basin, Colorado, Search and Discovery

Dirgantara F, Batzle ML, Curtis JB (2011) Maturity characterization and ultrasonic velocities of coals: 81st Annual International Meeting. SEG, Expanded Abstr 30:2308–2312

Dombrowski B, Dresen L, Rüter H (1994) Seismic coal exploration Part B: In-seam seismics: Elsevier Science Inc. Tarrytown

Gregory AG (1976) Fluid saturation effect on dynamic elastic properties of sedimentary rocks. Geophysics 41:895–921

Hart SB (2006) Seismic expression of fracture-swarm sweet spots, Upper Cretaceous tight gas reservoirs, San Juan Basin. AAPG Bull 90:1519–1534

Holditch SA (2006) Tight gas sands. J Petrol Technol 58 (6):86–93. https://doi.org/10.2118/103356-MS

Law BE (2002) Basin centred gas system. AAPG Bull 86:1891–1920

Mandal D, Tewari DC, Rautela MS (2004) Analysis of micro-fractures in coal for coal bed methane exploitation in Jharia coal field. In: 5th SPG conference, pp 904–909

NIkols DJ, Treasure S, Stuhec S, Goulet DE (1990) Coal bed methane in Alberta- what's it all about? Seminar proceedings in Alberta

Peng S, Chen H, Yang R, Gao Y, Chen X (2006) Factors facilitating or limiting the use of AVO for coal-bed methane. Geophysics, v 71(4):c49–c56. https://doi.org/10.1190/1.2217137

Ramos ACB, Davis TL (1997) 3-D AVO analysis and modeling applied to fracture detection in coal-bed methane reservoirs: Geophysics 62:1683–1695

Rodrigues CF, Laiginhas CM, Fernandes MJ, Lemos de Sousa Dinis MAP (2014) The coal cleat system: a new approach to its study. J Rock Mech Geotechn Eng 6 (3):208–218. https://doi.org/10.1016/j.jrmge.2014.03.005

Santos RG, Loh W, Bannwart AC, Trevisan OV (2014) An overview of heavy oil properties and its recovery and transportation methods. Braz J Chem Eng 31:571–590

Zaydullin R (2013) Thermal oil extraction, course work. Stanford University

Zhang X, Liu Q, Fan Z, Liu Q (2019) An in situ combustion process for recovering heavy oil using scaled physical model. J Petroleum Explorat Prod Technol 9:2681–2688

Shale Oil and Gas, Oil Shale and Gas Hydrates

Abstract

Shale oil and gas reservoirs have become one of the fastest growing economically viable energy resource. Traditionally considered as a source and cap rock for conventional hydrocarbon accumulations, shale by itself can be a reservoir by hosting the remnant part of oil and gas it generates which could not be expelled. Shale prospectivity is an arduous task for geoscientists to assess and more challenging for engineers to produce economically. Shale being a tight reservoir devoid of permeability, it requires hydraulic fracturing (fraking) to produce albeit at huge cost and environmental damage. Types of shale and their rock properties that make them potential prospects to produce hydrocarbon are analyzed. Seismic role in shale exploration by providing leads to shale plays, characterization of shale reservoirs and monitoring fracking for hydrocarbon production is deliberated.

Shale unconventional reservoirs include shale oil and gas and kerogen rich 'Oil Shale' sometimes slackly referred as 'shale oil'. It is basically different from shale oil; while shale oil produces natural oil from shale reservoirs, oil shale which contains kerogen, is to be treated to extract the 'synthetic oil' from it and is included in the chapter.

Methane gas hydrate, another unconventional reservoir, is a naturally occurring solid substance consisting predominantly of methane gas and water, in the form of ice-like crystals of water. Hydrates occur under conditions of low temperature and high pressure and are found in cold environments, in the ocean in deep-waters and on land beneath permafrost in arctic regions. Oceanic gas hydrates occur more commonly worldwide and are discussed in detail while the rare Permafrost hydrates are briefly outlined.

Seismic 'BSR' (bottom simulating reflector) plays an indispensable part in identifying and delineating the oceanic gas hydrates in offshore and its unique characteristics are discussed with seismic illustrations. The unconventional reservoirs of gas hydrates, with a massive prognostic resource, however, is in nascent stage with engineering technologies still evolving for economic production.

Technological advances and economic necessity have forced unconventional shale reservoirs to become economically viable energy resource, the shale oil and gas being the fastest growing resource. Shale oil and gas production in massive scale in USA and shale gas production in China in the last decade, have established it as feasible energy source, notwithstanding the high costs and ecological problems they cause. Shale oil and gas plays have since enticed exploration of unconventional oil and gas in many parts of the world.

N. C. Nanda, *Seismic Data Interpretation and Evaluation for Hydrocarbon Exploration and Production*, Advances in Oil and Gas Exploration & Production, https://doi.org/10.1007/978-3-030-75301-6_14

Shale Oil and Gas

Though shales are traditionally considered as source and cap rocks for oil and gas accumulations in conventional reservoirs, under some circumstances it can also behave as reservoir for hydrocarbon habitat. Hydrocarbons are generated by decomposition of kerogen in source rocks, under high pressure and temperature and expelled from the source (primary migration), migrate into reservoir rocks (secondary migration) in structural or stratigraphic traps for accumulation. However, a sizable part of the hydrocarbon generated, may not be expelled and continue to reside in the source, the shale. It thus behaves uniquely as the source, the reservoir and the cap rock and the self-contained hydrocarbon habitat is referred as unconventional shale reservoir.

Shale Reservoirs

Shale oil and gas, as mentioned earlier, are the remnant hydrocarbons trapped in the source rock. Hydrocarbon expulsion from the source is initiated and facilitated by fractures, created in shales due to increasing pore pressure of oil and gas generated by breaking of kerogen during thermal maturity, a process known as catagenesis (Chapter "Seismic Stratigraphy and Seismo-Tectonics in Petroleum Exploration"). For reasons, ranging from geological to geochemical, such as lack of nearby permeable reservoirs, inadequate high pore pressure to create sufficient fractures, the type of source under thermal maturity, all amount of oil and gas generated may not be able to be expelled. This leads to sizable amount of oil/gas being left behind, stuck in the shale. The trapped hydrocarbons in the shale remain adsorbed, similar to the process as in coal-bed methane reservoirs, onto the clay/kerogen particles and in free fluid state in the pore spaces and fractures. Because of poor matrix permeability, shale oil and gas are difficult to produce without stimulation, which is required to create fractures artificially in the host rock similar to that done to in tight reservoirs, for

extraction of hydrocarbon. The Shale oil/gas, for this reason, is referred sometimes as 'tight oil/gas' but the term can be misleading. Tight oil/gas refers to basically oil/gas occurring in conventional reservoirs such as sandstone, siltstone and carbonate formations which because of their very low permeability and porosity are called tight reservoirs. However, 'shale oil and gas' reservoirs, strictly should not be classified under 'tight reservoirs' as it is characteristically an unconventional reservoir and vary in several aspects from the conventional tight reservoirs. Shale gas reservoirs similar to conventional natural gas reservoirs can consist of mostly dry gas, methane or wet gas with higher compounds of hydrocarbon depending on stage of thermal maturity, metagenesis or catagenesis (Chapter "Seismic Stratigraphy and Seismo-Tectonics in Petroleum Exploration"). Shale reservoirs, unlike conventional reservoirs, do not require structural and/or stratigraphic trap for accumulation. Nonetheless, like conventional reservoirs they need preservation for not being destroyed by subsequent tectonic activities post accumulation.

Shale Prospect Appraisal

Shales are one of the most extensively deposited rocks found all over the world. However, all shales are not prospective as the potential hydrocarbon shales are limited to certain geologic factors. Since shale plays do not require structural or stratigraphic traps for accumulation they do not require conventional prospect appraisals. Evaluation of reservoir, cap and migration time and pathways, the crucial risk elements in prospecting for conventional oil and gas accumulations are immaterial. Despite these advantages and the fact that shale deposits are most widely pervasive and regionally extensive offering massive resource base, assessment of their potential may be an arduous task for the geoscientists. This is because it requires different kind of evaluation which is of the type and nature of shale rock and the depositional environment, its composition and minerology to assess physical and mechanical properties. More significantly, the shale prospects can be even more challenging for the engineers to produce oil and gas economically which is expensive and severely damaging to environment.

How and where does then an explorationist start looking for shale plays? It is important that firstly the shale depositional environment is assessed because some specific type of shales with requisite properties are only capable of producing oil and or gas. Shales are deposited under varied environments of fluvial, lacustrine, deltaic and marine and at shallow or deeper depths under oxic and anoxic conditions. Consequently, the shales vary widely in their rock properties and mineralogies. The depositional environment is important as it has direct and primary impact on the type and amount of organic matter (kerogen) the shale contains, to be considered good source of hydrocarbon generation. To be prospective reservoir, which needs fracturing for production, the shale rock must comprise of specific minerals that provide brittleness for facilitating fracturing under stimulation.

Potential oil/gas shales are essentially required to be rich in organic matters, contain minerals such as quartz, feldspar and carbonates that promotes brittleness and low in clay content for lesser ductility of the rock. Brittle minerals make the shale conducive to breakability, a necessary requisite for hydraulic fracturing (fracking) to produce hydrocarbon. The brittle minerals also make shales under tectonic stress, more amenable to develop natural fractures in random patterns that create swarm of fractures in promoting permeability.

Type of Shale

As mentioned, shale properties vary depending on their depositional environment and consequently in their degree of prospectivity. Nonmarine carbonaceous shales though usually have higher organic carbon (TOC) content than marine shales, the latter is considered better potential for shale prospectivity. High TOC indicates the organic richness but does not indicate the type or quality of the organic matter, the kerogen. The

amount of organic matter, the total organic carbon present and its quality (kerogen) influences the type, quality, and amount of hydrocarbons generated. These elements determine the source potential and rate them accordingly. Preservation of the organic matter without degradation (oxic conditions) is also an important factor for a quality source. Marine shales, deposited under anoxic condition are likely to contain high quality organic matter of type 1 and 2 kerogen and with high brittle minerals and low clay contents are generally considered better prospects.

Depth of Occurrence

The depth of occurrence is a factor for assessing the source generation potential for the prospective shale play. Hydrocarbon is generated by transformation of organic matter under sufficient temperature, a process known as thermal maturity which depends on depth of burial and ambient regional thermal gradient. Contingent to cooking history and type of organic matter, hydrogen generated can be oil or gas of thermogenic and biogenic nature. Biogenic gas is formed mostly in shallow depths by action of anaerobic micro-organisms during the early burial phase (diagenesis) without sufficient temperature. Oil and gas, on the other hand are formed when the source is buried deeper subjected to increased pressure and temperature during catagenesis. Further burial results in producing dry gas due to thermogenic breakdown of oil at greater depths and temperatures in the metagenesis stage (Chapter "Seismic Stratigraphy and Seismo-Tectonics in Petroleum Exploration").

Clay Content and Minerology

Shales mostly contain clay and the clay content with its minerology impact the physical and mechanical properties of shale in shale prospecting for hydrocarbon. Post deposit, tectonics, subsidence & diagenesis also affect shale properties by altering the clay minerals affecting prospectivity. Clay, is soft and compliant and high clay content tends to make shale ductile reducing its efficacy for fracturing. Clay-rich shales can also hinder production adversely due to the geomechanical properties of clay minerals. Clay minerals such as illite and montmorillonite being affable to contact with water are inclined to swell up during hydraulic fracturing which results in reduction of porosity and increase in tortuosity, and ultimately impeding permeability. Nonetheless, on the upside, clay has a huge positive effect in that more of clay in shale offers more storage space in the matrix for hydrocarbon to be adsorbed. The shale oil/gas production potential is dependent to large extent on the total pore space available in the shale and on pore-size distribution, all of which are linked to the amount of clay and the clay minerals present (Zhang et al. 2017). Clay, thus has an important part in shale prospecting, playing a dual role of conflicting nature; in one way promoting hydrocarbon storage space and at the same time hampering brittleness to fracture ensuing permeability reduction.

Though shale oil and gas reservoirs do not require traps, they may, however, need preservation of hydrocarbon. Many shale gas pools discovered in Sichuan basin in China were reported non-commercial because of lack of proper preservation linked to tectonic deformations. Multi-cycle tectonic stress has resulted in lateral variation of reservoir thickness posing challenges to fracturing the thin shale reservoirs (Zuqing et al. 2016).

Shale Oil/Gas Production

Primary production from shale reservoirs is not attainable and secondary recovery which is required is more difficult and expensive than of conventional oil. Unlike vertical wells drilled for conventional reservoirs, the shale reservoirs necessarily require horizontal drilling and hydraulic fracturing, known as fracking to retrieve hydrocarbon. Drilling horizontal well allows access to substantial volume of the tight reservoir while hydraulic fracturing induces fractures in the low porous - low permeable shale reservoir to facilitate fluid flow.

Fracking

Fracking is a reservoir stimulation process for secondary recovery in which a high-pressure water-based fluid is injected to the brittle rock to induce fractures as well as enlarge the pre-existing natural fractures. The fracturing fluid usually consists of water, proppants and some chemical additives as gelling agents. The induced fractures can extend up to hundreds of meters away from the wellbore in horizontal wells. The proppants commonly used are sand pellets which hold open the newly created fractures. Fracking effectively allows more pore space and inter-connectivity within the artificially created fracture network to allow fluid to flow. However, the stimulation process requires huge amount of water which after treatment is problematic for disposal and causes serious concerns of environmental damage.

Seismic Role

Shale play exploration is primarily driven by evaluation of depositional environment of shale in a basin and its tectonic history. Though shales may be pervasive covering over extensively large areas, it is required to identify the favourable locales for drilling the shale prospects. As mentioned earlier, shale prospectivity primarily and largely depends on evaluation of shale as the source which includes amount of organic matter, total organic carbon (TOC) and its type (Kerogen) and thermal maturity for generation. Characteristics of shale rock can vary laterally, particularly in nonmarine environment and influence source potential for hydrocarbon generation.

In virgin or less explored areas, the geology can be analysed with help of seismic data using seismic stratigraphy facies analysis and seismo-tectonic methods (Chapter "Seismic Stratigraphy and Seismo-Tectonics in Petroleum Exploration ") providing basin-scale overview of potential shale plays. Identification of prospective areas of shallow marine shale deposits under anoxic conditions linked to favourable kerogen type can lead to appropriate location for exploratory drilling to start. However, quantitative estimate of shale parameters can be done after drilling of wells by synthesising multidisciplinary information from geological, geochemical, petrophysical and core data obtained from the wells.

Shale Characterization

Shale is highly heterogeneous, anisotropic and complex reservoir which requires stimulation by hydraulic fracturing to produce hydrocarbon. Successful fracking necessitates proper characterization of shale reservoir, the physical and geomechanical properties including mineral composition of the shale and the clay. Estimates of elastic modulii and in-situ horizontal stress are especially important as they impact fracture efficacy. Shale characterization requires an integrated approach to analyse information from multiple disciplines of geology, geophysics, petrophysics, rock physics, geomechanics, geochemistry & engineering. 3D seismic constrained with well data can build rock physics models (SRM) to comprehensively understand the shale parameters at play. Bench-marked with log petrophysical parameters, seismic attributes can help predict the reservoir parameters and their vertical and lateral variations, away from the well bore. Characteristic log curves of a shale reservoir signifying low sonic velocity and density, very high gamma, resistivity and neutron porosity are shown in Fig. 1. Some of the key elements of shale play that can be analyzed from seismic to assist shale characterization are discussed below.

TOC and kerogen

Total organic carbon (TOC) indicates the richness of source and is the most important player in shale prospecting. However, the type of the organic carbon, the kerogen it contains is the key element which decides the type of hydrocarbon generated. The amount of TOC with its type of kerogen and the degree of thermal maturity controls the type, quality and quantity of hydrocarbon generation which is used to estimate

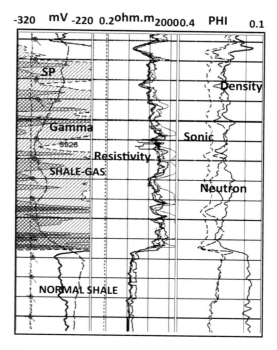

Fig. 1 Example of well log curves for a typical thick shale gas reservoir. It is characterized by extremely high Gamma, high Resistivity, low SP with low bulk density, and sonic velocity. The neutron and the sonic and density are shown In terms of derived porosity (%). Note the huge contrast in the all log motifs with those of normal shale seen below

volumetric reserves. TOC rich shale layers containing the important element kerogen can vary vertically and laterally, particularly in nonmarine environment and would need mapping to indicate priority locales for drilling. Kerogens show exceptionally low density ($\sim 1.1–1.4$ g/cc) and velocity similar to coal and TOC-rich shale layers are likely to exhibit low impedance. Such TOC layers embedded in thick shale formation can generate strong reflections with high negative amplitudes and low impedance seismic attributes. This is encouraging as several other attributes can be attempted from the strong amplitude reflection events..

TOC rich shales, besides P-velocity and density also influences shear velocities, Poisson' ratio, and anisotropy in the rock. Core samples from Woodford organic-rich black shales in

USA, measured in laboratory has shown Vp/Vs ratios decreasing with increasing TOC (Harris 2015). The TOC layers with strong amplitudes can then be validated by AVO. With negative contrasts in P-impedance and Poisson's ratio, the embedded TOC layers in shales would likely to show class 3 AVO. However, it is important the relationship between TOC and seismic impedance be established by rock physics modelling. TOC parameters derived from geochemical analysis and impedance measurements made in the lab on rock samples can indicate the empirical relationship which can be used to transform seismically derived impedance and Poisson's ratio volume into TOC volumes. Such volumes are useful as they indicate the lateral and vertical variation of TOC in the identification of the sweet spots.

Thermal Maturity

Thermal maturity indicates the transformation of organic matter to generate oil and gas under temperature and pressure (Chapter "Seismic Stratigraphy and Seismo-Tectonics in Petroleum Exploration"). Both temperature and pressure usually increase with depth when the source is buried deeper under successive layers of deposition of sediments. The burial depth and the rate of subsidence thus play an important role in thermal maturity. 3D seismic can indicate the depositional and tectonic history and help geochemists estimate the thermal maturity curves to indicate favorable prospects for drilling.

Anisotropy

Shales mostly exhibit some order of anisotropy (VTI, Chapter "Seismic Wave and Rock-Fluid Properties"). Large amount of organic matters deposited as layers parallel to bedding plane are likely to increase seismic anisotropy in the formation. High resolution 3D seismic with wide azimuth and long offset can detect anisotropy (seismic anisotropy) by detecting variations in amplitude and velocity with azimuth (AVAz, VVAz). However, to calibrate variance in anisotropy in terms of rich and poor shale may be limited (Chapter "Shear Wave Seismic, AVO and Vp/Vs Analysis").

Brittleness

Brittleness denotes the stiffness of a rock under external stress and is a requisite property of shale reservoir for hydraulic fracturing. Brittle shales with pre-existing natural fractures are considered more amenable to fracture in tensile and shear modes (Zhang et al. 2016). The degree of brittleness depends on the stiffness of rock and influences effectiveness of hydraulic fracking that ultimately impacts hydrocarbon recovery. Stiffness of a rock can be measured by its Young's modulus which is also known as stiffness modulus. Shear modulus also indicates stiffness in shear direction and both modulii can be estimated from seismic from the derived compressional and shear impedances from simultaneous inversion. However, it requires density which is usually difficult to obtain from seismic data. However, Sharma and Chopra (2015) have shown the product of Young's modulus and density, $E\rho$, which is a scaled version of $\mu\rho$ can be derived without determining the value of density Brittle shales would show high Young's modulus (stiffness)and shear modulus. E-Rho, Mu-rho and Poisson's ratio can also be computed from inversion to indicate rock stiffness and strength. While E-Rho and Mu-Rho are indicators of brittleness (stiffness) Poisson's ratio denotes strength of the rock (Chapter "Seismic Wave and Rock-Fluid Properties"). High E-Rho and Mu-Rho values complimented by low Poisson's ratio (Vp/Vs) which also does not involve density can help as indicators of brittleness. Figure 2 shows the attributes E-rho and Mu-rho, the increase indicates increasing brittleness. However, E-Rho is preferred as it is more sensitive.

Insitu Stress

In-situ stress is local confined stress in a rock and consists of the vertical effective pressure and the two orthogonal maximum and minimum horizontal tectonic stresses, (SH_{max}) and (SH_{min}). In brittle rocks, fractures would propagate in a random manner, if the rocks are not under any preferential stress orientation. However, fractures induced by fracking is influenced by the insitu pressure and as it varies from place to place, the

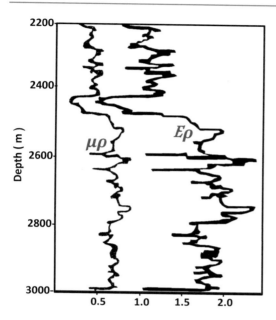

Fig. 2 Attribute curves of product of Young's modulus and density ($E\rho$) and shear modulus and density ($\mu\rho$) signifying stiffness of a rock. Both are similar and the product attributes do not need density value for their determination done from seismic inversion. Note the $E\rho$ is more sensitive and usually the preferred indicator of rock brittleness. Larger the Young's modulus higher is the brittleness(stiffness) of a rock. (after Sharma and Chopra 2015)

insitu stress needs to be determined. Zones with low stress are preferred where fractures are prone to be formed in random manner creating a fracture swarm conducive to conductivity. Insitu stresses can be estimated by mechanical earth modelling (MEM) prepared from seismic data (Chapter "Seismic Wave and Rock-Fluid Properties"). High Young's modulus and low stress areas are usually favored for fracking.

Microseismic Monitoring of 'Fracking'

However, in shale reservoirs with preexisting natural fractures/fissures, fracking may create fractures that are influenced by the natural fractures and associated local weakness planes and may not be optimal in desired dimensions and directions (Cornet and Valette 1984).It is important that fracking is carefully monitored

and controlled for fracture dimensions, azimuth and orientation confined to the reservoir only. This can be achieved by microseismic technology which has emerged as a means to effectively manage fracture operations.

Hydraulic fracturing process stresses the reservoir to crack which creates microseismic events. The microseismic events (disturbances) are recorded by sensitive detectors located in offset wells or on the surface in the form of arrays (Chapter "Borehole Seismic Techniques"). The challenge is usually to make sure that the fracture creation and growth is confined to the reservoir zones only, and make suitable modifications if required to ensure this. Microseismic monitoring is essentially to locate the microseismic events (the fractures) and their magnitude to measure the size and orientation of the fractures. Magnitude is measured by amplitudes recorded by the geophones which indicates the amount of energy released to interpret the fracture dimensions. The locations of the fractures is determined by the arrival time of the waves at the geophones which signifies the extent and orientation of the fractures created. Limitations of microseismic monitoring by seismic, however, suffers from the usual uncertainties of seismic amplitude and velocity.

Characterization of shale reservoirs is highly challenging and requires information from different disciplines such as geology, geophysics, petrophysics, rock physics, geomechanics and geochemistry & engineering. The critical properties defining a good shale reservoir are the amount and type of TOC (Kerogen), brittleness and thermal maturity which can be assessed and predicted from seismic. Clay content and minerology which play important role in impacting porosity, fracking and ultimately permeability are, however, difficult to quantify from seismic.

Oil Shale

Oil shale is a kerogen-rich shale and sometimes is slackly termed as 'shale oil' which is basically different from natural oil which is produced from shale reservoirs. Oil shale is different from shale oil in that it does not host oil as such, but contains kerogen, with the potential to extract 'synthetic shale oil' from it. As is well known, oil and gas is formed in nature by thermal cracking of kerogen, a solid organic compound in the organic material of decayed plant and animal remains, under heat and pressure over millions of years. Under unfavorable conditions such as lack of sufficient pressure and temperature, the kerogen may not crack and remain stored in the shale. Oil shale is thus a kerogen containing rock which can be cracked to crude oil artificially by applying intense heat without oxygen, a process known as pyrolysis. Heating can be done either above ground or while the oil shale is still underground (insitu) and pumped out the resulting oil. However, the extraction process so far seems to be uneconomical and oil shale is not considered as a feasible energy source. In contrast 'natural' shale oil and gases, are established unconventional energy source and are presently produced by USA and China in massive scale.

Gas Hydrates

Methane Gas hydrate is a solid, naturally occurring substance consisting predominantly of methane gas and water, in which gas molecules are trapped in ice-like crystals of water (clathrates) under requisite conditions of low temperature(<15 °C) and high pressure(>5 MPa). Gas hydrates are found primarily in two types of cold environments, in the ocean in deep-waters and beneath permafrost in arctic regions of Russia and Alaska. Oceanic gas hydrates are more common and distributed worldwide in deep-waters of continental margins whereas only a small fraction of natural gas hydrate is found on land in permafrost areas.

Oceanic Gas Hydrates

Methane gas is generated over long period of time by microorganisms which convert organic matters, the remains of the planktons living in the

ocean and buried in sediments. The methane gas is believed to be formed in the deep warm sediments and is transformed to methane hydrate in the cold upper sediment layers. As waters in the oceans up to the bottom of deep seabed are almost uniformly cold, with temperatures from 4 to 0 °C, the sea floor happens to be an ideal location for hydrate formation (Boswell and Dallimore 2014). In oceans, the temperature decreases from the surface with water depth to almost 0 °C at the sea floor and begins to rise with increasing sedimentary depth. Hydrates start forming and tend to become stable as temperature decreases with increase in pressure. Below a depth of about 350 m from the sea bottom, the zone where the temperature is <15 °C, and the pressure is adequate (>5 MPa), hydrates stabilize and occur mostly in this zone (Fig. 3). The

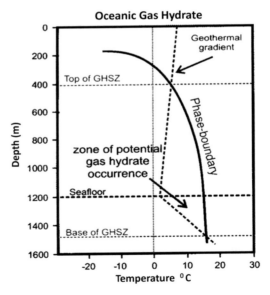

Fig. 3 Graphic illustrating temperature–pressure mechanism for formation of oceanic gas hydrate stability zone (GHSZ) in deep waters. Temperature continues to decrease below sea level till the sea floor and then starts increasing in the underlying sediments, while the pressure continues to increase. Hydrates are formed in the suitable zone of temperature less than 15 °C and pressure more than 5 MPa. It is dependent on the thermal gradient but is usually around 250–300 m below sea floor. The Phase boundary, top and bottom pf the GHSZ is shown. Beyond this depth the temperature increases more than 15 °C and hydrates break (after Amundsen and Landrø 2012, courtesy GEO ExPro)

hydrate stability zone (GHSZ), however, is limited to the phase boundary, a state of equilibrium existing between free gas-sea water (GHSZ top) and base of the gas hydrate(base of GHSZ). Below this depth, the temperature rises controlled by the geothermal gradient and averts stability ensuing in breakdown of hydrates. Hydrates also break if the water or the sea floor becomes warmer. Gas hydrates are sometimes underlain by free gas, believed due to hydrate recycling mechanism, a process of hydrates being dissociated and reformed. Gas is generated from hydrates by dissociation when the base of the GHSZ moves upward relative to hydrate-bearing sediment. Hydrate recycling is dominant where rapid rates of upward fluid flow and sea-bed uplift occur due to tectonics (RossHaacke et al. 2007).

However, according to Boswell and Collett (2006), hydrate stability zones may not be controlled only by a simple bond of uniform temperature and pressure. Gas Hydrate Stability Zones (GHSZ) are found to have a very complex geometry, with significant variability in occurrences due to lateral and vertical changes in pore water salinity and heat flow. Further, within the stability zone, the occurrence of gas hydrate is neither continuous nor random, but instead controlled by the complex interaction of factors such as temperatures, pressures, and geochemical regimes (Boswell and Collett 2006). This is important as the factor determine the mode of hydrate distribution within the stability zone that can have significant impacts on estimate of gas volume.

Occurrences

Oceanic methane hydrates occur mainly at water depths between 350 and 5000 m where the temperature and pressure conditions are usually suitable. They are found at or very close to the sea floor, as in Gulf of Mexico and many other parts of world including Pacific and Indian Ocean deep-waters. They are also known to occur buried deeply in sediments as in the Blake Ridge and Carolina gas hydrates, east of South Carolina and Georgia coast (Ruppel 2010). Gas hydrates are also found to occur as massive mounds, as in Blake Ridge accumulation, off-shore Carolinas, where the mounds lie exposed on the seafloor or beneath a very thin layer of sediment with unknown depth of extension (Boswell and Collett 2006). Oceanic gas hydrates occur in many countries, worldwide including India where the thickest and deepest gas hydrate stability zone near the Andaman Islands in the Bay of Bengal is reported (Smith 2009). Methane hydrates are not found in marginal seas and shelf areas because the pressure at the sea floor may not be sufficient for hydrate to stabilize.

Permafrost Gas Hydrates, Occurrences

Permafrost are sediments that remain permanently frozen because of profound cooling during glacial events that happened million years back. Since hydrates are primarily cold deposits, they occur in permafrost regions where requisite temperature - pressure condition prevails for the stability zone. In permafrost settings, the temperature, in contrast to in oceans, continues to increase from the surface with depth. Around 15 degrees Celsius, it meets the appropriate pressure conditions to limit the phase boundary for hydrate formation and thus the zone of potential hydrate occurrence happens to be much thicker (Fig. 4). Permafrost gas hydrates are believed to be probably formed when gas and water froze in place during ice-age cooling events. Generally, gas hydrates are more stable in fresh water than in salt water and are thicker, up to 4.5 times than the oceanic hydrates. This is because of the initial lower surface temperatures and the geothermal gradients being considerably lower compared to in the oceans (compare Fig. 3) and also due to presence of higher percentage of non-methane gases (Wanga and Lau 2020). The ambient temperature and the thickness of the frozen layer are important as these factors control formation of stable gas hydrate, their depth and thickness (Amundsen and Landrø 2012). The thickness of GHSZ decreases rapidly as the geothermal gradient increases. In polar continental regions, methane hydrate can occur at depths ranging from 150 to 2000 m, with a general temperature

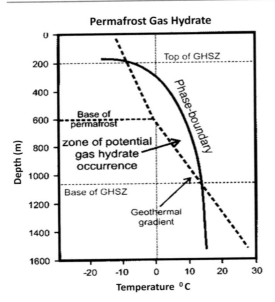

Fig. 4 Graphic illustrating temperature–pressure mechanism for permafrost gas hydrate stability zone (GHSZ) on land. Note the on land temperature continues to increases from the surface In contrast to thermal gradients in oceans. The requisite conditions of temperature, less than 15° and pressure more than 5 MPa to form the hydrate stability zone (GHSZ) in land permafrost varies depending on geothermal gradient. The zone of potential gas hydrate in permafrost is generally thicker compared to oceanic hydrates because of low temperature gradient. The phase boundary, top and bottom og GHSZ is shown (after Amundsen and Landrø 2012, Courtesy GEO ExPro)

ranging from −10 to 15 °C and can be expected to be thicker.

Hydrate occurrence can be onland as in Mallik accumulations or under shallow waters as found off continental shelf in the Mackenzie delta area, north Canada. Mallik hydrates occur in form of multiple layers, lying below 300–700 meter-thick permafrost at depths of 980–1020 m whereas in offshore the hydrates occur under water depths up to about 100 m in Beaufort shelf. In Mackenzie delta area the hydrates are predominantly thermogenic methane, generated by thermal maturity of organic material (Academic, Wikipedia). The Mallik hydrates being on land are better suited for researches and has become centre of worldwide attentions to understand hydrate behavior and experimenting techniques for commercial production.

Gas Hydrate Petroleum System

With recent ongoing researches to develop hydrates as an energy resource, it may be necessary to conceive a petroleum system to understand the hydrate plays like conventional hydrocarbon habitats. In addition to the critical temperature-pressure boundary conditions, the source, reservoir, trap and migration paths and timing and preservation also need to be considered.

Source

Worldwide studies indicate the methane gas may be biogenic or thermogenic or both. However, much of the offshore data points to more biogenic origin for the methane gas (Smith 2009). The permafrost hydrates, however are reported of thermogenic origin in Mackenzie delta area in Canada as mentioned earlier.

Reservoir

Hydrates occur in various type of reservoirs with varied forms, mode of distribution and concentration depending on their places of deposits, type of water and amount of methane gas available. The reservoirs may vary from good quality sands with intergranular porosity to fine grained and fractured muds and shales. Kurihara et al. (2011) have classified the methane hydrates broadly into three types - the pore-filling, naturally fractured and massive nodular. A representative sketch shows three types of the methane hydrate deposits (Fig. 5). Boswell and Collett (2006) had earlier classified the hydrate occurrences on similar lines and with details in a more comprehensive manner.

In Gulf of Mexico, the pore-filling types of hydrates (Fig. 5a) occur in good quality sand reservoirs with moderate-to-high concentrations, between 50 and 90% of the available pore space (BOEM 2013). Similar hydrate pore-filling accumulations in porous reservoir sands with

Types of Gas Hydrate Reservoirs

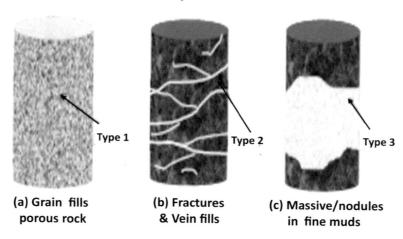

| (a) Grain fills porous rock | (b) Fractures & Vein fills | (c) Massive/nodules in fine muds |

Fig. 5 Showing representative types of methane gas hydrate reservoirs. (**a**) Hydrates filled in intergranular pores of porous sands with high saturation similar to conventional accumulations. (**b**) Hydrate-fills in fractures/veins and (**c**) massive/nodules in fine muds. Potential prospectivity of hydrate depends on its mode occurrence being the best in (**a**) (modified after Kurihara et al. 2011)

high concentrations are also found in Nankai trough, offshore Japan and offshore Vancouver Island (Boswell and Collett 2006) and onland Mallik site in Mackenzie Delta area, akin to conventional gas reservoirs. In Nankai trough the pore-filling gas hydrates mostly occur in highly porous sand layers with in saturation up to 70% of the pore space. The second type of hydrate accumulations is vein and fracture fills in naturally fractured reservoirs caused by structural disturbances under tectonics stress (Fig. 5b). The third type are hydrates occur as massive nodules encased in thick sections of fine-grained muds and shales (Fig. 5c).The hydrates occur in fine grained sediments with low saturation, distributed evenly in disseminated form or as nodules as typified by the Black Ridge accumulations. The low hydrate saturation may be due to the very small pore size and low permeability in clay-rich, fine grained mudrocks that hinder the mobility of both water and gas. A special type hydrate deposition as massive mounds that lie exposed on sea floor or under a thin veneer of sediments extending up to

unknown depths are also reported by Boswell and Collett (2006).

Gas hydrate reservoirs are complex and determination of reservoir parameters is a challenge, particularly with nodular or disseminated form of hydrates for estimating volumetric reserves. Production potential of the hydrate accumulations, except for pore-filling type, is poor and have the low priority for being considered as viable and sustainable energy resource. Even for hydrates occurring in multiple layers in sand reservoirs, where hydrates occupy matrix pores similar to conventional reservoirs, estimation of reservoir properties such as porosity and saturation from logs can be tricky (Boswell et al. 2017) due to the laminated hydrates (Fig. 6).

Trap

Most of the early explorations were carried out on structural highs for hydrates and particularly for the free gas below. However, recent

Fig. 6 Showing log motifs of multiple thin layers of porous reservoir sands saturated with hydrates, embedded in clastic formation. Note the laminar nature of the hydrate accumulations which poses challenge to estimate porosity and saturation for estimating reserves. (modified after Boswell et al. 2017)

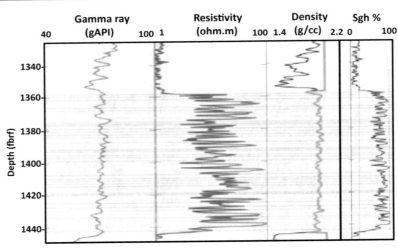

occurrences of gas hydrates show the trapping mechanism may be stratigraphic in nature.

Migration

Since gas hydrate is a solid comprising of gas and water, both must have migration paths to the reservoir to accumulate. Many hydrate deposits are associated with structural features where gas and water can migrate through a fracture or fault system. Hydrates found filling the pores of coarse-grained sands and vugs and fractures of fine grained sediments are corroborative evidences of the process of migration (Smith 2009).

Methane Production from Hydrates

Methane production from hydrates is essentially dissociating the methane and water from the hydrate in layers, pores and veins, and collect only methane. However, with dissociation and gas production, the reservoir temperature also decreases which makes it difficult to produce. As yet, no commercial production from hydrates are known. Several countries joined in forming a consortium, the MH21 Research Consortium, to test and experiment with different types of stimulation to hydrate reservoirs to arrive at a safe and workable method to extract methane

economically. Some important findings of the consortium are stated below to have a glimpse of tests and experiments carried out in onland Mallik hydrate reservoir site in Mackenzie delta, Canada. To restate the Mallik reservoir consists of fine-grained sandstone and conglomeratic rock units within the depth interval from 980 to 1020 m.

Once the dissociation from the hydrate starts and gas flows, production systems similar to that employed for developing natural gas fields can be deployed. The stable hydrates in GHSZ can be dissociated either by increasing the temperature by heating or decreasing the pressure (depressurization). Heating methods are similar to those deployed in stimulation of heavy oil reservoirs or as enhanced oil recovery (EOR) process for conventional resources. This includes steam flooding or cyclic steam stimulation (huff-n-puff) methods (see Chapter "Oil Sands, Heavy Oil, Tight Oil/Gas, BCGAs and CBM"). Tests carried out by MH21 Research Consortium with "hot water circulation method", exhibited the first ever production of methane from hydrate, though with poor rate. The use of depressurization method, however, showed many fold increase in productivity and proved to be a more effective way as hydrate inhibitor by injecting salt and alcohol into the reservoir to disturb the equilibrium and dissociate the hydrates in-situ (MH21 Research Consortium). Stimulation method for producing hydrate methane, however, depends largely on the kind of reservoir and associated hydrate accumulation type. Hydrates in sand reservoirs with high matrix porosity and permeability have well-based production concepts and are more credible for methane production similar to that from conventional reservoirs of gas as is demonstrated by pilots in Mallik hydrate accumulations.

Oceanic gas hydrates contain massive amount of methane and its exploitation is pursued by several countries as a future source of energy. However, their energy-resource potential depends on several factors including the reservoir type, hydrate saturation, reservoir volumetrics and depth of occurrence to produce economically and safely without environmental damage. Boswell and Collett (2006) have presented a gas hydrate pyramid model which succinctly describes the various types of hydrate deposits and their potential for production. Particularly economic recovery of natural gas from the highly disseminated gas hydrate accumulations in fine grained shale and muds, which remarkably forms the major portion of estimated resource base in the world, seems far remote with the current technologies under trial. At present no gas hydrate is exploited commercially as a source of natural gas. Because the resource is not yet proven as commercially viable, there are no known reserves of methane in gas hydrate (Boswell et al. 2017). Production of methane from hydrates continues to remain a huge challenge for engineers notwithstanding the odds of geomechanical effects that are likely to arise during production. The environmental problem of greenhouse effect can be a cause of concern also due to leakage from the oceans leading to increase in exposure of methane in the atmosphere.

Seismic Role

Oceanic gas hydrates can be easily identified in seismic by a unique reflection known as 'Bottom simulating reflector' (BSR). The reflection is characterized by (i) strong amplitudes, (ii) polarity opposite of sea-bottom reflection, (iii) reflection mimicking the sea bottom configuration and (iv) cutting across geologic strata (Fig. 7). The hydrate, the ice-like solid formation exhibits higher seismic velocity (~ 2.0–2.2 km/s) relative to the underlying sediments. Consequently, the reflection from the hydrate base is imaged with strong amplitude and with negative polarity opposite to that of the sea bottom reflection. The base of hydrate stability zone (GHSZ) runs parallel to the sea bottom in portions where no lateral change in the temperature- pressure relation

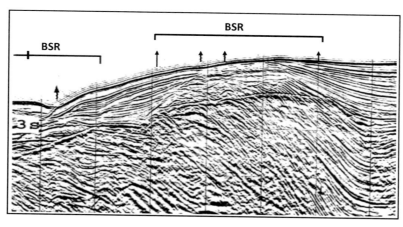

Fig. 7 Example of bottom simulating reflector (BSR), the seismic expression of oceanic gas hydrate. Note the typical characteristics of BSR, the reflection mimicking the sea bottom reflection (black), reverse polarity (white) with respect to that of sea bottom and cutting across stratal beds (Image: credit USGS)

occurs. The reflection from the base of GHSZ base, which marks the boundary between the gas-hydrates and the underlying sediments, accordingly follows the sea- bottom reflection, parallel to it, simulating its configuration and hence named bottom simulating reflection (BSR). Occurrence of free gas below hydrates are also reported which enhances the impedance contrast sharply causing an increase in the reflection strength of BSR. Reflection from the top of hydrate, however, may not be noticed because of its transitional nature as hydrates are typically more concentrated at the base and gradually decrease in concentration upwards.

Interestingly, however, BSRs are not always associated with hydrates. Seismic evidence of BSR did not lead to hydrates and conversely hydrates are found without the typical BSR signature imaged in seismic. Many BSR anomalies, after drilling, were found to have no hydrates. Though it is not quite clear as how the BSR is caused, conjectures are it may be either because of the too low concentration of hydrate due to disseminated form of occurrence or the reflection caused by other geologic reasons such as diagenesis of sedimentary layers. The latter hypothesis of diagenesis, however, does not explain the mimicking of sea bottom reflection unless the diagenesis in the sedimentary layer occurs parallel to the sea bottom, which seems unlikely. In contradistinction, in the Gulf of Mexico (GOM), hydrates with high saturation in porous sand layers were found in several places (BOEM 2013) showing no expression of classical BSR in seismic (Fig. 8). In GOM where hydrates occur in high saturation in porous sands, two kinds of variants of 'BSR', 'discontinuous' and 'pluming' types are seen, mostly in the northern part of GOM (Shedd et al. 2012). The geology of GOM is unique where most of the hydrate deposits are discrete and have seismic expression of discontinuous 'BSR's, which are basically widely

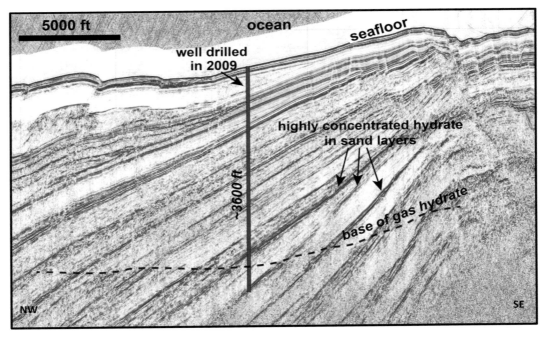

Fig. 8 Displaying a high resolution seismic segment in northern Gulf of Mexico which does not show BSRs but drilling for the high amplitude anomalies proved multiple layers of hydrate saturated porous sands. An imaginary dashed line joining the base of the hydrates (GHSZ) encountered in the discrete sand reservoirs seems broadly parallel to sea bottom and in conformity with pressure - temperature relation needed for hydrate stabilization. (image, credit USGS)

separated seismic events that can be perceived as aligning with the sea bottom. Lateral occurrence of hydrates with high saturation in porous sands within the GHSZ show strong reflections, of positive polarity similar to that of the sea bottom, occurring within the GHSZ. The base of these discrete hydrates, joined by an imaginary line aligns the base of GHSZ, broadly parallel to sea bottom configuration (Fig. 8). Boswell et al. (2016) have described the seismic signatures of hydrates which vary depending on the type of reservoir matrix, mode of occurrence of hydrate and its saturation, the top and the bottom lithologies.

Another variation of BSR, the 'pluming' type is more interesting, with seismic appearance of events 'bowed' towards the sea floor, continuous but not simulating the sea bottom. The relative abundance of discontinuous and pluming varieties of BSR are attributed to the strong lithologic and structural heterogeneity of the basin (Shedd et al. 2012).

Though seismic investigation for detecting hydrates plays the most important role in identifying and delineating the oceanic gas hydrates, its role in hydrate reservoir characterization may be challenging because of the nature of the complex reservoir and the wide varieties of types of hydrate accumulation and concentration. Without a reflection from hydrate top, seismic is limited to the amplitude attribute, the interfacial property and difficult to infer the thickness of column of hydrate and its saturation for characterization.

References

ACADEMIC, Wikipedia Mallik gas hydrate site

Amundsen L, Landrø M (2012) Gas hydrates part i: burning ice. GeoExpro 9(3)

Boswell R, Shipp C, Reichel T, Shelander D, Saeki T, Frye M, Shedd W, Collett TS, McConnell DR (2016) Prospecting for marine gas hydrate resources. Interpretation, pp SA13–SA21

Boswell R, Dallimore S2014) Methane hydrates in future energy, 2nd edn

Boswell R, Collett T (2006) The gas hydrates resource Pyramid. Methane Hydrate Newsl

Boswell R, Collett TS, Myshakin E, Ajayi T, Seol Y (2017) The increasingly complex challenge of gas hydrate reservoir simulation. Advances 7:5554–5577

Bureau of Ocean Energy Management (2013) New Insight on Gas Hydrates In Gulf of Mexico

Cornet FH, Valette B (1984) In situ stress determination from hydraulic injection test data. J Geophys Res: Solid Earth 89:11527–11537. https://doi.org/10.1029/JB089iB13p11527

Harris NB (2015) Shale velocity and density as functions of TOC and thermal maturity: Upper Devonian Woodford Shale, Permian Basin, Texas, Search and Discovery, Abstract, Article #51124

Kurihara M, Ouchi H, Narita H, Masuda Y (2011) Gas production from methane hydrate reservoirs. In: Proceedings of the 7th International Conference on Gas Hydrates, (ICGH 2011), Edinburgh, UK

MH21 Research Consortium, Japan, 2020, Production of gas from methane hydrate

RossHaacke R, Westbrook G, Hyndman R (2007) Gas hydrate, fluid flow and free gas: formation of the bottom-simulating reflector. Abstr, Earth Planet Sci Lett 261. https://doi.org/10.1016/j.epsl.2007.07.008

Ruppel C (2010) Ocean explorer. Gas Hydrates Offshore Southeastern, USA

Sharma RK, Chopra S (2015) Determination of lithology and brittleness of rocks with a new attribute, interpreter's corner. The Lead Edge, pp 936–941

Shedd W, Boswell R, Frye M, Godfriaux P, Kramer K (2012) Occurrence and nature of "bottom simulating reflectors" in the Northern Gulf of Mexico. Abstr, Mar Pet Geol 34

Smith T (2009) Gas hydrates-not so unconventional. GeoExpro 6(2)

Wanga J, Lau HC (2020) Thickness of gas hydrate stability zone in permafrost and marine gas hydrate deposits: analysis and implications. Fuel. https://doi.org/10.1016/j.fuel.2020.118784

Zhang D, Ranjith PG, Perera MSA (2016) The brittleness indices used in rock mechanics and their application in shale hydraulic fracturing: a review. J Pet Sci Eng 143:158–170

Zhang C, Ranjith PG, Perera MSA, Zhao J (2017) Characteristics of clay-abundant shale formations: use of CO_2 for production enhancement. Energies, pp 1–27. https://doi.org/10.3390/en10111887

Zuqing C, Hongfei Y, Jingbo W, Tianfa Z, Penggui J, Seguing L, Chao C (2016) Application of high-precision 3D seismic technology to shale gas exploration: a case study of the large Jiaoshiba shale gas field in the Sichuan Basin. Research article, Sci Direct, pp 117–128. https://doi.org/10.1016/j.ngib.2016.03.006

Fractured-Basement Reservoirs

Abstract

Fractured-basement reservoirs are igneous or metamorphic rocks having no matrix porosity and low secondary fracture porosity of ~ 2–3% and generally are devoid of adequate void space to hold sufficient volume of hydrocarbons for economic production. Nevertheless, several giant and major oil fields of fractured basement reservoirs are known to host substantial reserves and produce significant amount of hydrocarbons and are therefore categorized under unconventional reservoirs. The prospectivity of fractured basement reservoirs depends exclusively on the volume of rocks fractured and geometry of fractures which comprises the dimensions, densities and orientations of the fractures. The intensity of the fracture geometry ultimately defines the network it creates to host and produce oil and gas economically. Some such fractured basement fields in the world are discussed along with the challenges in exploring the fractured-basement reservoirs.

Traditionally, exploration of conventional hydrocarbon reservoirs are seismic driven, identification, delineation and characterization of prospects carried out by seismic. But its application is somewhat limited and conditional for fractured -basement reservoirs. The unconventional fractured-basement reservoirs are historically serendipitous finds all over the world. The difficulties and ambiguities involved in characterizing fracture geometry from seismic make basement exploration ventures highly uncertain and risky. Nevertheless seismic under certain favorable conditions can assist in evaluation of fractured-basement reservoirs and are indicated with limitations.

Traditionally, exploration for conventional reservoirs are based on identifying structural and high amplitude anomalies from seismic in the sedimentary formations to generate potential hydrocarbon prospects followed by test-drilling. Obviously the sedimentary fills in the basin are the most likely targets to look for source and porous reservoir rocks to exist in form of traps. Basement rocks being igneous in nature have little matrix porosity and permeability and prima-facie, are not considered as reservoirs for exploration. Often the import of drilling up to top of basement in wild-cat exploration to fathom the complete column of sedimentary section and their geology ends up in hydrocarbon indication in the basement. Most giant and major hydrocarbon fields are serendipitously discovered worldwide in a variety of basement rocks that are intensely fractured and host substantial reserves to produce significant amount of hydrocarbons. These reservoirs are categorized as unconventional, fractured-basement reservoirs.

Bulk of hydrocarbon reserves and their productivity depend solely on the volume of

N. C. Nanda, *Seismic Data Interpretation and Evaluation for Hydrocarbon Exploration and Production*, Advances in Oil and Gas Exploration & Production, https://doi.org/10.1007/978-3-030-75301-6_15

fractured rocks and the fracture geometry, i.e., the fracture dimensions, densities and orientations defining the intensity of the intertwined network. Unless the basement is severely tectonized to contain high degree of fractures it cannot have enough storage space to produce hydrocarbons efficiently and economically. The void spaces created by fractures and fissures in basement rock provide the porosity known as fracture porosity. Though fracture porosities are usually small, massive volume of fractured-basement rocks can host sizable amount of hydrocarbons and with fracture network providing high permeability for fluid to flow, fractured-basement reservoirs can be attractive exploration targets. Fractures, however, do not occur everywhere in the basement and obviously depend on the type and intensity of tectonic stress and the kind of basement rock, amenable to fractures. But how does one foresee the requisite fractures in the basement rocks and delineate and characterize them? Can seismic help image fractures?

Faults and Fractures, Tectonics and Basement Rocks

Faults and Fractures

Faults are essentially planar fractures or discontinuities in rocks with significant displacement in vertical and horizontal planes and can range from a few metres to several kilometers caused by horizontal tectonic stresses. Fractures such as joints, cracks and fissures besides external horizontal stress, are also caused by uplifts, weathering, erosion, heating and cooling of rocks and internal stresses within the rock. Fractures and fissures which are smaller in dimensions can be kilometers long laterally and extending hundreds of meters deep within the rocks. All of the above deformations can be considered broadly under the term fractures for the purpose of fractured-basement reservoirs.

Basement fractures are of small widths up to centimeters and are generally vertical to sub

vertical. Fractures are essentially of two types, shear or slip fractures and extension fractures depending on tectonic stress. Shear fractures show relative lateral displacements whereas extensional fractures are dilatational in nature. Extensional fractures include joints, veins and fissures and develop perpendicular to least stress direction while shear fractures develop oblique to the least stress, the angle depending on rock properties and the order of stress (Fig. 1). Faults and fractures, caused by tectonics are co-linked and though the terms are often used synonymously, their implications can be greatly different, especially in the context of fractured-basement reservoirs. It is important to stress that faults in a rock formation does not necessarily assure occurrence of fractures, it merely shows presence of tectonic stress and its type.

Tectonics

Tectonics play the key role in creating and enhancing fracture systems in the basement.

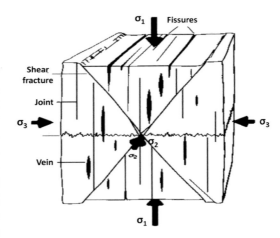

Fig. 1 Schematic diagram showing principal tectonic stresses and the resultant fracture types, the extensional and shear fractures. The extensional fractures include fissures, veins and joints. While extensional fractures open perpendicular to least horizontal stress σ_3, shear fractures are oblique depending mostly on rock properties and order of stress

Fracture development depends on the type of stress regime i.e., extensional, compressional and wrench tectonics. Fractures developed due to dilation under extensional tectonics are considered more favorable as they create more void space than fractures created under compressional tectonics. Moreover, compressional tectonics do not always involve the basement as in 'skin tectonics' and may not impact fracture development in the basement despite causing intense folds, reverse faults, thrusts and over thrusts in the overburden. Wrench tectonics, on the other hand, which necessarily involve the crustal basement, can cause two or more sets of faults; the intersecting conjugate radial faults and associated fractures that favor an effective network. The basement fractures are generally vertical to sub vertical, aligning typically parallel or perpendicular to normal or reverse faults and are in oblique associations with wrench faults. However, fracture orientations can change by later fault and block movements associated with varying polycyclic tectonic stress regimes over a very long period of geologic time in the basin.

Basement Rock Types

Basement rocks which form the base of sedimentary fills in a basin, are commonly igneous and metamorphic in nature. These rocks are void of porosity but can act as reservoirs if are fractured. While igneous and metamorphic rocks constitute the most part of the crustal basement worldwide, potential basement reservoirs are restricted to areas where fractures are present. Two factors essentially control fractures; the tectonic stress, its type and intensity and the basement with the kind of rocks having affinity to brittleness for developing intense fracture networks. Koning (2014) has graded different kind of basement rocks in order of preference for potential fractured-basement reservoirs. Hard and brittle crystalline igneous basement rocks such as quartzites and granites are the most suitable to develop faults and fractures under tectonic stress. Igneous metamorphic basement rocks such as gneisses and schists are considered less suitable

due to their ductility and are likely to develop planar fractures parallel to direction of foliation under tectonic stress. Likewise igneous rocks such as basalt flows, are usually not considered suitable for developing fractures. However, though weathered granites can be excellent reservoirs with leaching secondary porosity, weathered schists and gneisses with high mafic content may be unsuitable and less preferred.

Basement rocks are mostly complex and highly heterogeneous. The type and intensity of tectonic stress together with heterogeneity of kind of basement rock having diverse elastic properties, influence creation of fractures and their intensity. Basement rock mineralogy and grain orientations also play a part in facilitating fracture orientation in preferred directions. Dykes and sills emplacements in host granitic basement complex such as andesite and rhyolite also can create intense fracturing as in Gulf of Suez (Younes et al. 1998).

Hydrocarbon Accumulation in Fractured-Basement Reservoirs

Source

Like conventional reservoirs, the fractured-basement reservoirs require structural or stratigraphic traps with source rocks to host hydrocarbon. Usually, matured source rocks, juxtaposed as onlaps to the basement flanks expel hydrocarbon by updip migration to the fractured reservoirs. However, expulsion and downward migration of hydrocarbon from sources draping the basement to the reservoir beneath is also possible (Whaley 2016). The best example of this is the Cuu Long basin in southern shelf of Vietnam where several big oil fields including the giant Bach-Ho field are located. The granitic basement is directly overlain by widespread Upper Oligocene which is a prolific matured source that feeds hydrocarbon to the fractured-basement reservoirs underlying directly below in the basin (Hung and Le 2004). A representative geologic section of Bach-Ho (Koning 2014) illustrates the oil accumulation system in the giant

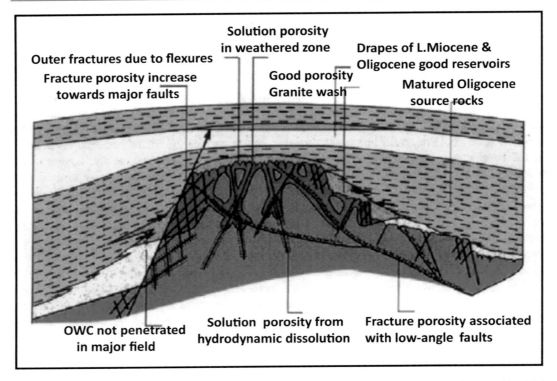

Fig. 2 A representative geologic section illustrating the hydrocarbon accumulation system in the giant Bach-Ho field, Viet Nam. The fractured-basement reservoir structure with fracture network is shown. The reservoir is overlain by the source rock from which downward migration of oil has occurred. Note the intense network of plethora of faults and fractures that provides high permeability. Fracture and other secondary porosities as annotated provide huge volume of void space to hold enormous amount of oil in the giant field (after Koning 2014)

Bach-Ho field with source overlying the fractured basement reservoir (Fig. 2). In areas where basement has been uplifted, it may be adjacent to a shallower source from where migration of hydrocarbon into the basement can occur.

Reservoirs

Basement reservoirs have little matrix and with low fracture porosity of usually 2–3%, usually have insufficient capacity to hold sizable volume of hydrocarbon for sustained economic production. However, discoveries of many giant and big size hydrocarbon fields in basement reservoirs have shown that huge volumes of enormously fractured basement rocks can hold significantly large amount of hydrocarbon stored in the voids created by the intensely faulted and fractured network in the rock (Belaidi et al. 2016). Massive volumes of basement rocks with interconnecting network of fault zones and swarms of fractures, fissures and microfractures, extending to considerable depths can provide large reserves to produce plentiful hydrocarbon economically for long period of time. A representative model of intense network of faults, fractures, joints and fissures in basement reservoir capable of holding and producing hydrocarbon economically for long period of time is shown in Fig. 3. Examples of such fractured-basement reservoirs with large oil columns are the giant fields, Bach Ho (1500 m), Lancaster, UK (620 m) and the Buried hill, China (400 m). Drilling horizontal wells for such thick reservoirs with intense fracture network greatly enhances productivity. Often under

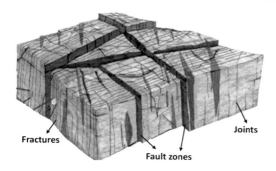

Fig. 3 Schematic model showing intensive network of faults, fractures, fissures and joints in basement that create enough capacity to store substantial amount of hydrocarbon and promote high permeability for production. Note the typical vertical fractures which can enhance productivity enormously by drilling horizontal wells (graphic after Hurricane energy/GeoExpro Magazine 2016)

favorable geologic conditions the porosity of the fractured reservoir can be augmented by solution drive, vuggy and weathering related porosities as is seen in the giant Bach Ho field (Refer Fig. 2).

While some reservoirs show that fractures can be dense and of considerable length as in the above reservoirs, despairingly many basement reservoirs are found devoid of fracture zones or with zones of sparse and disconnected fractures occurring at irregular intervals. For example, in Borholla-Changpang field, India, several discret

fracture zones of varying intervals of 20–140 m are encountered within the basement at different wells where the fractures vary in dimensions and densities and oriented differently. Also many of the wells, drilled on the domal basement high, encountered no or little fractures, though the map prepared from seismic and well data depicts pattern of intensely crisscrossing faults of sizable displacement (Fig. 4). This highlights the complexity in fractured-basement reservoirs that cannot be comprehended fully.

Most major fractured basement reservoirs in the world host hydrocarbon in igneous and metamorphic rocks such as granites, gneisses, schists and granodiorites. Metamorphic basement reservoirs may show secondary porosities other than fracture porosity as in the Buried Hill field in China. Weathered granites and volcanic rocks such as basalt (Deccan trap) flows, pyroclastics and metasediments can also be hydrocarbon bearing reservoirs as in Kura basin in Georgia, Tanjung, Indonesia and Padra in Cambay basin, India onland oil fields. The Deccan traps in Padra field are multiple layers of basalt flows which are massive at the bottom but grade upwards with altered and vesicular layers at the top. Fractures and the vesicles in the basalts behave as reservoir though in general basalts and its weathered products are found to be poor reservoirs.

Fig. 4 Structure map of basement top in Borholla field, Assam, India, mapped from well data and seismic. Despite the large number of intersecting faults with considerable displacement, many wells drilled on the high showed no or sparse fractures (dry wells not shown), highlighting the complexity and uncertainty in exploring fractured-basement reservoirs. (courtesy: ONGC, India)

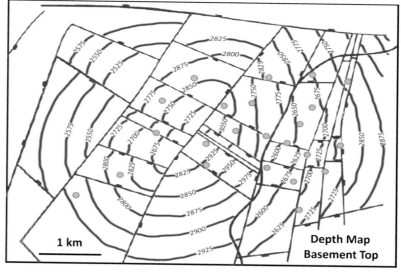

However, the above examples are stated to stress that basement reservoirs, can be diversely complicated as they vary lithologically, tectonically and structurally. Even in a single field, the reservoir comprising of diverse type of basement rocks, varying locally in composition can be found. For example, the "Buried Hill" Dangshenpuin field, China, having an oil column of 400 m, in Archean metamorphosed basement rocks consists of migmatic granites, granulites, diabases and hornblendes (Koning 2014). The Bombay high fractured basement reservoir in west offshore, India, with oil shows is another example where rock types encountered in wells are diverse rocks comprising granites, gneisses, schists, phyllites and Deccan trap basalts (Saran et al. 1993). Such locally limited varying basement rock types also influence fracture development.

Traps

Basement reservoirs are mostly structural highs but can also be stratigraphic traps. Oil is found outside of structural closures in Lancaster, UK and in the Northeast Oil pool in Central Sumatra where it is found associated with multiple water contacts (Koning 2019). In India, the Borholla field in Assam, oil water contacts are found at different depths in the wells drilled on the structure depending on presence of fractures and without structural play indicating the stratigraphic nature of the fractured-basement reservoir.

Reservoir Characterization-Fracture Geometry

Considering that the prime elements required for hydrocarbon accumulation such as matured source and structural traps are present in an area, the key to exploring basement hydrocarbon is the fractured reservoir. Successful commercial hydrocarbon for sustained production from basement depends on the volume of rocks intensively faulted and fractured creating swaths

of interconnected network. The network of faults, fractures, joints and fissures essentially provide adequate void space as capacity to store hydrocarbons for commercial production. Since fractures primarily determine the accumulation and production of hydrocarbons, characterization of basement fracture geometry becomes critical.

Fracture geometry involves estimating size (width and length) and shape of fractures, their density and orientation. This is usually a challenge and more so in highly heterogeneous basement rocks. As mentioned earlier the severity of fracturing in a rock depends on type and intensity of tectonic stress and the type of basement rocks, their composition and minerology. The type of tectonic stress and the ensuing strain, though, can be qualitatively assessed from geology, it remains difficult to define the fracture properties for evaluating hydrocarbon prospectivity reliably. Variations in basement rock composition locally within a prospect further add to uncertainty in estimating fracture geometry that can change from well to well and tend to be unreliable. For instance, in Borholla oil field in Assam, India, several discrete fracture zones are found at different depths with variable fracture density and lengths from 30 to 120 m and without any correlatable pattern. This is

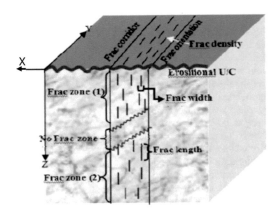

Fig. 5 Schematic model illustrating the complexities involved in characterizing basement fracture geometry in Borholla field, Assam, India. Note the variations in length, width, density and depth of occurrence of fractures which increase the uncertainties in estimation of fracture geometry. (after Sengupta and Nanda 2011)

incomprehensive and the fracture prediction becomes highly undependable. A representative sketch illustrates the problematic type of the reservoir in the Borholla field in Assam, India (Fig. 5).

Geologic assessment of fractures in basement from surface observation of faults, joints and fractures may not also be help to evaluate the reservoir as their pattern and behavior in the subsurface can be different and unpredictable. Outcrops are subjected to uplifts and weathering and the induced fractures can be non-representative of subsurface geometry. On another measure, fractures can be imaged in well logs and though can detect fracture attitude, spacing and orientation, the other important parameter, the fracture size and shape may be difficult to judge from these tools. This requires analysis of cores which can have technical and operational constraints in procuring them from wells. Large scale fracture studies based on geological, borehole imagery and oriented cores though help to a large extent in describing nature of fractures, it may not yet be the true representative of their network on a large field scale which ultimately controls production and more importantly the economics. The study also has inability to predict fracture geometry away from the well where significant variability in fracture properties exist in the basement reservoir.

Reserve Estimate and Productivity

Since fractures in the basement control the accumulation, distribution and flow of hydro-carbons, it is important that the fracture geometry is assessed properly. The most important parameters, the fracture length, signifying the hydrocarbon pay column and the density together with the area of the fractured rocks would pro-vide the effective volume of accumulation to estimate in-place hydrocarbon reserves. Thus delineating the basement reservoir and defining the fracture geometry are most crucial factors as uncertainties can lead to flawed estimate of reserves ensuing failed exploration endeavors.

Considering the nature of varying complicacies involved in basement fractures from well to well as discussed above, it can really be hard chal-lenges for an explorationist to predict prospec-tivity. In many unsuccessful ventures of fractured basement reservoirs, when initial encouraging production led to plan further exploratory inputs including drilling, the wells started reporting dwindling flows within a short period of time. The uncanny production behavior may be pri-marily because of inadequate storage volume due to insufficient fractures that could not be ade-quately defined due to lack of comprehension. Intensively fractured network can have large storage and permeability ranging up to thousands of millidarcies as in Bach-Ho giant field (Koning 2014).

Role of Seismic

Seismic Mapping of Faults and Fractures

Faults are 'big fractures' and are well imaged in seismic, whereas small microscopic and meso-scopic faults of sub-seismic scale, cannot be imaged directly. Fractures in rocks affect elastic properties, induce heterogeneity and anisotropy which impact seismic attributes and make the job of defining fracture geometry explicitly compli-cated and challenging (Chap. "Seismic Wave and Rock-Fluid Properties"). Lot of studies have gone to understand the geology of fracture properties and their seismic response including number of laboratory and field cases and are published (Special edition on fractures, The Leading Edge 2007). However, most of the work pertains to seismic delineation of fractures in sedimentary reservoirs. Mapping fractures in basement reservoirs is a different kind of play and is most challenging to characterize from seismic. Unlike in conventional sedimentary fractured reservoirs, a single reflection from the top basement is recorded and with no reflection from within or below the basement, it restricts utilizing interfacial attribute, the reflection amplitude and excludes scopes for other attributes to determine layer properties.

However, high density and high resolution (HDHR) multi-azimuth long offset 3D data, acquired and processed by sophisticated migration techniques can improve data and can bring out correlatable reflections from within the basement. Advanced seismic attribute techniques can extract information from such data and help qualitatively delineate the fault lineaments and define fracture swaths with their density and orientation. Nonetheless, credible fracture characterization would depend on an integrated multi-disciplinary approach by synthesizing seismic, geology, well logs, core analysis data and rock physics modelling and more importantly the imaginative skill of the analysts. Seismic techniques commonly used for detecting and defining fractures in a reservoir are velocity variation with azimuth, coherence, curvature and dip-azimuth attributes and are briefly mentioned below without repeating the details which are given in Chap. "Analysing Seismic Attributes". There are, however, limitations in application of these seismic techniques to define fractures in the basement and are discussed later under the head 'Seismic Limitations'

Velocity Variation with Azimuth (VVAz)

Fractures create anisotropy in rocks which yield differential seismic response depending on direction (seismic anisotropy) of the fractures in which the seismic wave propagates (Chap. " Seismic Wave and Rock-Fluid Properties"). The wave velocity is faster along the direction of fracture plane than across it. Long offset and wide azimuth 3D seismic data can measure the difference in azimuth varying travel-times. While the amount of time delay can be inferred in terms of magnitude and density of fractures, the recorded faster wave along the fractures would show their orientation. The effect is observed better in shear waves due to birefringence, the phenomenon of shear wave splitting to two orthogonal waves, travelling with different velocities in a rock along and across the orientation of fractures (Chap. "Shear Wave Seismic, AVO and Vp/Vs Analysis").

Coherence

Coherence is a measure of similarity between seismic reflection waveforms between traces along a horizon (strata). The reflection waveform depends on amplitude, frequency and phase of the wave and is controlled by rock properties. Dissimilarity in waveform, detected by coherency would signify change in the horizon property. Faults and fractures are discontinuities in a rock surface and the seismic coherence attribute can map them by detecting breaks in continuity or character of reflection horizons. No/poor reflection correlation is expressed by low coherence representing break in the horizon which can signify presence of faults and fractures (Chap. " Analysing Seismic Attributes"). The attribute is also known as variance attribute. Zones of lateral variance in reflection character (low coherence) can indicate gradational boundaries of fault-zone implying clusters of fractures. The cluster of subseismic fractures, with small Fresnel's zone (~ 10 m), though cannot be imaged directly, may be inferred from change in seismic reflection attributes by way of fracture lineaments or corridors. It may be mentioned that the seismic stacked trace represents an average of reflections from tens of meters of width comprising the Fresnel's zone and therefore may be considered to represent grossly the character of the zone of fractures rather than the individual fractures.

Curvature

Curvature is a measure of how bent a surface is at a particular point and defines the shape of geologic features. Curvature values determined from seismic are reciprocal of curvature and higher the curvature value, tighter is the bend. Positive curvatures conventionally signify anticlines and negative the synclines, whereas zero curvatures signify homoclines, the uniformly dipping planar beds. Variance in subtle structural forms caused by faults and fractures from the planar surfaces (horizons) are detected by curvature attribute and are also called variance attribute (Chap. " Analysing Seismic Attributes"). Faults at the slippage edge may cause subtle bends towards the hanging wall side due to drag and the antiform shapes thus formed can be picked by positive curvatures. Volume based curvature are sensitive attributes and emphasizing the most positive curvature, enables to identify zones of likely faults and fracture swaths.

Dip and Azimuth

Analysis of dip-azimuth attributes provides size and shape of geologic bodies, their continuity and trend. Sharp discontinuities in dip-azimuth help detect presence of small-scale faults and probable fracture corridors. More importantly, in the first step, the dip and azimuth attributes correlate the reflections in seismic 3D volume automatically driven by the volume data, which is the key input for extracting crucial discontinuity attributes for fracture mapping (Chap. " Analysing Seismic Attributes"). Combined analysis of coherence, curvature and dip-azimuth attributes facilitates mapping subtle deformations and discontinuities such as faults with small lateral offsets (strike slips) and fracture swaths, their density and orientation.

Ant-Tracking

Ant-tracking is a powerful technique often used for mapping in detail highlighting the faults and the fractures with their connected network (for details refer Chap. "Analysing Seismic Attributes"). The highly sophisticated intelligent algorithm tries automatically detecting and delineating fault and fracture planes in a target window by joining adjacent zones of low coherence and addresses the most vital issue, the connectivity of the fractures within the swath (Chap. "Analysing Seismic Attributes"). However, efficacy of this potent software is contingent to the quality of the input, the coherence or curvature cube which depends on quality of seismic data.

Seismic Limitations in Mapping Basement Fractures

Though seismic remains a principal tool used to map faults and fractures it may be noted that the techniques are best applicable in fractured sedimentary reservoirs. These are also used for mapping fractures in basements but the limitation of the techniques and the quality of data may be kept in mind, prior to an attempt to determine credible fracture geometry in basements. Azimuthal velocity variation, based on principle of seismic anisotropy need an interval for analysis. Coherence and curvature attributes though are volume based operations in 3D, they require target windows for display of reservoir zone to detect and delineate the fractures and more importantly the interconnecting path-ways in the network. In coherence and curvatures techniques, the most common fracture mapping tool, correlatable reflections from several closely spaced layers are either picked manually or by machine for detecting breaks or variance in reflections continuities. These are then delineated by showing their lateral and vertical extensions and orientation and would need more than one reflector for providing three dimensional configuration for display.

The basement reservoirs, however, may not meet these conditions. The basement top is mostly the only last correlatable reflection discernible in seismic and is often of poor to fair in quality due to several reasons. The basement top is usually an erosional unconformity, weathered with an irregular and curved surface that impedes reflection quality. The reflection generally varies in lateral amplitude and continuity often posing correlation problems across faults (Fig. 6). In geologic situations where high impedance rocks of old age overlie the basement, the impedance contrast at basement-top may be too poor to cause a reflection suitable for attribute extraction. Further, because of its monolithic nature, no coherent signals from within the crystalline basement rock are likely that can be locally correlated. Consequently a zone below the basement cannot be defined as the target interval for displaying and interpreting attributes. Faults, fractures and heterogeneity within basement usually create considerable scattering that are usually not processed and considered as noise. The reflection quality from top of basement and below can be worse on onland data due to statics and seismic wave attenuation problems. Under

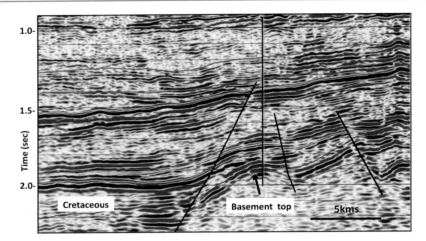

Fig. 6 A typical 3D seismic segment in Cauvery basin, India with Cretaceous formation overlying unconformably on the igneous basement. Note the poor character of the basement-top reflection (red), varying in amplitude and with patchy continuity. No correlatable reflection events are discernible below the basement which shows the prevailing noise (image courtesy, ONGC, India)

the circumstances, interpreting faults and fractures from the poor basement-top reflection and especially at deeper depths would be highly subjective and dubious.

Reliable estimation of fractures in basement, despite powerful and intelligent processing softwares largely depends on the quality of input. The two mainstay attributes for detecting fractures, the coherence or curvature are highly sensitive to noise. Utmost care is needed to sanitize data by reconditioning or reprocessing before application of these techniques. Otherwise, even using the most intelligent ant-tracking software for mapping fractures in poor and noisy data can be a futile exercise. However, without recorded reflection 'seed'-genuine primary reflection hodograph, advanced signal processing including powerful migration techniques may not deliver the true reflection event.

Meaningful application of seismic attributes for mapping fracture geometry based solely on the basement top reflection may be somewhat constrained and conditional. Discontinuity attributes may precisely detect the faults and fractures and their orientation with fair reliability from the single basement-top reflection where the quality is good and can be tagged to the basement top horizon, but with no reflection events from within the basement, the fracture geometry

may have to be extrapolated downward to depths. Herein lies the major uncertainty; since extension of fractures in depths signifies length of hydrocarbon column, extrapolations to unknown depths can be highly subjective and can have large impact on reservoir prospectivity.

However, there are offshore examples where the basement top reflection quality is excellent as in Cuu Long basin which hosts several fractured-basement fields including the giant Bach Ho and CNV (Fig. 7). The top basement reflection quality is excellent with well correlatable continuity. Below the reflection, events within the basement can be seen with details of the criss-crossing faults and the fault planes well imaged extending into deeper depths (Fig. 8). Seismic controlled beam PSDM migration has improved the data quality where the extracted seismic discontinuity attributes can be reliably interpreted and predicted.

Exploring Basement Reservoirs

Fractured-basement reservoirs are complicated geologically and difficult to be adequately characterized by seismic. The complexity in comprehending the reservoirs geologically and lack of dependable seismic prediction of fracture